Treatments for Adolescent Depression

Treatments for Adolescent Depression
Theory and Practice

Editor

Cecilia A. Essau

Professor of Developmental Psychopathology and
Director, Centre for Applied Research and Assessment in
Child and Adolescent Wellbeing (CARCAW);
School of Human and Life Sciences,
Roehampton University,
London, UK

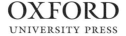

OXFORD
UNIVERSITY PRESS

OXFORD
UNIVERSITY PRESS

Great Clarendon Street, Oxford OX2 6DP

Oxford University Press is a department of the University of Oxford.
It furthers the University's objective of excellence in research, scholarship,
and education by publishing worldwide in

Oxford New York

Auckland Cape Town Dar es Salaam Hong Kong Karachi
Kuala Lumpur Madrid Melbourne Mexico City Nairobi
New Delhi Shanghai Taipei Toronto

With offices in

Argentina Austria Brazil Chile Czech Republic France Greece
Guatemala Hungary Italy Japan Poland Portugal Singapore
South Korea Switzerland Thailand Turkey Ukraine Vietnam

Oxford is a registered trade mark of Oxford University Press
in the UK and in certain other countries

Published in the United States
by Oxford University Press Inc., New York

British Library Cataloguing in Publication Data

Data available

Library of Congress Cataloging in Publication Data

Data available

Typeset in Minion by Cepha Imaging Private Ltd., Banglore, India
Printed in Great Britain
on acid-free paper by
the MPG Books Group

ISBN 978-0-19-922650-4

10 9 8 7 6 5 4 3 2 1

In loving memory of my parents

Essau Indit († 09.05.1992)
Runyan Megat († 26.05.1992)

Preface

Depression is one of the most common mental health problems in adolescence. Recent epidemiological studies report that up to 20% of adolescents in the general population meet criteria for major depression sometimes in their lives. It is associated with significant and persistent impairment in various life domains. Depression is characterized by a recurring course, with about one-third of adolescents having a further depressive episode within a five-year period. Of concern is also the association between depression and suicidal behaviour. Clearly, depression carries a significant individual and societal burden.

In response to the growing awareness of the significance of the problem associated with depression, various prevention and intervention programs for adolescent depression have been developed in recent years. Related to this recent development is the accumulating number of studies that has examined the effectiveness of these interventions for depression. Consequently, the literature on the various types of prevention and intervention programs for adolescent depression and the studies that examined the effectiveness of these programs has been accumulating at a very fast pace. Our aim is therefore to present the most common evidence-based interventions for adolescent depression in a single, comprehensive, and authoritative volume.

This volume is divided into five sections. Section 1 covers an introduction to the field of adolescent depression, including classification, epidemiology, comorbidity, course, risk, and vulnerability of depression in adolescents. The authors also review past work used to identify empirically supported psychosocial treatments for adolescents and discuss some critical issues relevant to this movement.

Sections 2–4 focus on individual and group prevention and intervention strategies (psychological intervention and pharmacotherapy) for adolescent depression, from various theoretical orientations. Section 2 contains four chapters on specific prevention and treatment strategies that are based on cognitive–behavioural therapy (CBT). By combining two distinct schools of psychotherapy (behaviour and cognitive therapy), these CBT-based prevention and treatment programs address the cognitive and behavioural deficits of adolescents with depression. Section 3 focuses on family factors that have been associated with elevated risk of depression, the mechanisms by which risk is transmitted, protective factors that are associated with adolescent resilience, and on various family-based approaches to the prevention and treatment of depression. Section 4 covers a chapter on pharmacotherapy, one chapter on interpersonal psychotherapy, and a chapter on how to deal with 'hard to treat' (i.e., use of interactive CD/DVD) depressed adolescents. Each of the chapters in these three sections begins with a description of theoretical background of the respective intervention programs, the therapeutic goals and methods, and the way in which the interventions are delivered. Available studies that examined the efficacy and their mechanisms of action is also presented and discussed. Section 5 contains a chapter on progress and unresolved issues in the treatment of adolescent depression and provides some recommendations for future studies in this field.

This book is written for advanced students, researchers, and clinicians that include psychologists, psychiatrists, social workers, paediatricians, counsellors, and other mental health professionals who are interested in adolescent depression, particularly on its treatment. The wealth of information concerning the risk factors and various types of treatment programs for adolescent depression will make this volume a valuable reference for both the novice and the expert, and to both the clinicians and the researchers interested in this field. It is hoped that this volume will not only serve to illustrate our current knowledge of various types of treatment for adolescent depression, but may stimulate and facilitate further progress in this field.

I am most grateful to the authors who have contributed to this volume, all of whom have made major contribution to the prevention and treatment of adolescent depression. I am especially honoured by their contributions and dedication to this book project. Without them, a comprehensive scholarly coverage of the various types of treatment for adolescent depression would not been so easily achieved. I would also like to acknowledge the support and patience of the staff at Oxford University Press.

Cecilia A. Essau

Contents

Preface *vii*

List of contributors *xi*

Part 1 **General issues**

1 Epidemiology, comorbidity, and course of
adolescent depression *3*
Cecilia A. Essau & Weining C. Chang

2 Risk and vulnerability in adolescent depression *27*
Elizabeth P. Hayden, Pamela M. Seeds, & David J.A. Dozois

3 Empirically supported treatments for adolescent depression *57*
Thomas H. Ollendick & Matthew A. Jarrett

Part 2 **Cognitive–behavioral therapy**

4 Challenges in school-based, universal approaches to the
prevention of depression in adolescents *83*
Susan H. Spence

5 Primary and secondary control enhancement training
(PASCET): Applying the deployment-focused model of
treatment development and testing *97*
Sarah Kate Bearman & John R. Weisz

6 Resourceful adolescent program: A prevention and early intervention
program for teenage depression *123*
Ian M. Shochet & Rebecca Hoge

7 Improving care for depression: Integrating evidence-based depression
treatment within primary care services *159*
Joan Rosenbaum Asarnow, James McKowen, & Lisa H. Jaycox

Part 3 **Family interventions**

8 Family-based approaches to the prevention of depression
in at-risk children and youth *177*
Catherine M. Lee & Veronica Asgary Eden

9 Attachment-based family therapy for depressed adolescents *215*
Guy S. Diamond, Suzanne A. Levy, Pravin Israel, & Gary M. Diamond

Part 4 **Other forms of treatment**

10 Pharmacotherapy *241*
Dara J. Sakolsky & Boris Birmaher

11 Interpersonal psychotherapy for adolescents *261*
Jami F. Young & Laura Mufson

12 'Working Things Out'—a therapeutic resource for
professionals working with young people *283*
Carol Fitzpatrick, Eileen Brosnan, & John Sharry

Part 5 **Epilogue**

13 Progress and unresolved issues in the treatment
of adolescent depression *313*
Cecilia A. Essau

Index *321*

List of contributors

Joan Rosenbaum Asarnow,
Semel Institute for Neuroscience &
Human Behavior,
University of California,
Los Angeles, CA, USA

Veronica Asgary Eden,
School of Psychology,
University of Ottawa,
Ottawa, Ontario, Canada

Sarah Kate Bearman,
Judge Baker Children's Center,
Harvard Medical School,
Boston, MA, USA

Boris Birmaher,
University of Pittsburgh
Medical Center,
Pittsburgh, PA, USA

Eileen Brosnan,
Mater Child and Adolescent Mental
Health Service & Department
of Psychiatry, University College
Dublin, Ireland

Weining C. Chang,
Nanyang Technological University,
School of Humanities &
Social Sciences,
Division of Psychology, Singapore

Gary M. Diamond,
Department of Psychology,
Ben Gurion University, Israel

Guy S. Diamond,
University of Pennsylvania School of
Medicine & Center for Family
Intervention Science,
Children's Hospital of Philadelphia,
Philadelphia, PA, USA

David J.A. Dozois,
Department of Psychology,
Faculty of Social Science,
The University of Western Ontario,
London, Ontario, Canada

Cecilia A. Essau,
Professor of Developmental
Psychopathology and Director,
Centre for Applied Research and
Assessment in Child and Adolescent
Wellbeing (CARCAW);
School of Human and Life Sciences,
Roehampton University, London, UK

Carol Fitzpatrick,
Mater Child and Adolescent Mental
Health Service & Department of
Psychiatry, University College
Dublin, Ireland

Elizabeth P. Hayden,
Department of Psychology,
Faculty of Social Science,
The University of Western Ontario,
London, Ontario, Canada

Rebecca Hoge,
School of Psychology and Counselling,
Queensland University of Technology,
Carseldine, Australia

Pravin Israel,
Stavanger University Hospital,
Department of Child and Adolescent
Psychiatry, Stavanger, Norway

Matthew A. Jarrett,
Child Study Center,
Department of Psychology,
Virginia Polytechnic Institute and
State University,
Blacksburg, VA, USA

Lisa H. Jaycox,
RAND,
Arlington, VA, USA

Catherine M. Lee,
School of Psychology,
University of Ottawa,
Ottawa, Ontario, Canada

Suzanne A. Levy,
Center for Family Intervention Science,
Children's Hospital of Philadelphia,
Philadelphia, PA, USA

James McKowen,
Family Development and Treatment Lab,
Boston University, Boston, MA, USA

Laura Mufson,
Columbia University College of
Physicians and Surgeons,
New York State Psychiatric Institute,
New York, NY, USA

Thomas H. Ollendick,
Child Study Center,
Department of Psychology,
Virginia Polytechnic Institute and
State University,
Blacksburg, VA, USA

Dara J. Sakolsky,
University of Pittsburgh Medical Center,
Pittsburgh, PA, USA

Pamela M. Seeds,
Department of Psychology,
Faculty of Social Science,
The University of Western Ontario,
London, Ontario, Canada

John Sharry,
Mater Child and Adolescent Mental
Health Service & Department
of Psychiatry, University College
Dublin, Ireland

Ian M. Shochet,
School of Psychology and Counselling,
Queensland University of Technology,
Carseldine, Australia

Susan H. Spence,
Griffith Psychological Health
Research Centre,
Griffith University, QLD,
Australia

John R. Weisz,
Judge Baker Children's Center,
Harvard Medical School,
Boston, MA, USA

Jami F. Young,
Graduate School of Applied and
Professional Psychology,
Rutgers University,
New Brunswick, NJ, USA

Part 1

General issues

Chapter 1

Epidemiology, comorbidity, and course of adolescent depression

Cecilia A. Essau & Weining C. Chang

Until recent years, depression in adolescents had received little research attention. Indeed, there was a prevailing assumption that depressive disorders rarely occurred in children and adolescents. This view stems from the theoretical notion that children and adolescents are too cognitively immature to be depressed, and the concept that psychopathological manifestations and difficulties represent normal developmental processes of childhood and adolescence (Rie, 1966). Nevertheless, a handful of investigators of depression in adolescence during the late 1970s and early 1980s had not only established the presence of depression at this developmental stage, but their work had also delineated some of the psychosocial impairments associated with depression. The late 1970s was also associated with an increasing recognition that children and adolescents exhibit the essential features of adult depression. This change in viewpoints is reflected in the use of the same adult criteria for depressive disorders in children and adolescents in the third edition of the Diagnostic and Statistical Manual of Mental Disorders (DSM-III; American Psychiatric Association; APA, 1980) and its subsequent revisions (DSM-III-R; APA, 1987; DSM-IV; APA, 1994).

Depressive disorders are characterized by the presence of depressed moods along with a set of additional symptoms, persisting over time, and causing disruption and impairment of function. In DSM-IV (APA, 1994), depressive disorders fall under the category of major depressive disorder, dysthymic disorder, and depressive disorder not otherwise specified.

Major depressive disorder (MDD) denotes a severe, acute form of depressive disorder (DSM-IV; APA, 1994). The disorder is diagnosed when the adolescent has experienced at least five of the following nine symptoms nearly every day for at least a two-week period at a level that represents a change from previous functioning: depressed mood (or can be irritable mood in children and adolescents); markedly diminished interest or pleasure in all, or almost all activities; significant weight loss or weight gain, or decrease or increase in appetite (in children, consider failure to make expected weight gains); insomnia or hypersomnia; psychomotor agitation or retardation; fatigue or loss of energy; feelings of worthlessness or excessive or inappropriate guilt; diminished ability to think or concentrate, or indecisiveness; and recurrent thoughts of death, recurrent suicidal ideation without a specific plan, or a suicide attempt or a specific plan for committing suicide. At least one of the two core symptoms, depressed mood (or irritable mood in children and adolescents) or loss of interest or pleasure must be present for the diagnosis to be made (APA, 1994).

Dysthymic disorder is a chronic, but a less severe form of depressive disorder (DSM-IV; APA, 1994). Adolescents are diagnosed with this disorder when they have had a period of at least one year in which they have shown depressed or irritable moods every day without more than two symptom-free months. In addition to irritable or depressed mood, at least two of the following symptoms must be present: poor appetite or overeating, insomnia or hypersomnia, low energy or fatigue, low self-esteem, poor concentration or difficulty making decisions, and feelings of hopelessness.

Epidemiology

Major depression (MDD) is one of the most frequent disorders in adolescence. The point prevalence of MDD in adolescents is about 5% (Fergusson et al., 1993; Lewinsohn et al., 1993), whereas the lifetime rate is about 10% (range from 6.8 to 24%) (Essau et al., 2000; Lewinsohn et al., 1993; Reinherz et al., 1999) (Table 1.1). Dysthymic disorder has been the focus of less investigation in adolescence. According to some studies, lifetime prevalences of dysthymic disorder have been estimated to range from 0.1 to 8% (Essau et al., 2000; Fergusson et al., 1993; Lewinsohn et al., 1993; McGee & Williams, 1988; Whitaker et al., 1990). Overall, the prevalence rates for depressive disorders among adolescents are comparable to those reported in recent epidemiological studies of adult population (e.g., Kessler et al., 1993).

Incidence rates (i.e., refer to the emergence of new cases of disorder over a specified period of time) seemed to be the highest during mid- to late adolescence. In the Oregon Adolescent Depression Project (OADP), the 1-year incidence rate for MDD was 7.14% for girls, 4.35% for boys, and 5.72% for total sample (Lewinsohn et al., 1993); the incidence rate for dysthymic disorder was 0.07%. In a study by Garrison and colleagues (1997), a 1-year incidence of MDD was 3.4%.

In addition to the high prevalence of MDD in adolescence, this disorder also appears to be increasing among the younger generation (Lewinsohn et al., 1993). For example, Lewinsohn et al. (1993) found the presence of an age cohort effect when comparing adolescents who were born between 1968 and 1971 with those who were born between 1972 and 1974. Specifically, by age 14, 7.2% of the more recent adolescent birth cohort had experienced a depressive episode; the rate found among adolescents in the earlier birth cohort (1993) was 4.5%. While there is no clear explanation for this finding, several factors have been proposed, including (for review, see Fombonne, 1995) changes in family life (e.g., single-parent families), which expose children and adolescents to more frequent and earlier challenges; an earlier onset of puberty; presence of negative events (e.g., parental divorce); and chronic stressors (e.g., increased educational demands) (Table 1.2).

Gender: About twice as many girls than boys met the diagnostic criteria for MDD sometimes in their lives (Anderson et al., 1987; Cohen et al., 1993; Essau et al., 2000; Lewinsohn et al., 1993; Reinherz et al., 1993). This gender difference seems to emerge around puberty (Cohen et al., 1993; Essau et al., 2000; Petersen et al., 1991), and then

Table 1.1 Prevalences of MDD in adolescents

Authors (years)	No. of subjects	Age of adolescents	Informants	Diagnostic instrument/ (diagnostic criteria)	Depressive disorders	Major depression	Dysthymic disorder
Canino et al. (1987)	295	11–24	Adolescent	DIS/DSM-III		2.6%**	0%
Kashani et al. (1989)	150	14–16	Adolescent, parent	DICA/DSM-III, with impairment		4.7%*	3.3%*
Velez et al. (1989)	456	12–20	Adolescent, mother	DISC/DSM-III-R, with severity criteria		3.1%*	
McGee et al. (1990)	943	15	Adolescent, parent	DISC/DSM-III-R, with severity criteria		1.2%*	1.1%*
Cohen et al. (1993)	508	14–16	Adolescent, parent	DISC/DSM-III-R		7.6%*	
Cohen et al. (1993)	446	17–20	Adolescent, parent	DISC/DSM-III-R		2.7%*	
Lewinsohn et al. (1993)	1710	14–18	Adolescents	K-SADS-E/ DSM-III-R	2.9** 18.4***	M = 1.7%* F = 3.4%*	0.5%*
Goodyer & Cooper (1993)	1068	11–16	Adolescents	DISC/ DSM-III-R		6.0****	
Reinherz et al. (1993)	386	18	Adolescents	DIS-III-R/ DSM-III-R	6.0** 9.4***		
Reinherz et al. (1999)	375	21	Young adults	DIS/DSM-III-R		10%***	
Reinherz et al. (2003)	354	18–26	Adolescents and young adults	DIS/DSM-IV		23.3%***	
Feehan et al. (1994)	340	18	Adolescents	DIS-III-R/DSM-III-R	16.7%****		
Newman et al. (1996)	961	21	Adolescents	DIS/DSM-III-R, with impairment		M = 11.2%***** F = 22.6%*****	3.0%*****
Verhulst et al. (1997)	780	13–18	Adolescents	DISC/ DSM-III-R		2.8%**	1.5%**

(continued)

Table 1.1 (continued) Prevalences of MDD in adolescents

Authors (years)	No. of subjects	Age of adolescents	Informants	Diagnostic instrument/ (diagnostic criteria)	Depressive disorders	Major depression	Dysthymic disorder
Kessler et al. (1998)	1769	15–24	Adolescents and young adults	CIDI/DSM-III-R		15.3%*** 12.4%****	
Wittchen et al. (1998)	3021	14–24	Adolescents	M-CIDI/DSM-IV		M = 3.3%**** F = 7.2%****	2.9%****
Essau et al. (2000)	1035	12–17	Adolescents	CAPI/DSM-IV	17.9%***		

Note: %, prevalence rates; DIS, Diagnostic Interview Schedule; DISC, Diagnostic Interview Schedule for Children and Adolescents; K-SADS-E, The Kiddie Schedule for Affective Disorders and Schizophrenia; CAPI, The computer-assisted personal interview of the Composite International Diagnostic Interview; CIDI, The Composite International Diagnostic Interview; M-CIDI, The computer-assisted personal interview (CAPI) of the Munich version of the Composite International Diagnostic Interview; * current; ** 6-month; *** lifetime; **** 12-month.

Table 1.2 Factors related to a negative course and outcome of depressive disorders

Authors	Factors related to negative course
Asarnow et al. (1993)	High expressed emotion.
Beardslee et al. (1993)	Parental depression, early onset of depression, comorbid disorders.
Hammen et al. (1990)	Maternal depression.
Goodyer et al. (1997)	Moderate/poor friendship after the onset of depression.
Kovacs et al. (1994)	Comorbid dysthymic disorder.
Lewinsohn et al. (1994)	Earlier age of onset from the first episode, suicidal ideation, seeking treatment for depression.
Rao et al. (1995)	Low socioeconomic status.
Warner et al. (1992)	Early onset of depression (below 13 years old), parents who were divorced and had multiple depressed episodes, prior comorbid diagnosis of dysthymic disorder, problem social functioning.
Dunn & Goodyer (2006)	Severe impairment, having a longer depressive episode before starting treatment, an early psychiatric history.
Essau (2007)	Parental alcohol problems, suicidal behaviour and ideation, negative life events and negative coping, presence of substance use disorders.

remain throughout adulthood (Weissman et al., 1996). Petersen et al. (1991), for example, showed that girls were significantly more depressed than boys by grade 12, with gender differences emerging around grade 8, and increasing over time. In Essau et al.'s study (2000), no significant gender differences could be found before the age of 14; however, after that age, girls had a constant and almost a linear increase in depression compared to boys.

Although gender difference is well established, the reason for this gender difference is unclear. Various biological and psychosocial explanations for women's greater vulnerability to depression have been offered. These include divergent socialization practices concerning power and control, victimization, management of feelings and sex role orientation, as well as differences in the biological changes of puberty (Petersen et al., 1991). Another explanation is that girls experience more challenges in early adolescence than boys (Petersen et al., 1991), and that they are more affected than boys by stressful life events (Petersen et al., 1991). Others (Aro, 1994) suggested that the coping styles of girls are less effective and more dysfunctional compared to boys. Cyranowski et al. (2000) presented the so-called model of 'correlated consequences' to explain the emergence of gender differences in depression in adolescence. According to this model, (i) intensified 'affiliative need' (i.e., preference for close emotional communication, intimacy and responsiveness within interpersonal relationships) experienced in combination with (ii) adolescent transition difficulty may create an increased likelihood that (iii) negative life events trigger the onset of a depressive episode.

Age and Puberty: In some studies, there is a significant relationship between prevalence of MDD and age (Essau et al., 2000; Kashani et al., 1989), but not in others (Lewinsohn et al., 1993). For example, in the Isle of Wight Study, there was a tenfold increase in depression when the 10-year-old children were reinterviewed four years later (Rutter, 1986). Significantly, more postpubertal than prepubertal boys had depressed feelings, indicating that an increase in depression is linked to puberty instead of age. In the Garber et al.'s study (1997), early and late maturing girls compared to girls with a normal pubertal onset time had significantly elevated rates of MDD. In boys, the rate of MDD did not differ as a function of pubertal onset; however, early and late maturation tended to have other problems such as emotional reliance on others. In the Great Smoky Mountain study, girls showed an increase of depression after the age of 12, whereas in boys there was a decrease after the age of 9 years (Angold et al., 1998). Their findings showed pubertal status to better predict the emergence of female preponderance than did age. That is, girls were more likely than boys to be depressed after the transition to mid-puberty (Tanner stage III and above). Boys, by contrast, had higher rates of depression than girls before Tanner Stage III. Among adolescents in the 5th through 8th grades, Hayward et al. (1999) found pubertal status as a better predictor of depressive symptoms than chronological age in Caucasian, but not African-American or Hispanic girls. It was argued that girls in these two ethnic groups attach different meaning of weight-related bodily changes. That is, the consequence of increasing body fat during puberty is interpreted as less negative in African-American than in Caucasian girls.

Depression and Culture: There seems to be a general agreement on the core symptoms of depression in adolescents across different cultural communities. However, the specific meaning and manifestations of such symptoms seem to vary from one culture to another (Tseng & Streltzer, 1997). This has posed serious problems in terms of cross-cultural comparisons both in diagnosis and treatment of depression. Practically, it is difficult to use the same diagnostic criteria for calculating the prevalence rate for cross-cultural comparison. With a better understanding of how these basic mental health problems are conceptualized and manifested in different cultures, a common strategy might be derived at how to conduct cross-cultural comparison of these mental health conditions.

The world has become smaller and different cultural communities are increasingly interdependent with each other. A comprehensive understanding of these common human problems is becoming necessary. Natural calamities and human catastrophes, wars, earth quakes, famine, and pandemic diseases observe no cultural boundaries. Migration and population fluxes have made cultural boundaries increasingly blur. An understanding of cross-cultural differences in these human conditions is only the first step towards mutual understanding and integration in the global village.

We would like to apply the framework of cultural psychology to our presentation of worldwide perspective of depression in adolescence. This framework postulates that human behaviour, healthy or unhealthy, is embedded within the context of culture. The manifested behaviours and subjective experiences of psychological processes are interpreted within the meaningful framework that is made of the shared values, beliefs, and practices of the community (Geertz, 1973). In other words, each culture produces its own symptomatology for the manifestation of and the 'explanation model' with which to explain mental health problems that might be common to human beings (Kleiman, 1986). Within each cultural community, these shared meanings and manifestations give rise to the culture's unique 'idiom of distress' (Nichter, 1981) whereby the problem is communicated within the community. Finally, each cultural community would have its own 'tried and true' means of managing its mental health problems, however they might be labeled.

The relationship between stress, anxiety, and depression is well established. Across different cultural communities not only the manifestations of depression are different, the stressful conditions experienced by youth in different parts of the world are also different. The following is a list of the stress often mentioned in today's mental health literature: disintegration of traditional social support systems, cultural transition and cultural clashes brought by voluntary and involuntary migrations, violence in daily lives, socially oriented pressures, and pressure for individual success. These stressors are not evenly distributed across nations in the world: within different geopolitical regions, the specific configurations of historical, economic, and political situations formulated different challenges of life. Within these different cultures, such environmental challenges would be understood in ways that are consistent with the prevailing beliefs and values, and reacted to with the commonly acceptable behavioural strategies. The same stressor might be understood with different meanings and managed with different strategies.

Many studies have been conducted in the bio-medical models of depression. These studies have yielded evidence to support the notion that adolescence is a period when the individual is biologically predisposed to emotional volatility. These conditions would pre-dispose the adolescent to depression. Psychologically, this is a period of time when one is developing one's individuated identity and how this individuated identity might integrate into the environment to which one belongs (Erickson, 1968). These critical developmental tasks might be conceptualized and experienced differently in different cultures, as reflected in the different 'coming of age' rituals reported in anthropological studies (Geertz, 1973).

Age of onset

The first depressive episode is generally late childhood or early adolescence, with the mean age of onset being 15 years (Essau & Petermann, 1997; Giaconia et al., 1994; Lewinsohn et al., 1994). An earlier age of onset has been reported among adolescents in clinical than in epidemiological settings (Kovacs et al., 1984), and in children of depressed compared to children of non-depressed parents (Weissman et al., 1984). An early onset was also associated with a female gender (Giaconia et al., 1994; Lewinsohn et al., 1994; Reinherz et al., 1993), with females reporting the onset of their depression at an average of about two years earlier than males (Giaconia et al., 1994). The ages of onset for dysthymic disorder have been reported to range from 6 to 13 years (Kovacs et al., 1984).

The age at which the adolescents experienced their first depressive episode seemed to be important for the course and outcome of the depression. As reported by several authors, early onset of MDD was also associated with suicide (Harrington et al., 1990), more depressive episodes, a more protracted course of the disorder (Kovacs et al., 1984), and psychosocial impairment including interpersonal problems and having high emotional and behavioural problems. The reason for this association is unclear, although an early onset of MDD may represent severe forms of this disorder (Weissman, 1988). It could also be that adolescents with an early onset had more time to experience additional episodes, and that the younger they become depressed, the less likely that they have the coping resources to ameliorate depression. Thus, their emotional and intellectual immaturity could prolong the course of depression (Kovacs et al., 1984). Yet, others argued that early onset may signal a vulnerability that could be genetically, perinatally, and/or constitutionally determined and/or precipated by environmental adversity (Kovacs et al., 1984). Regardless of the validity of these explanations, an early onset of depression may signal the beginning of multiple occurrences of major depressive episodes, and not simply a single episode with little developmental significance (Giaconia et al., 1994). Thus, previous assumption that the presence of MDD in adolescents was a mere reflection of transient difficulties is no longer valid (Kutcher & Marton, 1989).

Comorbidity

Frequency and pattern of comorbidity

MDD shows substantial comorbidity with many psychiatric disorders, especially anxiety, eating, and conduct disorders. Comorbidity is so common that it is regarded as the rule rather than the exception (Nottelmann & Jensen, 1999). As reported by Anderson and colleagues (1987), about 60% of children and adolescents with a diagnosable condition have two or more additional disorders. After reviewing six community studies, Angold and Costello (1993) concluded that the presence of depression in children and adolescents increased the probability for another disorder by at least 20 times. In a study by Essau et al. (1999), 42.2% of all the depressed adolescents had MDD only; 40.1% had one additional, and 17.9% had at least two other disorders.

In almost all studies, the most common comorbidity is with anxiety disorders, followed by conduct disorder, and substance use disorders. Specifically, 25–75% of the depressed cases had anxiety disorders, 21–50% had comorbid conduct disorder, and about 25% had comorbid alcohol and drug abuse (Cohen et al., 1993; Goodyer & Cooper, 1993; Kashani et al., 1987). For most depressed cases with a comorbid anxiety disorder, the anxiety preceded the onset of MDD (Kovacs et al., 1989; Reinherz et al., 1989; Rohde et al., 1991). In a recent study by Essau (2003), 72% of the adolescents with both anxiety and depression had anxiety before that of depression, 12% had depression before anxiety, and 16% reported the onset of these disorders within the same year. Within the anxiety disorders, half of those with agoraphobia, anxiety NOS (not otherwise specified), and generalized anxiety disorder first had these disorders before MDD. All of those with social and specific phobia first had these two subtypes of anxiety disorders before depression. About half of those with panic disorder and depression experienced the onset of these disorders within the same year.

The frequent comorbidity of depression and anxiety has led to the development of two broad models. One model proposed that depression causes anxiety, and vice versa. The model is based on comparing the age of onset of both depression and anxiety. Another model posits that common or shared aetiological processes account for the comorbidity between anxiety and depression. Specifically, depression and anxiety are thought to be manifestations of the same underlying processes (Andrews, 1996; Tyrer, 2001). The tripartite model (Clark & Watson, 1991) has also been influential in explaining the comorbidity between depression and anxiety disorders. According to this model, depression and anxiety have both shared and unique factors. The shared factor is the presence of high level of negative affectivity. Unique factors include the presence of low level of positive affectivity in depression, and the presence of high level of physiological arousal in anxiety.

There seem to be gender differences in the type of comorbid disorders with MDD. Depression is more frequently comorbid with anxiety disorders in girls than in boys. By contrast, depression is comorbid more frequently with antisocial behaviour and conduct disorder in boys than in girls (McGee & Williams, 1988). MDD also comorbid frequently with alcohol use disorder (Rohde et al., 1996), and among those with both disorders, 58.1% of them reported the occurrence of depression before that of alcohol (Rohde et al., 1996). Similar finding has been reported by Hovens et al. (1994), in that 53% of the adolescents with dysthymia and alcohol use disorders reported dysthymia preceding alcohol use disorder.

Impact of comorbidity

Comorbidity of depression and psychiatric disorders is of significance to health services, health care providers, adolescents, and their family members both because of its frequency and its negative impact. The presence of comorbidity has been found to be associated with a greater number of past depression episodes (Rohde et al., 1991) and with more impairment and distress (Essau et al., 1999). In the OADP cohort, adolescents with MDD only compared to depressed adolescents with another mental disorder were much more likely to have received treatment, showed poor global functioning, to have elevated rate of suicide attempts, and to show evidence of academic problems (Lewinsohn et al., 1994). However, the impact of comorbidity seemed to be affected by gender. Specifically, males who had depression only had very low probability of being in treatment. The presence of a comorbid disorder increased treatment especially if the boy had a substance use disorder. In girls, those with depression only were more likely, whereas those who had a comorbid disruptive behaviour disorder were less likely to receive treatment. The highest use of mental health services was observed in depressed adolescents with substance use disorders. Depression also seemed to predict escalation in adolescent drug use (Henry et al., 1993) and correlates positively with severity of drug use (Riggs et al., 1995).

In Harrington et al.'s study (1990), the depressed adolescents with conduct disorder were more impaired in all areas of functioning (social dysfunction at work, love relationships, friendship, non-intimate social contacts, negotiations, and daily coping) compared to those with depression only. The authors interpreted these findings as showing some continuity between depression that had an onset during adolescence and adult depression.

Psychosocial impairment

Adolescent depression has been linked to psychosocial impairment across multiple domains. Adolescents with MDD have impaired social functioning and family relations, decreased self-esteem, and low academic achievement (Geller et al., 2001; Giaconia et al., 2001; Rao et al., 1995; Reinherz et al., 1999). Increased dysfunction from depression was also associated with early onset and greater severity of disorder, and increased number of recurrent episodes.

According to several longitudinal studies, depressed adolescents showed impaired psychosocial functioning at follow-up investigations (Fleming et al., 1993; Harrington et al., 1990; Puig-Antich et al., 1993). Data from the Ontario Child Health Study showed that about one-quarter of the depressed adolescents had problems with their family and friends, half had dropped out of school, and one-third had been involved with the police or court at a 4-year follow-up investigation (Fleming et al., 1993). Adolescent depression is also associated with school drop-out and occupational difficulties in young adulthood (Bardone et al., 1996; Fergusson & Woodward, 2002; Kessler et al., 1997). Puig-Antich et al. (1985) reported that after the depressive episodes, the formerly depressed adolescents as compared to normal controls remained significantly inferior in their communication skills with mothers, tension in relationship with fathers, and being teased by peers. These findings seem to suggest that some social deficits related to adolescent depression may be a reflection of enduring characteristics of adolescents who are prone to be depressed. Depression during adolescence also predicts early marriage and marital distress in young adulthood (Gotlib et al., 1998), and that they have an earlier transition to parenthood (Bardone et al., 1996). This finding is of great concern due to the association between parental and offspring depression (Beardslee et al., 1998). Lewinsohn et al. (2003) examined psychosocial functioning of young adults who have experienced and recovered from MDD during adolescence. In unadjusted analyses, young adults who had experienced depressive episodes during adolescence reported being impaired in various domains of psychosocial functioning such as impairment in occupational performance, interpersonal functioning, quality of life, and physical well-being. However, when the specificity of these associations was examined, only reduced life satisfaction was associated with adolescent depression. This finding was interpreted as showing that having experienced depression in adolescence tended to be associated with subsequent and enduring reductions in life satisfaction.

Depressed adolescents with comorbid disorders seemed to have the most impaired psychosocial functioning. As reported by Fombonne et al. (2001), among individuals with childhood depression, those with comorbid conduct disorder had higher rates of suicide attempt, criminal offences, and more pervasive social dysfunction in adulthood. In Rao et al.'s study (1995), depressed adolescents with a recurrent course, compared to those with no disorders, were significantly impaired in the overall degree of functioning (based on the GAF Scale), and in relationship with friends, and satisfaction with life and global functioning. During a depressive episode, both the depressed adolescents with a recurrent course and the adolescents with new onset of depression had significant impairment at work, interpersonal relationships, and social/leisure activities. These findings showed substantial continuity and specificity of affective problems from adolescence to adulthood.

In addition to the high level of psychosocial impairment, depressed adolescents also reported substantial levels of suicidal ideation and attempts (Reinherz et al., 1995). As many as 17.9% of depressed adolescents reported having had concrete plan for suicide, and 9.7% even had tried to commit suicide (Essau et al., 1999). In a study by Kovacs et al. (1993), the likelihood of a suicide attempt was about four- to fivefold higher for children with a history of MDD compared with those who did not have affective disorders but other psychiatric disorders. At follow-up, 32% of the children who met the diagnosis of MDD and/or dysthymia had attempted suicide compared to 11% of those whose index diagnosis was adjustment disorder with depressed mood and 8% of those with nonaffective disorders.

Health services utilization

According to the World Health Organization Global Burden of Disease Study (Murray & Lopez, 1996), MDD is the leading disease that causes disability among the 15–44 year olds in developed countries. Given the findings that depression generally begins early in life (i.e., in childhood or adolescence), which often continues into adulthood, there is a need to focus on early intervention. However, the few studies that have examined help-seeking behaviour among depressed adolescents showed that only a small proportion of these adolescents use mental health services. The few existing studies have reported much variation in the use of mental health services for MDD, with rates ranging from 15% to 65% (Cuffe et al., 2005; Offord et al., 1987). This difference may reflect methodological differences or real cultural differences among samples, or differences in health care systems in different countries. In Lewinsohn et al.'s study (1998), 60% of the adolescents with MDD had received any mental health treatment. The most commonly used treatment was individual outpatient psychotherapy (60.1%). Inpatient treatment was rare, and was generally given to those whose depression co-occurred with substance use disorders. Mental health services utilization was significantly associated with the presence of comorbid mental disorders, a history of suicide attempt, academic problems, a non-intact family, female gender, severity of depression, and the number of previous depressive episodes. Nine percent received pharmacotherapy, mostly antidepressant (4.2%) and antianxiety (3.7%) medication. Using data from the Dunedin Multidisciplinary Health Development Study, Feehan et al. (1994) reported strong association between depression and self-medication. The most common point of entry for adolescent seeking health services are the schools (Farmer et al., 2003).

In a recent study by Essau (2005), 23% of the adolescents with MDD received mental health services sometime in their lives. The majority of adolescents with depression sought mental health services treatment in the outpatient setting (62%), mostly from school psychologists. About 12% had sought treatment through other social services. The number of those who had received treatment in inpatient settings (19%) was higher than that of those with anxiety disorders. The only factor significantly associated with mental health services utilization was the presence of a past suicide attempt.

The use of mental health services seemed to influence the stability of MDD. For example, Essau (2005) reported that a high majority of the adolescents with depression at both the index and follow-up interview did not receive any mental health services. In the Lewinsohn et al.'s study (1998), adolescents who received treatment were not less likely to experience a new depressive episode at young adulthood. Their findings showed that among formerly depressed males (but not among females) previous treatment was associated with greater relapse. In two other longitudinal studies, depressed adolescents showed an increased likelihood of seeking professional help (Kashani et al., 1987), being prescribed psychotropic medication, attending psychiatric services, and being hospitalized for mental illness (Harrington et al., 1990) at a follow-up investigation.

Long-term course and outcome

Little is known about the course and outcome of MDD in adolescence. However, according to the few longitudinal studies of depressed adolescents (Anderson & McGee, 1994; Beardslee et al., 1996; Emslie et al. 1997; Fleming et al., 1993; Geller et al., 1994; Kovacs et al., 1994; Lewinsohn et al., 1994; Harrington et al., 1990; Hammen et al., 1990; Rao et al., 1995; Warner et al., 1992; Weissman et al., 1992), depression in these age groups does not reflect mild and short-lived or transient disturbances as previously thought (Rie, 1966). Depressed adolescents are not only at risk of having recurrent and/or continuing MDD in adulthood, but they have sustained impairments in various life domains such as at work, social activities, academic functioning, and interpersonal relationship (Kovacs et al., 1984; Harrington et al., 1990). These adolescents are also at an increased risk for attempted and completed suicide, anxiety disorders, and substance use disorders (Kovacs et al., 1993; Rao et al., 1995).

In considering studies on the course and outcome of depression, several indices have been used, including

1. Episode (i.e., meeting the full syndromal criteria of MDD for at least 14 days; APA,1994),
2. Remission (i.e., period in which the adolescent is asymptomatic or has minimal symptoms independent of treatment; Emslie et al., 1997),
3. Recovery (i.e., no mental state abnormalities; Goodyer et al., 1991),
4. Relapse (i.e., return of symptom that satisfy the full syndrome criteria for an episode that occurs during the remission period, but before recovery; Emslie et al., 1997), and
5. Recurrence (i.e., development of a new depressive episode that occur after recovery; Emslie et al., 1997).

These indices are based on depressive symptomatology such as symptom severity or the number of symptoms. Several other studies have used psychosocial outcome measures like academic performance, family relations, peer relations, drug and alcohol abuse, and suicide. The inconsistent and lack of uniform use of the indices of course and outcome make it difficult to interpret and compare findings across studies.

Duration of episodes

The mean length of major depressive episode in community samples is about 30 weeks (ranging from 23 to 36 weeks), and for dysthymic disorder 134 weeks (Lewinsohn et al., 1993); the average length of dysthymic disorder in clinical sample is about 3 years (Kovacs et al., 1984). In both epidemiological and clinical settings, between 21% and 41% of the depressed children and adolescents were still depressed after one year, and between 8% and 10% after 2 years (Kovacs et al., 1984; Lewinsohn et al., 1994; McCauley et al., 1993). In 83.5% of their subjects, the duration of MDD before the index interview was less than 2 years, and most were severely impaired (Geller et al., 1994). The results of the Sanford study indicated that one-third of the cases reported persistent MDD at follow-up. The average time to remission of MDD from the initial evaluation was 59.5 days (range 14–246 days) (Emslie et al., 1997). The mean duration of dysthymia in community study was 134 weeks (Lewinsohn et al., 1993), and in clinical study, dysthymia persisted for three years (Garber et al., 1988).

Factors associated with a longer index depressive episode include being female, greater episode severity, more dysfunctional family environment, early onset (before age 15), the presence of suicidal ideation, and having received treatment for the disorder (Lewinsohn et al., 1994). The length of depression was not affected by comorbid anxiety disorder, when depression was the primary diagnosis. However, when MDD was the secondary diagnosis and when it comorbid with anxiety and dysthymia, the MDD had a shorter duration (Kovacs et al., 1989). It was suggested that the combination of 'double depression' (i.e., major depression and dysthymia) and anxiety disorders may represent a 'neurotic', labile, or unstable depression that influence rapid recovery. In a recent study by Dunn and Goodyer (2006), depressed adolescents in the clinical setting had significantly longer index episodes than those in the community setting. Predictors of longer index episodes were severe impairment, having a longer depressive episode before starting treatment, and an early psychiatric history.

In the Sanford et al.'s study (1995), the predictors of MDD persistence was the presence of comorbid substance use, anxiety disorder, low involvement with father, poor response to mother's discipline, and older age at interview; however, age of onset of MDD failed to predict its persistence and remission. Since older age at interview was a predictor for MDD persistence, the authors suggest the importance of considering developmental stage when assessing psychopathology. Understanding factors related to protracted length of disorder is important because the longer an episode persists the greater the risk for negative effects on healthy developmental processes (Goodyer et al., 1997).

Birmaher and his colleagues (2004) compared the course of MDD in children and adolescents. Their results showed no significant differences between children and adolescents in the duration and relapse and recurrence rates of depression. In both groups, the average index depressive episode was 17 months. Longer duration was predicted by one depressive symptoms 'guilt', but not by severity of depression, comorbid disorder, and parental psychiatric history. At follow-up, 85% of the children and adolescents recovered from their depression, and 4% reported having had at least one recurrence after recovery. Factors that predicted a lower rate of recovery were child's history of MDD and father MDD. Increased risks of recurrence were predicted by father's MDD and being female, whereas having mothers with behavioural disorders were significantly related to higher recovery rate.

Recovery

The rates of recovery vary tremendously across studies, partially due to differences in the definition of recovery and the length of follow-up. In Garber et al.'s study (1988), 64% of the depressed adolescents had at least one major depressive episode at follow-up; 36% even had more than one episode. About 40% of the children developed a subsequent depression and none had recovered more than 2 years before experiencing their first remission (Kovacs et al., 1989). Within 5 years of entering adulthood, 40% had a depressive episode (Harrington et al., 1990). Emslie et al. (1997) similarly found that almost all subjects (98%) recovered with one year of initial evaluation, although there was also a high rate of recurrence. Among those with recurrence, 47.2% had it within a year of follow-up and 69.4% by 2 years.

In Lewinsohn et al.'s study (1994), 336 of the 362 adolescents who had experienced a MDD recovered from the episode at follow-up. The likelihood for recovery decreased as the episode duration lengthened. That is, about 25% of the subjects were recovered by 3 weeks, 50% by 8 weeks, and 75% by 24 weeks. About 5% of the recovered adolescents relapsed within 6 months, 12% developed a recurrent depressive episode within a year, and one-third became depressed within 4 years. Eighty-four of the 316 adolescents who recovered from a major depressive episode developed a second-episode before the follow-up investigation.

However, the rates of recovery seemed to be affected by informants used. As reported by Goodyer et al. (1991), about 43% of the depressed children considered themselves as being recovered at follow-up; the recovery judgement made by their mother was 53% and by the psychiatrists 50%. This difference in judgement may be due to the parent's inability to detect the child's internal emotional and cognitive symptoms.

Predictors of recovery in clinical and high-risk studies include first affective disorder at or before the age of 13, having been exposed to multiple parental depression, having a moderate/poor friendship after the onset of depression, and having parents with high expressed emotion. In a community study by Lewinsohn et al. (1994), those who took longer to recover from MDD had an earlier age of onset from the first episode, had suicidal ideation, and had been seeking treatment for the mood disorder. In the Goodyer et al.'s study (1991), none of the social factors examined, such as undesirable life events, friendship, and recent social achievement, predicted recovery at a 12-month follow-up investigation. Negative outcome of depression was related to having a moderate/poor friendship after the onset of depression. It was argued that adolescents who are not recovered may over-report undesirable experiences and difficulties.

Asarnow et al. (1993) reported that adolescents whose parents were rated as having low expressed emotion were significantly more likely to recover compared to those whose parents have high expressed emotion. That is, at a one-year follow-up interview, none of the adolescents in the high expressed emotion group recovered, compared to 53% of the adolescents in the low expressed emotion group. This result remained after controlling for the adolescent's sociodemographic factors (gender, age, socioeconomic status, single versus dual parent family) and clinical factors such as treatment during the follow-up period (i.e., psychosocial interventions versus psychosocial and pharmacologic interventions), depressive subtype (major depression, dysthymic disorder, double-depression), comorbidity with disruptive behavioural disorder, and chronicity (Asarnow et al., 1993). The authors argued that the 'affective climate' at home is an important predictor of outcome in depression. It was argued that children tend to be dependent on their families, especially when they are depressed and prone to withdraw from peers and other social activities.

In a recent study by Essau (2007), 24.4% of the adolescents with MDD met the diagnosis of this disorder at both the index and follow-up interviews. About half of the adolescents (48.9%) with a MDD at index interview no longer meet the diagnostic criteria of any psychiatric disorders at follow-up. In the remaining cases, the depression was replaced by other disorders such as anxiety, substance, and somatoform disorders. This finding suggested the heterogeneous pattern of depression in that sample. The presence of parental alcohol problems, suicidal behaviour and ideation (i.e., past suicidal attempt, suicidal thought, concrete suicidal plans), negative life events and negative coping, and the presence of substance use disorders significantly predicted the stability of depression.

Relapse

Relapse occurs at a high frequency after recovery for adolescents with MDD (Kovacs et al., 1984; Garber et al., 1988). Within one year of recovery, 26% of the treated depressed patients had a new depressive episode, which in most cases resulted in rehospitalization (Kovacs et al., 1984). In Lewinsohn et al.'s study (1994), 50% of those who recovered had relapsed within 6 months, 12% developed a recurrent/depressive episode within a year, and about one-third become depressed within 4 years. Kovacs and her colleagues also reported a 72% risk of relapse within 5 years after the initial episode, with the children with 'double depression' having a greater probability of relapse. Several studies (Fleming et al., 1993; Lewinsohn et al., 1994) have shown a recurrence rate of up to 70% by five years after the index episode and that adolescents with MDD face a 2- to 4-fold greater risk for depression as young adults (Pine et al., 1998).

Shorter time to relapse with MDD was associated with a history of suicide ideation and attempt during the first major depressive episode, greater severity of first major depressive episode, later age of first onset, and shorter first episode duration (Lewinsohn et al., 1994), as well as the presence of comorbid dysthymic disorder (Kovacs et al., 1984). The finding that MDD that occurred early during childhood had longer durations was interpreted as supporting the hypothesis that early-onset depression differ from depression that occurs later in life.

In another publication of the OADP data (Lewinsohn et al., 2003), factors identified during adolescence that predicted recurrence of depression at young adulthood included specific features of adolescence (e.g., elevated depressive symptoms, excessive emotional reliance on others, lower social competence, daily hassles), features of adolescent MDD episode (e.g., long duration, multiple episodes, severity, history of suicide attempt), and having family members with MDD. Pettit et al. (2006) recently examined the association between the first depressive episode and the presence of a recurrent episode among adolescents and young adults. Two of the MDD's criteria—depressed mood and increased appetite—predicted recurrence. The finding that depressed mood predicted depression was interpreted as supporting depressive mood as being central to MDD. Thus, MDD without depressive mood is not only uncommon, but it may follow a unique and less recurrent course.

In Warner et al.'s study (1992), adolescents with an early onset (below 13 years old) and whose parents were divorced and had multiple depressed episode had significantly more protracted time to recovery. The strongest predictor of recurrent depression in these adolescents was a prior comorbid diagnosis of dysthymic disorder, followed by problem in social functioning. That is, those whose first episode occurred before the age of 13 years took an average of 74 weeks to recover, whereas those who had experienced 2 or more bouts of parental depression took an average of 79 weeks to recover. Additionally, the mean number of weeks to recovery was 54 in children of depressed parents, and 23 in children of non-depressed parents; within the 2-year period, 87% of these children had recovered. These authors suggested that MDD in adolescents could have different predictors of incidence, recurrence, and time to recovery.

Conclusion and future direction

In this chapter, we have reviewed findings on the epidemiology, comorbidity, and course of depression in adolescents. There has been tremendous interest in adolescent depression in recent years, and consequently, our knowledge about depression in this age group has substantially increased. MDD is a common disorder that affects about 10% of the adolescents in the general population. Recent studies have shown high comorbidity and impairment associated with depression, and low level of mental health services utilization.

The course of MDD is chronic, with the average length of depressive episodes among adolescents in the community setting being about 30 weeks and for dysthymic disorder being 134 weeks. Relapse occurs frequently, with a high percentage of the depressed patients experiencing a new depressive episode a year after recovery. Given the frequency, chronicity, and severity of MDD experienced by adolescents, these disorders should not be viewed as a normal part of development. However, a major challenge is the question of whether our current classification system of MDD, designed for adults, is valid for use with adolescents. Another challenge is to reach the depressed adolescents who need professional help the most. Many depressed adolescents who seek treatment usually do so from a general practitioner (e.g., Essau, 2005). Because general care practitioners differ in their ability to detect depressive and other mental disorders (usually they tend to under-diagnose depression in their patients), efforts are needed to develop an assessment instrument for depression to allow its accurate and early detection. However, to be useful, they have to meet some specific requirement, including (Wittchen & Essau, 1990) (i) being brief so that they will not be time-consuming to administer or interact significantly with the time constraints in primary care, (ii) require only minimal training, and (iii) have a high sensitivity and specificity to allow early detection and treatment.

Although numerous studies have been focused on the comorbidity of depression and other disorders, the meaning of comorbidity for classification and aetiological mechanism is unclear. To progress further in this issue, future studies need to rule out chance, referral bias, population stratification, and overlapping diagnostic criteria. It would also be helpful to investigate comorbidity patterns across developmental stages to determine the extent to which specific comorbid disorders may represent subtypes of depression (Avenevoli et al., 2007). Furthermore, to solve the issues of diagnostic specificity and aetiologic mechanisms in MDD, future studies need to explore the temporal relationship of the disorders by examining their age of onset. Given the findings that depression with different age of onset tend to have different pathways to adult depression and health, an area of future research would be to compare the course of depression based on age of onset (i.e., child-, prepubertal-, and adolescent-onset depression).

To conclude, although our knowledge about adolescent depression has increased over the last decade, there is much more to learn before we can assert that we fully understand their onset, course, and long-term sequels.

References

Anderson, J.C. & McGee, R. (1994). Comorbidity of depression in children and adolescents. In W.M. Reynolds & H.F. Johnston (Eds.), *Handbook of depression in children and adolescents* (pp. 581–601). New York: Plenum Press.

Anderson, J.C., Williams, S., McGee, R., & Silva, P.A. (1987). DSM-III disorders in preadolescent children. Prevalence in a large sample from the general population. *Archives of General Psychiatry, 44*, 69–76.

Andrews, G. (1996). Comorbidity and the general neurotic syndrome. *British Journal of Psychiatry Supplement, 30*, 76–84.

Angold, A. & Costello, E.J. (1993). Depressive comorbidity in children and adolescents: Empirical, theoretical, and methodological issues. *American Journal Psychiatry, 150*, 1779–1791.

Angold, A., Costello, E.J., & Worthman, C.M. (1998). Puberty and depression: The roles of age, pubertal status and pubertal timing. *Psychological Medicine, 28*, 51–61.

American Psychiatric Association (1987). *Diagnostic and statistical manual of mental disorders* (3rd rev. ed.). Washington, DC: American Psychiatric Association.

American Psychiatric Association (1980). *Diagnostic and statistical manual of mental disorders, Third edition (DSM-III)*. Washington, DC: American Psychiatric Association.

American Psychiatric Association (1994). *Diagnostic and statistical manual of mental disorders, Fourth edition (DSM-IV)*. Washington, DC: American Psychiatric Association.

Aro, H. (1994). Risk und protective factors in depression: A developmental perspective. *Acta Psychiatrica Scandinavica (Suppl. 377)*, 59–64.

Asarnow, J.R., Goldstein, M.J., Tompson, M., & Guthrie, D. (1993). One-year outcomes of depressive disorders in child psychiatric in-patients: Evaluation of the prognostic power of a brief measure of expressed emotion. *Journal of Child Psychology and Psychiatry, 34*, 129–137.

Avenevoli, S., Knight, E., Kessler, R.C., & Merikangas, K.R. (2007). Epidemiology of depression in children and adolescents. In J.R. Abela & B.L. Hankin (Eds.), *Handbook of depression in children and adolescents* (pp. 6–32). New York: The Guilford Press.

Bardone, A.M., Moffitt, T.E., Caspi, A., Dickson, N., & Silva, P.A. (1996). Adult mental health and social outcomes of adolescent girls with depression and conduct disorder. *Development and Psychopathology, 8,* 811–829.

Beardslee, W.R., Keller, M.B., Seifer, R., Lavori, P.W., Staley, J., Podorefsky, D., et al. (1996). Prediction of adolescent affective disorder: Effects of prior parental affective disorders and child psychopathology. *Journal of the American Academy of Child and Adolescent Psychiatry, 35,* 279–288.

Beardslee, W.R., Keller, M.B., Lavori, P.W., Staley, J., & Sacks, N. (1993). The impact of parental affective disorder on depression in offspring: A longitudinal follow-up in a non referred sample. *Journal of the American Academy of Child and Adolescent Psychiatry, 32,* 723–730.

Beardslee, W.R., Versage, E.M., & Gladstone, T.R.G. (1998). Children of affectively ill parents: A review of the past 10 years. *Journal of the American Academy of Child and Adolescent Psychiatry, 37,* 1134–1141.

Birmaher, B., Bridge, J.A., Williamson, D.E., Brent, D.A., Dahl, R.E., Axelson, D.A., et al. (2004). Psychosocial functioning in youths at high risk to develop major depressive disorder. *Journal of the American Academy of Child and Adolescent Psychiatry, 43,* 839–846.

Canino, G.J., Bird, H.R., Schrout, P.E., Rubio-Stipec, M., Bravo, M., Martinez, R., et al. (1987). The prevalence of specific psychiatric disorders in Puerto Rico. *Archives of General Psychiatry, 44,* 727–735.

Clark, L.A. & Watson, D. (1991). Tripartite model of anxiety and depression: Psychometric evidence and taxonomic implications. *Journal of Abnormal Psychology, 100,* 316–336.

Cohen, P., Cohen, J., Kasen, S., Velez, C.N., Hartmark, C., Johnson, J., et al. (1993). An epidemiologic study of disorders in late childhood and adolescence: I. Age- and gender-specific prevalence. *Journal of Child Psychology and Psychiatry, 34,* 851–867.

Cuffe, S.P., McKeown, R.E., Addy, C.L., & Garrison, C.Z. (2005). Family and psychosocial risk factors in a longitudinal epidemiological study of adolescents. *Journal of the American Academy of Child and Adolescent Psychiatry, 44,* 121–129.

Cyranowski, J.M., Frank, E., Young, E., & Shear, M.K. (2000). Adolescent onset of the gender difference in lifetime rates of major depression: A theoretical model. *Archives of General Psychiatry, 57,* 21–27.

Dunn, V., & Goodyer, I.M. (2006). Longitudinal investigation into childhood- an adolescence-onset depression: Psychiatric outcome in early adulthood. *British Journal of Psychiatry, 188,* 216–222.

Emslie, G.J., Rush, A.J., Weinberg, W.A., Kowatch, R.A., Hughes, C.W., Carmody, T., et al. (1997). A double-blind, randomized, placebo-controlled trial of fluoxetine in children and adolescents with depression. *Archives of General Psychiatry, 54,* 1031–1037.

Erickson, E.H. (1968). *Identity, youth and crisis.* New York: W. W. Norton.

Essau, C.A. (2003). Comorbidity of anxiety disorders in adolescents. *Depression and Anxiety, 18,* 1–6.

Essau, C.A. (2005). Use of mental health services among adolescents with anxiety and depressive disorders. *Depression and Anxiety, 22,* 130–137.

Essau, C.A. (2007). Course of depressive disorders in adolescents. *Journal of Affective Disorders, 99,* 191–201.

Essau, C.A., Conradt, J., Groen, G., Turbanisch, U., & Petermann, F. (1999). Kognitive Faktoren bei Jugendlichen mit depressiven Störungen: Ergebnisse der Bremer Jugendstudie. *Zeitschrift für Klinische Psychologie, Psychiatrie und Psychotherapie, 47,* 51–72.

Essau, C.A., Conradt, J., & Petermann, F. (2000). Frequency, comorbidity, and psychosocial impairment of depressive disorders in adolescents. *Journal of Adolescent Research, 15*, 470–481.

Essau, C.A. & Petermann, F. (Eds.) (1997). *Developmental psychopathology: Epidemiology, diagnostics, and treatment*. London: Harwood Academic Publishers.

Farmer, E.M., Burns, B.J., Phillips, S.D., Angold, A., & Costello, E.J. (2003). Pathways into and through mental health services for children and adolescents. *Psychiatric Services, 54*, 60–66.

Feehan, M., McGee, R., Nada-Raja, S., & Williams, S. M. (1994). DSM-III-R disorders in New Zealand 18-year-olds. *Australian and New Zealand Journal of Psychiatry, 28*, 87–99.

Fergusson, D.M., Horwood, L.J., & Lynskey, M.T. (1993). Prevalence and comorbidity of DSM-III-R diagnoses in a birth cohort of 15 year olds. *Journal of the Academy of Child and Adolescent Psychiatry, 32*, 1127–1134.

Fergusson, D.M. & Woodward, L.J. (2002). Mental health, educational, and social role outcomes of adolescents with depression. *Archives of General Psychiatry, 59*, 225–231.

Fleming, J.E., Boyle, M.H., & Offord, D.R. (1993). The outcome of adolescent depression in the Ontario child health study follow-up. *Journal of the American Academy of Child and Adolescent Psychiatry, 32*, 28–33.

Fombonne, E. (1995). Depressive disorders: Time trends and possible explanatory mechanisms. In M. Rutter & D. J. Smith (Eds.), *Psychosocial disorders in young people: Time trends and their causes* (pp. 544–615). Chichester: Wiley.

Fombonne, E., Wostear, G., Cooper, V., Harrington, R., & Rutter, M. (2001). The Maudsley long-term follow-up of child and adolescent depression: 2. Suicidality, criminality and social dysfunction in adulthood. *British Journal of Psychiatry, 179*, 218–223.

Garber, J., Kriss, M.R., Koch, M., & Lindholm, L. (1988). Recurrent depression in adolescents: A follow-up study. *Journal of the American Academy of Child and Adolescent Psychiatry, 27*, 49–54.

Garber, J.A., Lewinsohn, P.M., Seeley, J.R. & Brooks-Gunn, J. (1997). Is psychopathology associated with the timing of pubertal development? *Journal of the American Academy of Child and Adolescent Psychiatry, 36*, 1768–1776.

Garrison, C.Z., Waller, J.L., Cuffe, S.P., McKeown, R.E., Addy, C.L., & Jackson, K.L. (1997). Incidence of major depressive disorder and dysthymia in young adolescents. *Journal of the American Academy of Child and Adolescent Psychiatry, 36,* 458–465.

Geertz, C. (1973). *The interpretation of culture*. New York: Basic Books.

Geller, B., Fox., L.W., & Clark, K.A. (1994). Rate and predictors of prepubertal bipolarity during follow-up of 6- to 12-year-old depressed children. *Journal of the American Academy of Child and Adolescent Psychiatry, 33*, 461–468.

Geller, B., Zimmerman, B., Williams, M., Bolhofner, K., & Craney, J.L. (2001). Adult psychosocial outcome of prepubertal major depressive disorder. *Journal of the American Academy of Child and Adolescent Psychiatry, 40*, 673–677.

Giaconia, R.M., Reinherz, H.Z., Paradis, A.D., Hauf, A.M.C., & Stashwick, C.K. (2001). Major depression and drug disorders in adolescence: General and specific impairments in early adulthood. *Journal of the American Academy of Child and Adolescent Psychiatry, 40,*1426–1433.

Giaconia, R.M., Reinherz, H.Z., Silverman, A.B., Pakiz, B., Frost, A.K., & Cohen, E. (1994). Age of onset of psychiatric disorders in a community population of older adolescents. *Journal of the American Academy of Child and Adolescent Psychiatry, 33*, 706–717.

Goodyer, I. & Cooper, P.J. (1993). A community study of depression in adolescent girls. II: The clinical features of identified disorder. *British Journal of Psychiatry, 163*, 374–380.

Goodyer, I., Germany, E., Gowrusankur, J., & Altham, P. (1991). Social influences on the course of anxious and depressive disorders in school-age children. *British Journal of Psychiatry, 158*, 676–684.

Goodyer, I.M., Cooper, P.J., Vize, C.M., & Ashby, L. (1993). Depression in 11–16-year-old girls: The role of past parental psychopathology and exposure to recent life events. *Journal of Child Psychology and Psychiatry, 34*, 1103–1115.

Goodyer, I.M., Herbert, J., Secher, S.M., & Pearson, J. (1997). Short-term outcome of major depression: I. Comorbidity and severity at presentation as predictors of persistent disorder. *Journal of the American Academy of Child and Adolescent Psychiatry, 36*, 179–187.

Gotlib, I.H., Lewinsohn, P.M., & Seeley, J.R. (1998). Consequences of depression during adolescence: Marital status and marital functioning in early adulthood. *Journal of Abnormal Psychology, 107*, 686–690.

Hammen, C., Burge, D., Burney, E., & Adrian, C. (1990). Longitudinal study of diagnoses in children of women with unipolar and bipolar affective disorder. *Archives of General Psychiatry, 47*, 1112–1117.

Harrington, R., Fudge, H., Rutter, M., Pickles, A., & Hill, J. (1990). Adult outcomes of childhood and adolescent depression: I. Psychiatric status. *Archives of General Psychiatry, 47*, 465–473.

Hayward, C., Gotlib, I.H., Schraedley, P.K., & Litt, I.F. (1999). Ethnic differences in the association between pubertal status and symptoms of depression in adolescent girls. *Journal of Adolescent Health, 25*, 143–149.

Henry, B., Feehan, M., McGee, R., Stanton, W., Moffitt, T.E., & Silva, P. (1993). The importance of conduct problems and depressive symptoms in predicting adolescent substance use. *Journal of Abnormal Child Psychology, 21*, 469–480.

Hovens, J.G.F.M., Cantwell, D.P., & Kiriakos, R. (1994). Psychiatric comorbidity in hospitalized adolescent substance abusers. *Journal of the American Academy of Child and Adolescent Psychiatry, 33*, 476–483.

Kashani, J.H., Carlson, G.A., Beck, N.C., Hoeper, E.W., Corcoran, C.M., McAllister, J.A., et al. (1987). Depression, depressive symptoms, and depressed mood among a community sample of adolescents. *American Journal of Psychiatry, 144*, 931–934.

Kashani, J.H., Rosenberg, T.K., & Reid, J.C. (1989). Developmental perspectives in child and adolescent depressive symptoms in a community sample. *American Journal of Psychiatry, 146*, 871–875.

Kessler, R.C., Olfson, M., & Berglund, P.A. (1998). Patterns and predictors of treatment contact after first onset of psychiatric disorders. *American Journal of Psychiatry, 155*, 62–69.

Kessler, R.C., McGonagle, K.A., Swartz, M., Blazer, D.G., & Nelson, C.B. (1993). Sex and depression in the National Comorbidity Survey: I. Lifetime prevalence, chronicity and recurrence. *Journal of Affective Disorders, 29*, 85–96.

Kessler, R.C., Zhao, S., Blazer, D.G., & Swartz, M. (1997). Prevalence, correlates, and course of minor depression and major depression in the National Comorbidity Survey: I. Lifetime prevalence, chronicity and recurrence. *Journal of Affective Disorders, 45*, 19–30.

Kleinman, A. (1986). *Social origins of stress and disease: Depression, neurasthenia, and pain in modern China.* New Haven: Yale University Press.

Kovacs, M., Akiskal, H.S., Gatsonis, C., & Parrone, P. (1994). Childhood-onset dysthymic disorder: Clinical features and prospective naturalistic outcome. *Archives of General Psychiatry, 51*, 365–374.

Kovacs, M., Feinberg, T.L., Crouse-Novak, M., Paulauskas, S.L., Pollock, M., & Finkelstein, R.F. (1984). Depressive disorder in childhood: II. A longitudinal study of the risk for a subsequent major depression. *Archives of General Psychiatry, 41*, 643–649.

Kovacs, M., Gatsonis, C., Paulauskas, S.L., & Richards, C. (1989). Depressive disorders in childhood: IV. A longitudinal study of comorbidity with and risk for anxiety disorders. *Achives of General Psychiatry, 46*, 776–782.

Kovacs, M., Goldston, D., & Gatsonis, C. (1993). Suicidal behaviors and childhood-onset depressive disorders: A longitudinal investigation. *Journal of the American Academy of Child and Adolescent Psychiatry, 32*, 8–20.

Kutcher, S.P. & Marton, P. (1989). Parameters of adolescents depression: A review. *Psychiatric Clinics of North America, 12*, 895–918.

Lewinsohn, P.M., Clarke, G.N., Seeley, J.R., & Rohde, P. (1994). Major depression in community adolescents: Age at onset, episode duration, and time to recurrence. *Journal of the American Academy of Child and Adolescent Psychiatry, 33*, 809–818.

Lewinsohn, P.M., Hops, H., Roberts, R.E., Seeley, J.R., & Andrews, J.A. (1993). Adolescent psychopathology: I. Prevalence and incidence of depression and other DSM-III-R disorders in high school students. *Journal of Abnormal Psychology, 102*, 133–144.

Lewinsohn, P.M., Rohde, P., Seeley, J.R., Klein, D.N., & Gotlib, I.H. (2003). Psychosocial functioning of young adults who have experienced and recovered from major depressive disorder during adolescence. *Journal of Abnormal Psychology, 112*, 353–363.

Lewinsohn, P.M., Rohde, P., & Seeley, J.R. (1998). Treatment of adolescent depression: Frequency of services and impact on functioning in young adulthood. *Depression and Anxiety, 7*, 47–52.

McCauley, E., Myers, K., Mitchell, J., Caleron, R., Schloredt, K., & Treder, R. (1993). Depression in young people: Initial presentation and clinical course. *Journal of the American Academy of Child and Adolescent Psychiatry, 32*, 714–722.

McGee, R., Feehan, M., Williams, S., Partridge, F., Silva, P.A. & Kelly, J. (1990). DSM-III disorders in a large sample of adolescents. *Journal of the American Academy of Child and Adolescent Psychiatry, 29*, 611–619.

McGee, R. & Williams, S. (1988). A longitudinal study of depression in nine-year-old children. *Journal of the American Academy of Child Psychiatry, 27*, 342–348.

Murray, C.L. & Lopez, A.D. (Eds.) (1996). *The global burden of disease: A comprehensive assessment of mortality and disability from diseases, injuries, and risk factors in 1990 and projected to 2020.* Cambridge, MA: Harvard University Press.

Newman, D.L., Moffitt, T.E., Caspi, A., & Magdol, L. (1996). Psychiatric disorder in a birth cohort of young adults: Prevalence, comorbidity, clinical significance, and new case incidence from ages 11–21. *Journal of Consulting and Clinical Psychology, 64*, 552–562.

Nichter, M. (1981). Idioms of distress: Alternatives in the expression of psychosocial distress: A case study from South India. *Culture, Medicine and Psychiatry, 5*, 397–408.

Nottelmann, E.D. & Jensen, P.S. (1999). Comorbidity of depressive disorders in children and adolescents: Rates, temporal sequencing, course and outcome. In C.A. Essau & F. Petermann (Eds.), *Depressive disorders in children and adolescents: Epidemiology, risk factors, and treatment.* Northvale, NJ: Jason Aronson.

Offord, D.R., Boyle, M.H., Szatmari, P., Rae-Grant, N.I., Links, P.S., Cadman, D.T., et al. (1987). Ontario Child Health Study: Six-month prevalence of disorder and rates of service utilization. *Archives of General Psychiatry, 44*, 832–836.

Petersen, A.C., Sarigiani, P.A. & Kennedy, R.E. (1991). Adolescent depression: Why more girls? *Journal of Youth and Adolescence, 20*, 247–271.

Pettit, J.W., Lewinsohn, P.M., & Joiner, T.E. (2006). Propagation of major depressive disorder: Relationship between first episode symptoms and recurrence. *Psychiatry Research, 141,* 271–278.

Pine, D.S., Cohen, P., Gurley, D., Brook, J., & Ma, Y. (1998). The risk for early-adulthood anxiety and depressive disorders in adolescents with anxiety and depressive disorders. *Archives of General Psychiatry, 55,* 56–64.

Puig-Antich, J., Kaufman, J., Ryan, N.D., Williamson, D.E., Dahl, R.E., Lukens, E., et al. (1993). The psychosocial functioning and family environment of depressed adolescents. *Journal of American Academy of Child and Adolescent Psychiatry, 32,* 244–253.

Puig-Antich, J., Ryan, N.D., & Rabinovich, H. (1985). Affective disorders in childhood and adolescence. In J.M. Wiener (Ed.), *Diagnosis and psychopharmacology of childhood and adolescent disorders* (pp. 151–178). New York: John Wiley.

Rao, U., Ryan, N.D., Birmaher, B., Dahl, R.E., Williamson, D.E., Kaufman, J., et al. (1995). Unipolar depression in adolescents: Clinical outcome in adulthood. *Journal of the American Academy of Child and Adolescent Psychiatry, 34,* 566–578.

Reinherz, H.Z., Giaconia, R.M., Hauf, A.M.C., Wasserman, M.S., & Silverman, A.B. (1999). Major depression in the transition to adulthood: Risks and impairments. *Journal of Abnormal Psychology, 108,* 500–510.

Reinherz, H.Z., Giaconia, R.M., Pakiz, B., Silverman, A.B., Frost, A.K., & Lefkowitz, E.S. (1993). Psychosocial risks for major depression in late adolescence: A longitudinal study. *Journal of the American Academy of Child and Adolescent Psychiatry, 36,* 1155–1163.

Reinherz, H.Z., Giaconia, R.M., Silverman, A.B., Friedman, A., Pakiz, B., Frost, A.K., et al. (1995). Early psychosocial risks for adolescent suicidal ideation and attempts. *Journal of the American Academy of Child and Adolescent Psychiatry, 34,* 599–611.

Reinherz, H.Z., Paradis, A.D., Giaconia, R.M., Stashwick, C.K., & Fitzmaurice, G. (2003). Childhood and adolescent predictors of major depression in the transition to adulthood. *American Journal of Psychiatry, 160,* 2141–2147.

Reinherz, H.Z., Stewart-Berghauer, G., Pakiz, B., Frost, A.K., Moeykens, B.A., & Holmes, W.M. (1989). The relationship of early risk and current mediators to depressive symptomatology in adolescence. *Journal of the American Academy of Child and Adolescent Psychiatry, 28,* 942–947.

Rie, H.E. (1966). Depression in childhood: A survey of some pertinent contributions. *Journal of the American Academy of Child Psychiatry, 5,* 653–685.

Riggs, P.D., Baker, S., Mikulich, S.K., Young, S.E., & Crowley, T. (1995). Depression in substance-dependent delinquents. *Journal of the American Academy of Child and Adolescent Psychiatry, 34,* 764–771.

Rohde, P., Lewinsohn, P.M., & Seeley, J.R. (1991). Comorbidity of unipolar depression: II. Comorbidity with other mental disorders in adolescents and adults. *Journal of Abnormal Psychology, 100,* 214–222.

Rohde, P., Lewinsohn, P.M., & Seeley, J.R. (1996). Psychiatric comorbidity with problematic alcohol use in high school adolescents. *Journal of the American Academy of Child and Adolescent Psychiatry, 35,* 101–109.

Rutter, M. (1986). The developmental psychopathology of depression: Issues and perspectives. In M. Rutter, C.E. Izard, & P.B. Read (Eds.), *Depression in young people* (pp. 3–30). New York: Guilford Press.

Sanford, M., Szatmari, P., Spinner, M., Muroe-Blum, H., Jamieson, E., Walsh, C., et al. (1995). Predicting the one-year course of adolescent major depression. *Journal of the American Academy of Child and Adolescent Psychiatry, 34,* 1618–1628.

Tseng, W.S. & Streltzer, J. (1997). *Culture and psychopathology: A guide to clinical assessment.* New York: Brunner/Mazel, Publishers.

Tyrer, P. (2001). The case for cothymia: Mixed anxiety and depression as a single diagnosis. *British Journal of Psychiatry, 179*, 191–193.

Velez, C.N., Johnson, J., & Cohen, P. (1989). A longitudinal analysis of selected risk factors for childhood psychopathology. *Journal of the American Academy of Child and Adolescent Psychiatry, 28*, 851–864.

Verhulst, F.C., van der Ende, J., Ferdinand, R.F., & Kasius, M.C. (1997). The prevalence of DSM-III-R diagnoses in a National sample of Dutch adolescents. *Archives of General Psychiatry, 54*, 329–336.

Warner, V., Weissman, M.M., Fendrich, M., Wickramaratne, P., & Moreau, D. (1992). The course of major depression in the offspring of depressed parents: Incidence, recurrence, and recovery. *Archives of General Psychiatry, 49*, 795–801.

Weissman, M.M. (1988). Psychopathology in the children of depressed parents: Direct interview studies. In D.L. Dunner, E.S. Gershon, & J. Barret (Eds.), *Relatives at risk for mental disorder* (pp. 143–159). New York: Raven Press.

Weissman, M.M., Bland, R.C., Canino, G.J., Faravelli, C., Greenwald, S., Hwu, H.G., et al. (1996). Cross-national epidemiology of major depression and bipolar disorder. *Journal of American Medical Association, 276*, 293–299.

Weissman, M.M., Fendrich, M., Warner, V., & Wickramaratne, P. (1992). Incidence of psychiatric disorder in offspring at high and low risk for depression. *Journal of the American Academy of Child and Adolescent Psychiatry, 31*, 640–648.

Weissman, M.W., Gershon, E.S., Kidd, K.K., Prusoff, J.F., Leckman, E., Dibble, E., et al. (1984). Psychiatric disorders in the relatives of probands with affective disorders. *Archives of General Psychiatry, 41*, 13–21.

Whitaker, A., Johnson, J., Shaffer, D., Rapoport, J.L., Kalikow, K., Walsh, B.T., et al. (1990). Uncommon troubles in young people: Prevalence estimates of selected psychiatric disorders in a nonreferred population. *Archives of General Psychiatry, 47*, 487–496.

Wittchen, H.-U. & Essau, C.A. (1990). Assessment of symptoms and psychological disabilities in primary care. In N. Sartorius et al. (Ed.), *Psychological disorders in general medical settings* (pp. 111–136). Bern: Hogrefe & Huber Publishers.

Wittchen, H.-U., Nelson, C.B., & Lachner, G. (1998). Prevalence of mental disorders and psychosocial impairments in adolescents and young adults. *Psychological Medicine, 28*, 109–126.

Chapter 2

Risk and vulnerability in adolescent depression

Elizabeth P. Hayden, Pamela M. Seeds, & David J.A. Dozois

There are many reasons why research on adolescent depression is uniquely equipped to shed light on issues critical to both theory and practice. It is arguable that depression is, in many respects, a disorder of adolescence; those who experience the greatest impact of the disorder, by virtue of having recurrent or chronic mood symptoms, often have a first onset of depression in adolescence (Golan et al., 2005). Adolescence is also a period in which rates of the disorder show a marked and rapid increase. In preadolescent samples, prevalence estimates of depression using both lifetime and past-year prevalence are generally less than 3% (Costello et al., 2006; Garber & Horowitz, 2002). In contrast, prevalence estimates in adolescence range from 5–6% (Costello et al., 2006) to 8% (Lewinsohn et al., 1998), and longitudinal studies similarly suggest that rates of depression increase dramatically during adolescence (Hankin et al., 1998). Additionally, adolescence is when the female preponderance of depression emerges; while male children may actually show slightly higher rates of depression than girls (Angold & Rutter, 1992), over the course of early adolescence, cases of depression in females increase and eventually double those in males (e.g., Angold et al., 1998; Cairney, 1998; Hankin et al., 1998). The sequelae of depression in adolescence are serious, and include persistent problems with mental disorders (Dunn & Goodyer, 2006) and poor interpersonal functioning (Gotlib et al., 1998a) in adulthood. Finally, as this developmental stage is rife with significant biological (Hayward & Sanborn, 2002) and psychosocial changes (Blyth et al., 1983), studying depression in adolescence can provide important clues about vulnerability and aetiological processes. Thus, from a preventative standpoint, studying adolescents could potentially elucidate mechanisms of plasticity or malleability with regard to vulnerability to depression.

In this chapter, we review the large literature relevant to vulnerability to adolescent depression from several perspectives, focusing on cognitive, contextual, and genetic and biological models of the disorder. There are important reasons why these models have become as influential as they are in the field. In addition to characterizing the thinking patterns associated with depression, cognitive models of depression have spurred the development of safe and effective treatments for this highly debilitating disorder. Regarding context, robust associations have been repeatedly found between stress, social support, and depression. Finally, given that all behaviour is rooted in biological processes, any contemporary formulation of depression is incomplete without an account of biological factors implicated in the disorder. However, it is unfortunate that these models are often juxtaposed with one another as competing accounts of the origins of the disorder, especially given the almost certain aetiological heterogeneity of the disorder. In the context of a literature review, the need to treat these models as distinct processes is not intended to be reductionistic, as biological factors in depression occur within environmental contexts that often play a profound role in determining the long-term impact of putatively endogenous predispositions. Furthermore, although genetic/biological and environmental factors are often treated as orthogonal processes in theoretical models and study designs, the independence of the effects of the two in terms of predicting adverse outcomes in depression is likely exaggerated (e.g., Caspi et al., 2003; Kendler & Karkowski-Shuman, 1997). Increasingly, investigators are recognizing the likely false dichotomy of the nature–nurture debate with respect to the aetiology of depression, and are incorporating this recognition into novel study designs to examine the interplay between biological and contextual influences.

With these caveats, in order to coherently present a review of factors implicated in depression in adolescence, decisions must be made about how to organize the vast literature relevant to this topic. Therefore, we have divided this chapter into three broad sections that reflect several predominant lines of research in this field. In the first section, cognitive models of depression vulnerability are reviewed. In the second section, the literature on stress, coping, and social support is discussed. In the final section, we consider genetic and biological (hormonal & neurotransmitter system) factors that appear to play a role in depression.

Cognitive vulnerability to depression

Cognitive theories of depression explain the disorder in terms of individual differences in maladaptive thinking and biased appraisals in response to life stress (Abramson et al., 2002; Beck, 1967; Hankin & Abramson, 2001; Ingram et al., 1998). These theories are diathesis–stress models, in that 'under ordinary conditions, people who are vulnerable to the onset of depression are indistinguishable from nonvulnerable people. . .[it is only] when confronted with certain stressors do cognitive differences between vulnerable and nonvulnerable people emerge, which then turn into depression for those who are vulnerable' (Ingram et al., 2006, p. 64). Premises of two of the major cognitive theories, Beck's cognitive theory (1967, 1976) and the hopelessness model of depression (Abramson et al., 1989), have been tested in adolescent samples.

Beck's cognitive model and hopelessness theory

According to Beck's cognitive model (Beck, 1963, 1964, 1967, 2005; Beck et al., 1979; Clark et al., 1999), an individual's emotions and behaviours are influenced by his or her perception or appraisal of events. Schemas, information processing/intermediate beliefs (including dysfunctional rules, assumptions, and attitudes), and automatic thoughts make up the three primary levels of cognition emphasized in this theory.

Conceptually, schemas are viewed as central to the model and are defined as 'relatively enduring internal structures of stored generic or prototypical features of stimuli, ideas, or experience that are used to organize new information in a meaningful way thereby determining how phenomena are perceived and conceptualized' (Clark et al., 1999, p. 79; also see James et al., 2007). A self-schema is a well-organized perceptual set that forms the basis of core beliefs about self. According to Beck, the development and structure of a maladaptive self-schema occurs in early childhood but remains dormant until it is activated by negative life circumstances (see Beck et al., 1979). Individual differences in the relative value placed on different classes of life events are also important to understanding vulnerability (Beck, 1983). For example, individuals who rely on interpersonal approval and acceptance for their self-worth (referred to as sociotropy/dependency) are especially prone to depression when they experience negative life events in a relevant interpersonal domain. In contrast, autonomous or self-critical individuals are predicted to be more vulnerable to depression following the experience of threats to independency and personal control.

Once activated, schemas are thought to influence the filtering, encoding, storage, retrieval, and interpretation of information in a negative and schema-congruent fashion (Beck et al., 1979; Ingram et al., 1998). An individual who is susceptible to depression, for example, may have an underlying core belief that (s)he is worthless and unlovable. When this schema is later activated by relevant negative life events (e.g., peer or partner rejection), this individual may exhibit negatively biased processing (e.g., selectively attending to or recalling negative information to the exclusion of positive or neutral information) and demonstrate errors in thinking (e.g., overgeneralization, personalization). These processes, in turn, increase the probability that the individual will experience automatic thoughts in the form of a negative view of self, the world, and the future (a negative cognitive triad), the proximal catalyst of depression (Beck et al., 1979; Clark et al., 1999).

According to hopelessness theory (Abramson et al., 1989), the tendency to attribute negative life events to stable (i.e., persistent across time) and global causes (i.e., present in multiple domains) leads to depressive symptoms and hopelessness (Abramson et al., 2002; Alloy et al., 2000). Like Beck's model, this model can be viewed as a diathesis–stress framework; in the absence of negative life events, individuals who exhibit such an inferential explanatory style will be no more likely than individuals without this style to develop hopelessness or depression.

Empirical status of negative thinking in depression

There is a voluminous body of research attesting to the association between negative thinking and depression in adult (Clark et al., 1999), child (Garber & Flynn, 2001b; Hammen & Rudolph, 2003), and adolescent (e.g., Garber et al., 1993) populations. Depression is consistently associated with dysfunctional attitudes, negative automatic thoughts, pessimism, hopelessness, low perceived self-worth, negative explanatory styles, and irrational beliefs. Studies that have assessed negative cognition through information processing measures also tend to support the tenet that depression is associated with biases of memory, attention, and interpretation (see Mathews & MacLeod, 2005). Notwithstanding support for the relationship between negative thinking and depression, studies on the causal aspects of these theories have, until recently, yielded equivocal results.

The stability of negative thinking

One strategy for attempting to address the issue of vulnerability to depression has been to compare negative thinking in individuals who have experienced depression in the past but are no longer depressed to individuals who have never experienced depression (but see Just et al., 2001, for a conceptual critique). These designs have, for the most part, failed to find reliable differences between adults or adolescents with remitted depression and those with no history of psychiatric problems (see Garber & Flynn, 2001b; Ingram et al., 1998, for reviews).

The stability of negative cognition (specifically for interpersonal content) in previously depressed adults has been examined (e.g., Dozois, 2007; Dozois & Dobson, 2001; Joorman & Gotlib, 2007). Dozois and Dobson (2001), for example, tested the structure of the self-schema using a computerized task in which participants rated self-referential adjectives on a grid, based on their self-descriptiveness and valence. The assumption underlying this task is that the way individuals organize adjective content is reflective of the degree of schema consolidation or interconnectedness. A sample of depressed females was assessed on this task and was also administered information processing tasks measuring attention to and recall of positive and negative interpersonal information. Participants were retested 6 months later when half of the sample had remained depressed and the other half was remitted. Negative information processing was evident only during episodes and appeared to remit once depressive symptoms improved. In contrast, negative cognitive organization remained stable across time, irrespective of concurrent symptomatology. A subsequent study found that the stability of negative cognitive organization was specific to interpersonal content (Dozois, 2007). In a dot-probe task using photos of facial expressions, Joorman and Gotlib (2007) found that previously depressed individuals showed a heightened attention to sad faces, whereas nonpsychiatric controls avoided sad faces and preferentially attended to happy faces. These findings suggest that negative (and in particular interpersonal) self-structures may be vulnerability factors for depression and its recurrence.

In contrast to these findings, other studies have shown that negatively biased thinking, present in a mood-disordered state, improves once depression subsides, raising the issue of whether negative cognition might operate more as a state marker of depression than as a vulnerability factor (e.g., Haaga et al., 1991). However, the fact that depressive schemas are thought to be latent until activated under stress has not been adequately incorporated into many of early studies of cognitive vulnerability (Scher et al., 2005). Indeed, most of the early studies of cognitive vulnerability did not examine vulnerability by stress interactions or attempt to activate the self-schema prior to assessment, which is particularly important when assessing cognitive products (e.g., self-report) and processes (e.g., attention, memory) in depression. More recent studies using a mood challenge procedure or naturally occurring dysphoric mood have consistently found that previously depressed persons show an increase in dysfunctional attitudes, irrational beliefs, or information processing that is absent in never-depressed controls (e.g., Hedlund & Rude, 1995; Ingram et al., 1994; Ingram & Ritter, 2000; Miranda & Persons, 1988; Segal et al., 1999; Soloman et al., 1998; Teasdale & Dent, 1987). This effect has also been found in studies of high-risk

(Murray et al., 2001; Taylor & Ingram, 1999) and previously depressed (Timbermont & Braet, 2004) children. Recently, Segal et al. (2006) investigated whether such mood-linked changes in dysfunctional attitudes were predictive of relapse in adults treated for major depressive disorder, finding that individuals treated with antidepressant medication showed greater cognitive reactivity (increased dysfunctional attitudes) to a negative mood manipulation than did patients treated with cognitive–behavioural therapy. In addition, and irrespective of treatment modality, patients who showed cognitive reactivity were at increased risk for relapse of depression at 18 months follow-up. These results provide support for the predictive role of cognition in depression.

Negative thinking in at-risk populations

Studies of remitted samples do not elucidate mechanisms related to initial onset, which may be quite different from those related to relapse or recurrence of depression (Dobson & Dozois, 2004). To address this issue, cognitive vulnerability has also been studied in at-risk individuals who are not currently depressed. One common strategy has been to assess children of depressed mothers (e.g., Garber & Martin, 2002; Goodman & Gotlib, 1999; Goodman & Gotlib, 2002; Malcarne et al., 2000; Murray et al., 2001; Taylor & Ingram, 1999), since children of depressed parents are at significantly greater risk for depressive disorders than are the offspring of nonpsychiatric controls (e.g., Dierker et al., 1998; Downey & Coyne, 1990; Goodman & Gotlib, 1999; Halligan et al., 2007; Hammen, 2002; Hammen et al., 1990). The risk conferred by having a depressed parent appears somewhat nonspecific to depression, as other types of disorders, such as behavioural problems and medical dysfunction, are also elevated in children of depressed parents (Beidel & Turner, 1997; Hammen, 1991; Leschied et al., 2005; Weissman et al., 1997). However, lack of specificity notwithstanding, there are also important developmental reasons to examine the young offspring of depressed parents. For example, positive and negative beliefs about the self develop greatly during childhood and adolescence (Bruce et al., 2006), beliefs that may serve as vulnerability (or protective factors) for depression later in life (Ingram, 2001; Ingram et al., 1998). For example, Dweck and colleagues (Burhans & Dweck, 1995; Smiley & Dweck, 1994) proposed that a child's global perception of him or herself as 'good' or 'bad' is acquired early in life (also see Bruce et al., 2006; Cicchetti et al., 1997; Ingram et al., 2006).

Only a handful of studies have assessed the cognitions of offspring of depressed parents. These studies have demonstrated that children of depressed mothers do exhibit depressive attributional styles (e.g., attributing negative events to internal, stable, and global factors; attributing positive events to external, unstable, and specific factors), greater hopelessness, and lower perceived self-worth than do children of nonpsychiatric mothers (Garber & Flynn, 2001a; Garber & Horowitz, 2002; Garber & Robinson, 1997; Goodman et al., 1994; Stark et al., 1996). The information processing of high-risk children also seems to be depressotypic. Taylor and Ingram (1999), for instance, compared offspring of depressed and nondepressed mothers on a self-referent encoding task. The high-risk children who underwent a mood induction procedure endorsed fewer positive words than did high-risk children in the neutral condition or the low-risk children in either condition. These individuals also recalled significantly more negative words than did the high-risk children in the neutral condition. Joorman et al. (2007) found that never-depressed daughters of recurrently depressed mothers selectively attended to negative facial expressions, following a negative mood prime, whereas low-risk daughters selectively attended to positive facial stimuli.

Longitudinal studies of cognitive vulnerability

Some prospective research with adults, adolescents, and children indicates that depressogenic attributional styles (e.g., Abela, 2001; Abela & D'Alessandro, 2002; Hankin et al., 2001, 2004, 2005) and dysfunctional attitudes (e.g., Hankin et al., 2004; Joiner et al., 1999; Kwon & Oei, 1992; Lewinsohn et al., 2001) interact with stress to predict depressive symptoms. However, other research has produced only mixed or limited support for cognitive vulnerability to depression (see Hankin & Abela, 2005, for review). One complicating factor is that the prediction of depressive symptoms by the interaction of attributional style and negative life events appears to be stronger in older (ages 13–19 years) than in younger (ages 8–12 years) children (e.g., Lakdawalla et al., 2007), possibly due to genuine developmental change in the ability of children to engage in abstract reasoning about the self and future (Abela, 2001; Garber & Robinson, 1997; Lakdawalla et al., 2007). Alternatively, conceptual, methodological, and statistical limitations of past research have been identified (see Lakdawalla et al., 2007) that might account for the age differences. For example, Murray et al. (2001) argued that much of the research on cognitive vulnerability in young children is limited due to its reliance on self-report measures. These researchers examined negative cognition in a sample of 5-year-old children of depressed and nondepressed mothers. The children were assessed in the context of a competitive card game and their positive or negative verbalized thoughts coded. When the outcome of the game was positive, the two groups did not differ in their expressed cognitions. When the outcome of the game was negative, however, the children who were exposed to maternal depression during their lifetime were more likely to express hopelessness, pessimism, and low self-worth than were children without exposure to maternal depression. It is therefore possible that cognitive vulnerability is present at younger ages, although researchers may need to use developmentally sensitive measures.

The Temple-Wisconsin Cognitive Vulnerability Project (CVP) has provided a rich source of data that has supported the idea that negative cognition represents an important vulnerability factor for depression (Alloy et al., 2000, 2006a, 2006b). Alloy et al. (2006b), for instance, followed up cognitively high- and low-risk college students over a period of two and a half years. Participants who scored in the upper quartile on a composite index of the Dysfunctional Attitudes Scale and the Cognitive Style Questionnaire were labeled high-risk, whereas those participants who scored in the bottom quartile on these instruments were defined as low-risk. High-risk persons were 3.5–6.8 times more likely than were low-risk participants to experience major, minor, and hopelessness depression. Moreover, negative cognitive styles predicted the onset of depression (both major depression and hopelessness depression) and its recurrence even after controlling for initial depressive symptomatology and previous history of depression. These findings provide compelling support for cognitive models of vulnerability to depression.

Stress and social support

Stressful life events

Researchers and clinicians in search of clues regarding the aetiology of depression have long attributed explanatory power to the occurrence of adverse life events. As in adults, stressful/negative life events have been shown to increase the risk for developing depressive symptoms in adolescence (Cole et al., 2006; Ge et al., 1994), and may also play a key role in precipitating the onset of a depressive episode (Compas et al., 1994; Goodyer et al., 2000).

Stressful life events have been examined as a way to potentially account for the emerging female preponderance of depression in adolescence. Adolescent girls are exposed to higher levels of stressful life events than boys (Compas & Wagner, 1991; Dornbusch et al., 1991; Larson & Ham, 1993; Siddique & D'Arcy, 1984) and show greater reactivity to stressors, especially if they are interpersonal in nature (Shih et al., 2006; Simmons et al., 1987). One study found that with increasing age, adolescents, especially adolescent girls, were more likely to experience stressful life events in various domains (Ge et al., 1994). This is significant, as adolescents may be at especially high risk for developing depression when they concurrently encounter several stressful situations across various life domains (DuBois et al., 1992; Petersen et al., 1991; Simmons et al., 1987).

Maltreatment also appears to play a role in adolescent depression; Brown et al. (1999) reported that adolescents with a history of maltreatment were three to four times more likely to become depressed than those without such a history. Similarly, Kaplan et al. (1998) reported that adolescents with a history of physical abuse had a significantly increased risk of a current and lifetime diagnosis of major depression, and another study found that early care lacking in emotional support prospectively predicted adolescent depressive symptoms (Duggal et al., 2001). Egeland (1997) conducted a prospective, longitudinal study, finding that childhood experiences of sexual abuse, physical abuse, and psychological unavailability of caregivers were strongly associated with various forms of adolescent psychopathology, notably major depression.

Relatively minor stressors (often referred to as 'daily hassles'), such as poor parent–child relations and academic stressors (Compas et al., 1987; Daniels & Moos, 1990; Kanner et al., 1987), have also been examined with respect to depression. Depressive symptoms in adolescence are strongly associated with exposure to ongoing stressors (Compas, 1987; Daniels & Moos, 1990; Robinson et al., 1995), and minor life events have also been shown to be associated with the severity of depression among adolescents (Reinecke & DuBois, 2001). Not surprisingly, more severe, ongoing problems, such as poor quality friendships (Goodyer et al., 1989) or family dysfunction (Goodyer et al., 1998), can also contribute to the onset and maintenance of internalizing disorders. Some evidence suggests that adolescent boys may experience greater amounts of chronic stress (especially in the academic and close friendship domains) compared to adolescent girls, and that boys may be more reactive to chronic stress in social domains (Shih et al., 2006). In contrast, other research has found that adolescent girls experience more stressors than boys in various domains (e.g., family, peer, romantic) and react with more depressive symptoms than boys in the face of these stressors (Hankin et al., 2007). Thus, the extant literature on stress and stress reactivity is somewhat mixed with respect to elucidating the adolescent gender difference in depression.

Stress generation

In contrast to the stress exposure model, which would conceptualize depression as a reaction to stress (e.g., Ge et al., 1994; Hilsman & Garber, 1995), dynamic models that capture the possibility of reciprocal relations between depression and stress have been formulated. Within stress-generation models (Hammen, 1991, 1992), individuals with depressive symptoms and the associated impairments create stressful situations, which further exacerbate and maintain their depressive syndrome. Hence, stress is conceptualized as both an aetiological factor and a consequence of depression within this model.

Prospective and cross-sectional evidence supports the stress-generation hypothesis in adolescent depression (Cohen et al., 1987; Rudolph & Hammen, 1999). Depressed adolescents, especially those with comorbid externalizing problems, may behave in ways that elicit stressful events and circumstances (Rudolph et al., 2000). In a prospective longitudinal study, Cole and colleagues (2006) explored both the stress exposure and stress-generation hypotheses in children using self-reports of stressful life events and depressive symptoms, finding evidence for both hypotheses. Moreover, they found that across development, the impact of depression on the occurrence of stressful life events increased, indicating that the interaction between the individual and stressful life events is not static across development. Further adding to the complexity of stress-generation models, some literature (e.g., Hammen, 1991) indicates that symptoms of depression do not fully account for the stress generation seen in this disorder, suggesting that other characteristics, such as temperament/personality, may be involved. In support of this notion, neuroticism has been found to predict the onset of stressful life events (Kendler et al., 2003), and introversion is related to lower social support (Swickert et al., 2002). Along similar lines, another recent study (Safford et al., 2007) found associations between negative cognitive styles and the occurrence of 'dependent' stressful life events (i.e., stressors viewed as resulting from the individual's own behaviour). Much of this work has been conducted in adult samples, however, so investigations of stress generation in adolescence that account for the role of individual differences are warranted.

Social relationships and social support
Parent–child relations

Factors such as parental acceptance, family cohesion, pattern of communication, parental psychological control, degree of conflict, parental support/nurturance, and parental rejection are associated with depression in adolescence (Garber et al., 1997; Lau & Kwok, 2000; Nolan et al., 2003; Vazsonyi & Belliston, 2006). Adolescents in families characterized by a lack of parental support, high levels of conflict, poor communication, over-controlling behaviour, and increased rejection are at an increased risk for depressive symptoms (Burt et al., 1988; Feldman et al., 1988; Garber et al., 1997; Lau & Kwok, 2000; Nolan et al., 2003; Vazsonyi & Belliston, 2006). This may be particularly true for adolescent girls, who may display more depressive symptoms in face of problematic parenting behaviour than boys (Ge et al., 1994). At least one recent study provided evidence that lower parental support, not peer support, was predictive of increases in depressive symptoms and onset of a major depressive episode in adolescent girls (Stice et al., 2004).

As the relationships between adversity and psychopathology are complex, researchers have proposed mediational pathways through which impaired child–parent relationships lead to depression. For example, the relationship between a negative parenting style and depressive symptoms could be mediated via effects on child self-esteem or self-worth. In terms of empirical support for this model, Garber et al. (1997) found that the relationship between maternal acceptance and maternal psychological control and depressive symptoms was partially mediated through perceived self-worth in children. Conversely, positive parenting may protect against negative circumstances or promote emotional wellness. Adolescents who perceive a high degree of family support report fewer symptoms of depression than those with lower levels of perceived family support (Holahan et al., 1994; Licitra-Kleckler & Waas, 1993; Wolfradt et al., 2003). As well, a warm and supportive parenting environment has been shown to moderate the effect of negative life events on adolescents (e.g., DuBois et al., 1992; Hauser et al., 1985; Petersen et al., 1991; Zimmerman et al., 2000). Parental warmth, in particular, may be important in protecting the developing youth in the face of stress (Wagner et al., 1996), especially in helping to moderate the relationship between independent stressful life events and depressive symptoms in females (Ge et al., 1994).

Peer relationships

Peer relationship quality is related to depressive symptoms in youths (Altmann & Gotlib, 1988; Eberhart & Hammen, 2006; Rudolph et al., 1994; reviewed in Hammen & Rudolph, 1996). Peer rejection is a stronger and more consistent predictor of depressive symptoms than academic impairment (Blechman et al., 1986; Patterson & Stoolmiller, 1991). Peers may be especially important when familial support is low, as adolescents from abusive families are more likely turn to their peers for instrumental and emotional support (Bao et al., 2000). There may also be gender differences in how adolescents respond to difficulties in peer relations. For example, girls tend to be more sensitive to relationship disruptions than boys, which may increase the likelihood of emotional problems when relationships falter (Simmons et al., 1987). Finally, prospective research has shown that a history of peer victimization predicts self-reported symptoms of depression in adolescence (Bond et al., 2001; Klomek et al., 2007), as well as peer-reported internalizing symptoms and peer rejection (Hodges & Perry, 1999). Thus, both peer rejection and aggression from peers have implications for the emergence of depressive symptoms in adolescence. It is also important to recall that, as in the case of stressful life events, seemingly exogenous variables such as social relationships and support are undoubtedly related to individual characteristics, such as personality (Swickert et al., 2002). Greater attention to the mechanisms by which adolescent social support develops may provide a more precise understanding of the likely complex relationships between the individual, social support, and depression.

Genetic and biological vulnerability

Genetics of depression and depression endophenotypes

The notion that depression vulnerability is rooted in biological or inborn factors is literally an ancient one, dating back to antiquity (Jackson, 1986). Much of the relevant literature to date has focused on adults with depression. However, adolescence may be an especially important and informative time to study biological and genetic processes in depression. At least some evidence suggests that depressive symptoms emerging during adolescence are more heritable and under relatively greater genetic control than symptoms emerging earlier in development (Harrington et al., 1997; Thapar & McGuffin, 1994). Furthermore, since prevalence rates of depression show a marked and rapid increase during adolescence, research on samples in this age group may help disentangle biological processes important to the initial onset of disorder from those implicated in recurrence.

Twin studies

Research on genetic influences on depression has consisted primarily of quantitative twin studies and, more recently, molecular genetic approaches examining the association of specific candidate genes with depression. Quantitative twin studies consistently indicate at least moderate heritable effects on the disorder (e.g., Goldberg, 2006; Sullivan et al., 2000). Recently, Lau and Eley (2006) examined genetic and environmental effects on depressive symptoms in a sample of adolescent twins at three time points. Consistent with the extant literature, moderate genetic effects were found at each time point, accounting for almost half of the phenotypic variance. Unique environmental effects were also moderate across development. However, shared environmental effects, significant at the first assessment during early adolescence, declined appreciably with age. This does not necessarily mean that family-wide influences such as family conflict or disruption are less important in later adolescence, only that individual sensitivity to the effects of these influences may become increasingly important (Rutter et al., 1997).

Association studies

The significant heritability estimates from twin studies suggest the possibility of identifying specific genes that increase depression risk. Several candidate genes for depression have attracted attention largely on the basis of what is known about the pathophysiology of depression or the mechanisms of therapeutic drugs for the disorder; hence, genes associated with neurotransmitter systems, such as the serotonin transporter gene and the dopamine receptor genes, have received the greatest attention. However, the literature examining associations between these candidates and depression has produced ambiguous findings to date (Jones et al., 2002), possibly because major depression is most likely a polygenic disorder, determined by multiple genes of small individual effect. Unfortunately, few studies have examined multiple genes and their interactive effects on depression (see Kaufman et al., 2006, for an exception).

On the other hand, single genes may show a strong association with depression within relevant environmental contexts. For example, seminal research by Caspi and colleagues (2003) examined the effects of a polymorphism in the serotonin transporter promoter region (5-HTTLPR), in conjunction with stressful life events, on rates of depression. This paper provided evidence that individuals with putative genetic vulnerability to depression, as evinced by having short alleles of the 5-HTTLPR gene, developed depression more frequently in the context of stressful life events than those without this genotype. Several replications have been published, as have failures to replicate (for a review, see Zammit & Owen, 2006).

Similar studies have been conducted in adolescent samples, with mixed results. For example, Kaufman et al. (2006) examined the interactive effects of maltreatment history and 5-HTTLPR genotype on depressive symptoms in a sample comprised of child and adolescent participants. These investigators replicated the finding of Caspi et al. (2003), reporting that association between the 5-HTTLPR genotype and depression was strongest in participants with a history of maltreatment, albeit with a different classification of genotype than the Caspi group. Eley and colleagues (2004) also replicated Caspi and colleagues' finding in an adolescent-aged sample, but only within the female participants; there was no evidence for a gene–environment interaction in predicting depression in males. In a genetically informative twin sample, Rice et al. (2006) found that children and adolescents with genetic vulnerability to depression were most likely to experience depression when exposed to family conflict. Measures of depression and environmental stress differ considerably across these studies, which may account for the variability in findings. Also, it has been previously reported that depressive episodes subsequent to the first in adolescence are less strongly associated with stressors (Daley et al., 2000; Monroe et al., 1999). This would be consistent with the possibility that the nature of the relationship between genetic vulnerability and environmental stress changes across episodes, and suggests the important of distinguishing between first and subsequent onsets of depression in terms of delineating vulnerability processes in adolescence (Angold, 2003).

Endophenotypes

It has been argued that what is inherited in depression is a constitutional vulnerability to the disorder, rather than the disorder per se (Silberg & Rutter, 2002). This concept, as well as the absence of consistent findings regarding specific candidate genes for depression, suggests the potential value in examining the genetic bases of endophenotypes for depression. Endophenotypes are traits associated with the disease that are heritable, precede disease onset, and are present in unaffected relatives (Gottesman & Gould, 2003); their study may inform our understanding of genetic risk for psychopathology for several reasons. First, endophenotypes may have a relatively simple genetic basis compared to complex diagnostic categories. Also in contrast to psychiatric diagnoses, endophenotypes are usually dimensional constructs, which lends increased statistical power to data analyses and may better map onto underlying genetic mechanisms than a dichotomous phenotype. Finally, compared to the phenotypes to which they are linked, endophenotypes often show greater continuity across the lifespan, and can therefore be examined across multiple developmental periods. This characteristic allows for the examination of continuities and discontinuities across maturation, and may also prove useful in prevention strategies in that validated endophenotypes may help identify those at risk relatively early in life. In the case of depression, various endophenotypes have been proposed for research attention, including impaired reward responsivity, diurnal variation, and stress sensitivity (Hassler et al., 2004). While little is known about these endophenotypes in adolescent samples, applying this strategy represents a promising approach to delineating genetic influences on depression vulnerability.

Temperament traits, which are typically viewed as rooted in individual differences in biological systems, may also prove to be informative endophenotypes for the genetic dissection of depression vulnerability. A potentially useful temperamental endophenotype for depression is positive emotionality (PE), the trait-like predisposition to experience positive emotions and to be sensitive to environmental signals of reward. Related concepts include Gray's behavioural approach system (BAS; Gray, 1972, 1990, 1994), also described as a behavioural activation system (Fowles, 1994) and a behavioural facilitation system (Depue & Collins, 1999); these systems are thought to regulate appetitive behaviour aimed at acquiring desirable stimuli in the environment and the accompanying emotional experiences of excitement and elation. Individuals who are constitutionally lower on these continuous traits are thought to possess a diathesis for depression (Clark, Watson, & Mineka, 1994), especially early-onset, chronic forms of the disorder (Meehl, 1975).

Findings from a study of children and adolescents indicate that self-reported PE predicts changes in depressive symptoms over time (Lonigan et al., 2003). Low PE in childhood has been linked to familial depression (Durbin et al., 2005) and the subsequent development of cognitive vulnerability to depression (Hayden et al., 2006). Importantly, in contrast to other temperament traits, low PE appears to plays a relatively specific role in depression vulnerability (Clark et al., 1994). However, the genetic bases of PE and related constructs are poorly understood to date, although animal models suggest some potentially useful avenues for future investigation (Peciña et al., 2003) and genes that influence dopaminergic neurotransmission are logical candidates (Depue & Collins, 1999). Twin studies indicate that PE is heritable (Jang et al., 1998) and preliminary evidence suggests that unaffected family members of depressives may tend to exhibit lower levels of PE-like traits (Hecht et al., 1998). Thus, although research on specific genes is lacking, preliminary evidence supports the notion that this trait is indeed a genetically based vulnerability marker for the disorder.

Negative emotionality (NE) is another temperament trait linked to depression, although its relationship to the disorder appears to show less specificity (Clark et al., 1994). Lonigan et al. (2003) recently reported that self-reported levels of NE predicted variation in both anxious and depressive symptoms longitudinally in a sample of children and adolescents. Recently, Goldston et al. (2006) found that trait components of NE were a strong predictor of adolescent suicide attempts, supporting the importance of this construct in terms of its linkages to clinically meaningful outcomes. The moderate heritability of NE has been established (Jang et al., 1998). Furthermore, unlike PE, multiple studies have examined the effects of candidate genes on NE, especially the 5-HTTLPR polymorphism described earlier. The short alleles of this gene were linked to higher self-reported avoidance, a facet of NE, in a recent meta-analysis (Munafò et al., 2003).

Temperamental vulnerability to depression may be shaped by both genetic and environmental factors that interact to predict liability. High behavioural inhibition, a facet of NE reflecting wariness and reticence in novel situations involving unfamiliar people or stimuli, has been linked to depression vulnerability in several studies (e.g., Kochanska, 1991). Fox and colleagues (2005) reported that children with short alleles of the 5-HTTLPR were more likely to display higher levels of BI when their mothers reported low levels of social support. This suggests the intriguing possibility that the effects of specific genes, along with aspects of the early home environment, interact to produce temperamental vulnerability to depression

BAS activity is thought to influence electroencephalographic (EEG) measures of asymmetry in anterior cortical regions. Authors have hypothesized that activity in left frontal regions reflects BAS-related behaviours, such as appetitive, approach-directed emotional responses (Davidson, 1998). A pattern of EEG asymmetry reflecting left frontal hypoactivation refers to decreased alpha power in electrodes over the left frontal region, relative to the homologous electrodes in the right hemisphere. This pattern of anterior activity is associated with current (Thibodeau et al., 2006) and lifetime history of depression (Gotlib et al., 1998b; Henriques & Davidson, 1990; although see Pizzagalli et al., 2002; Reid et al., 1998 for inconsistent findings). These data suggest the possibility of treating EEG measures of frontal asymmetry as an endophenotype for genetic studies.

Genetic study of temperament traits linked to depression is an important next step toward understanding genetic vulnerability to depression. However, it is important to note that the mechanisms by which temperamental factors increase depression vulnerability are probably complex and are currently poorly understood. Complex models of the relationship between traits and depression have been proposed (Klein et al., 2002a), and are beyond the scope of the present review. Further longitudinal research is needed to understand the effects of the aforementioned temperament traits on depression and how these processes unfold during adolescence.

Neurotransmitter and neuroendocrine systems

Neurotransmitters

The monoaminergic neurotransmitters include serotonin, norepinephrine, and dopamine, which regulate basic functions that are disturbed in mood disorders, such as sleep, energy, and appetite. Following the recognition that symptoms of depression can be improved by agents that mechanistically increase synaptic concentrations of monoamines, the monoamine theories of mood disorders were developed (Thase et al., 2002). While the earliest iterations of these theories were overly simplistic, investigation continues into more complex aspects of the relationship between these neurotransmitters and various measures of depression and depression vulnerability.

Manipulation of dietary tryptophan, as a precursor of serotonin, can be used to examine serotonergic neurotransmission. Response to tryptophan depletion procedures is thought to index depression vulnerability in that the procedure causes a brief depressive-like episode in remitted adult depressives. However, responses of children and adolescents to such procedures are mixed (see Kaufman et al., 2001 for a review). Understanding the role of serotonergic functioning in adolescent depression is important, as abnormal serotonergic activity has been linked to suicidal behaviour, possibly through its association with impulsive aggression (Spirito & Esposito-Smythers, 2006). Pandey and colleagues (2002) reported abnormal serotonin transporter binding in the ventral prefrontal cortex of postmortem brains of adolescent suicide victims, consistent with the notion that impaired executive functioning related to abnormal serotonin transporter binding contributes to increased suicidality in adolescents. Similarly, lower plasma serotonin levels have been associated with increased severity of suicidality in an adolescent patient sample (Tyano et al., 2006). Of course, these findings must be considered in light of the fact that not all adolescents who attempt suicide are depressed; thus, these findings may be more relevant to impulsivity or aggression than depression per se.

Investigators have also been interested in dopaminergic functioning in depression (Nestler & Carlezon, 2006; Thase et al., 2002), since dopamine appears to be critical to incentive-reward motivation (Depue & Collins, 1999), which is typically impaired in depressive episodes. It is important to note that chronic stress has been shown to downregulate both dopaminergic and serotonergic functioning (Weiss & Kilts, 1998; Willner, 1995). This suggests that variation in these neurotransmitter systems that may have relevance for depression can be either inherited or acquired through adverse circumstances, and indicates that integrative models are called for toward understanding these processes.

Growth hormone

Decreased secretion of growth hormone in response to pharmacological challenge has been reported in depressed adolescents, compared to control participants (Dahl et al., 2000). Growth hormone secretion in adolescents may remain abnormal even after recovery from a depressive episode (Dahl et al., 2000), suggesting that this biaological phenomenon is either a risk marker or a 'scar' of the experience of depression. A high-risk study of children and adolescents indicated that growth hormone secretion is a risk marker for depression by showing that the high-risk group secreted less growth hormone after a challenge than those at low risk (Birmaher et al., 2000). Although the nature of the relationship between growth hormone and depression is not well understood, it appears to be a marker of central noradrenergic and serotonergic functioning.

Gonadal hormones

Puberty is associated with major morphological and hormonal changes. While both may have implications for the development of depression, few studies have used the methodology needed to disentangle the unique influences of the two (Hayward & Sanborn, 2002). An exception is the study of Angold and colleagues (1999), which used Tanner stage ratings of pubertal status derived from physical characteristics, and also collected assays of testosterone, follicle stimulating hormone, luteinizing hormone, and estradiol in a sample of girls aged 9–15 years old. When hormones were added to a model predicting depression, the effects of Tanner stage were nonsignificant, while the effects of testosterone and estrogen remained significant after controlling for Tanner stage.

Hypothalamic–pituitary–adrenal (HPA) axis and cortisol

HPA axis activity is a feedback loop by which signals from the brain trigger the release of hormones needed to respond to stress, including corticotrophin-releasing hormone, adrenocorticotropin, epinephrine, norepinephrine, and cortisol. Normally, cortisol exerts a feedback effect to shut down the stress response when it is no longer necessary. The ability of the HPA axis to shut down when not needed is important, as cortisol may exert harmful effects on the brain, especially the hippocampus (Gubba et al., 2000). Typically, levels of cortisol in the bloodstream display diurnal variation such that concentrations of cortisol vary throughout a 24-hour period, with levels at their highest in the early morning and at their lowest around midnight.

In adults, depression is associated with two abnormalities in cortisol excretion: more cortisol is excreted in general (hypercortisolism) and diurnal variation is reduced, such that cortisol is excreted continuously. Interestingly, males appear to show greater HPA axis responses to stress, which would seem inconsistent with the female preponderance of depression; however, some have argued that this would be consistent with adaptive aspects of stress reactivity for males but not females (Altemus, 2006). Findings from adolescent samples are less consistent, and the development of HPA axis activity across puberty is not well understood (Hayward & Sanborn, 2002). In general, hypercortisolism has not been observed in studies of depressed adolescents, but cortisol is often found to be elevated around sleep onset, in contrast to normal patterns (Angold, 2003). Goodyer et al. (2003) reported that elevated morning cortisol relative to dehydroepiandrosterone (DHEA, an agent that may buffer the harmful effects of cortisol) was associated with persistent major depression in a sample of adolescents. Cortisol/DHEA levels were not associated with remitted, nonchronic cases of depression in this sample. Interestingly, this same group reported that high evening cortisol/DHEA levels predicted disappointing life events in an adolescent sample; in this study, both cortisol/DHEA ratio and negative life events had independent effects on depression (Goodyer et al., 1998). Granger et al. (1994) reported that increased cortisol in response to a parent–offspring conflict task was associated with social withdrawal and negative attributional styles in a sample of children and adolescents, suggesting that cortisol activity may index problematic social behaviours that may eventuate in depression.

The dexamethasone suppression test is a method used to assess the integrity of HPA feedback system in terms of its ability to 'shut down' when activation is no longer adaptive. Dexamethasone is a synthetic glucocorticoid, which normally suppresses the pituitary gland's secretion of hormones for 24 hours. Impaired HPA feedback results in early 'escape' from the suppression caused by dexamethasone administration, and are characteristic of many adults with depression. Depressed and suicidal children appear similar to depressed adults, commonly failing to suppress in response to a dose of dexamethasone (Kaufman et al., 2001). Early exposure to stress may permanently alter HPA regulation (Shea et al., 2005), suggesting that vulnerability to depression stemming from HPA axis dysregulation can be either inborn or acquired.

Conclusions and future directions

A broad overview of three approaches to understanding vulnerability to depression has been provided in this chapter. It may be apparent from this review that future research will greatly benefit from the use of transactional models of depression vulnerability that integrate multiple perspectives; process-oriented questions are unlikely to be answered by research focused on narrowly defined aspects of depression vulnerability. The relationship between many 'endogenous' variables (e.g., cognitive styles, biological factors, or measured genes) and 'exogenous' variables (e.g., stressful life events) is highly complex; for example, gene–environment correlations appear to be widespread (Jaffee & Price, 2007), although an understanding of how such relationships operate in depression is limited. Top–down levels of analysis that examine how depression vulnerability unfolds over time in relevant environmental contexts is needed. Although such studies are expensive and require expertise in diverse research areas, complex designs are required when insight into complex processes is sought. For example, exciting models measuring the associations between genes and depression in relevant environmental contexts are being successfully explored in studies of depression (e.g., Caspi et al., 2003). Including environmental factors in genetic studies may be especially enlightening when examining genes of small effect, which may achieve penetrance only when considered in conjunction with environmental factors. The vast research on psychosocial influences on depression can be drawn upon for useful starting points for further studies integrating genetic and biological processes with environmental influences. Such research may also possibly identify environmental targets for intervention (Jaffee & Price, 2007).

The heterogeneity of depression on multiple levels (e.g., clinical, aetiological) is widely acknowledged, and there is a long research tradition aimed at uncovering more homogenous subgroups. Adolescent depression may be especially aetiologically complex, given the myriad psychosocial challenges experienced during this developmental stage. Recurrence of adolescent depression appears to be an important marker of greater familiality of the disorder (Klein et al., 2002b), and may distinguish cases with a stronger psychosocial basis from those stemming from a stronger genetic liability. Age of depression onset is also an important consideration, as onset during different developmental stages may reflect diverse underlying genetic and environmental influences (e.g., Bland et al., 1986; Kupfer et al., 1989; McGuffin et al., 1987). Adolescents have been grouped with both adult and child samples for the purposes of research; whether they form a more homogenous group with children or adults is unclear to date (Kaufman et al., 2001), and likely depends on the nature of the question at hand. Certainly, an awareness of issues particularly relevant to adolescence and depression vulnerability (e.g., pubertal status, Ge et al., 1996; Ge et al., 2001) is critical, both when designing studies and interpreting findings.

It is also important that research on adolescent depression and vulnerability pays close attention to issues of measurement. A literature examining the relationship between self- and parent-reports of adolescent symptoms indicates low convergence between these measures (e.g., Youngstrom et al., 2000). The limited agreement between various measures of child depression strongly suggests that it is critical to use multiple measures of constructs of interest in this research. Similarly, agreement is frequently low between different measures of constructs thought to be related to depression vulnerability (e.g., Hayden et al., 2005; Roberts et al., 2005); this would indicate that research aimed at identifying vulnerability factors for depression cannot afford to rely on a single measure of the construct of interest.

Future studies of the genetics of depression may benefit from using phenotypes of both increased specificity and increased breadth. For example, studies may wish to examine subgroups of depression based on factors such as early age of onset (Zubenko et al., 2003) or the presence of comorbid anxiety disorders. Conversely, expanding genetic studies of depression to include novel endophenotypes is an exciting approach worthy of further expansion. Interesting and potentially informative endophenotypes for depression include circadian rhythm disruption, temperament, cortisol, and cognitive styles (e.g., Beevers et al., 2006), among others. A fuller understanding of the genetic bases of depression will require more specific insights into the mechanisms by which genes increase the likelihood of developing this disorder. Answers to such process-related questions will likely involve longitudinal research examining genetic associations with neuroimaging data, psychophysiological measures, hormonal assays, cognitive measures, and early-emerging emotional behaviour. Expanded investigations of process-oriented endophenotypes may also contribute toward this important goal. Furthermore, identification of such process-related variables will have tremendous implications for prevention and early intervention approaches.

Regarding cognitive models of depression, additional research on cognitive vulnerability would benefit from examining more refined components of diathesis–stress models. Abela and Sarin (2002), for example, found that it was an adolescent's 'weakest link' (i.e., the most depressogenic inferential style rather than his or her overall negative inferential style) that interacted with subsequent negative events to predict depressive symptomatology. Researchers have also begun to test diathesis–stress interactions in more proximal ways to understand the predictive utility of cognitive vulnerability. Employing multiple assessments periods (e.g., using daily diary methodologies) and more sophisticated data analytic techniques (e.g., hierarchical linear modeling), for instance, may better capture the dynamic nature of cognitive vulnerability–stress interactions as they unfold during adolescence (cf. Hankin et al., 2005).

An empirical literature has also emerged on the potential buffering effects of positive thinking (e.g., Taylor & Brown, 1988). Although research in depression has focused almost exclusively on pathological facets of cognition, the study of positive psychology and its implications for mental health has gained considerable momentum in recent years. Clearly, mental health is more than simply the absence of mental illness (Keyes, 2007), and researchers are increasingly identifying protective cognitive factors (e.g., optimism, the perception that one has mastery over one's environment, the belief that one has purpose in life, the fostering of autonomy, self acceptance) as important elements of mental well-being (Keyes, 2007). For example, Valle et al. (2006) recently reported that hope is a key protective factor in youth, finding that adolescents who reported higher levels of hope at baseline had lower risk for internalizing problems and poor life satisfaction when confronted with adverse life events over one-year follow-up. Positive psychology has also begun to make its way more explicitly into psychotherapeutic and preventative interventions (e.g., Ingram & Snyder, 2006). With respect to protection from depression in the face of stressful life events, less is known, although even brief interventions can increase optimistic explanatory styles in adolescents/young adults (Seligman et al., 2007). It seems reasonable to expect that positive cognitive styles could promote greater resiliency from negative life events and could stave off the onset of depression through a variety of mechanisms, such as by decreasing guilt and self-blame for negative events, or by enhancing coping skills and active problem-solving, among others.

On a related, final note, while a vast literature relevant to vulnerability to adolescent depression has accumulated from multiple perspectives, far less work has been done toward identifying factors that may protect against depression, whether from a biological, cognitive, or interpersonal/contextual perspective. Furthermore, a good understanding of how protective factors relate to risk factors is lacking (Essau, 2004); in other words, high resilience may result from a different set of underlying processes than low vulnerability. For example, psychological well-being and resilience may be linked to a different cognitive set than the thinking patterns linked to depression vulnerability. The implications of research on resilience for targeted preventative work cannot be overemphasized (Dozois & Dobson, 2004); thus, such work poses an important challenge to researchers over the next decades.

Acknowledgement

The authors gratefully acknowledge the support of the Ontario Mental Health Foundation.

References

Abela, J.R.Z. (2001). The hopelessness theory of depression: A test of the diathesis–stress and causal mediation components in third and seventh grade children. *Journal of Abnormal Child Psychology, 29,* 241–254.

Abela, J.R., & D'Alessandro, D.U. (2002). Beck's cognitive theory of depression: A test of the diathesis–stress and causal mediation components. *British Journal of Clinical Psychology, 41,* 111–128.

Abela, J.R., & Sarin, S. (2002). Cognitive vulnerability to hopelessness depression: A chain is only as strong as its weakest link. *Cognitive Therapy and Research, 26,* 811–829.

Abramson, L.Y., Alloy, L.B., Hankin, B.L., Haeffel, G.J., MacCoon, D.G., & Gibb, B.E. (2002). Cognitive vulnerability–stress models of depression in a self-regulatory and psychobiological context. In I.H. Gotlib & C.L. Hammen (Eds.), *Handbook of depression* (268–294). New York: Guilford.

Abramson, L.Y., Metalsky, G.I., & Alloy, L.B. (1989). Hopelessness depression: A theory-based subtype of depression. *Psychological Review, 96,* 358–372.

Alloy, L.B., Abramson, L.Y., Hogan, M.E., Whitehouse, W.G., Rose, D.T., Robinson, M.S., et al. (2000). The Temple-Wisconsin Cognitive Vulnerability to Depression Project: Lifetime history of Axis I psychopathology in individuals at high and low cognitive risk for depression. *Journal of Abnormal Psychology, 109,* 403–418.

Alloy, L.B., Abramson, L.Y., Safford, S.M., & Gibb, B.E. (2006a). The cognitive vulnerability to depression (CVD) project: Current findings and future directions. In L.B. Alloy, & J.H. Riskind (Eds.), *Cognitive vulnerability to emotional disorders* (pp. 33–61). Mahwah, NJ: Erlbaum.

Alloy, L.B., Abramson, L.Y., Whitehouse, W.G., Hogan, M.E., Panzarella, C., & Rose, D.T. (2006b). Prospective incidence of first onsets and recurrences of depression in individuals at high and low cognitive risk for depression. *Journal of Abnormal Psychology, 115,* 145–156.

Altemus, M. (2006). Sex differences in depression and anxiety disorders: Potential biological determinants. *Hormones and Behavior, 50,* 534–538.

Altmann, E.O., & Gotlib, I.H. (1988).The social behavior of depressed children: An observational study. *Journal of Abnormal Child Psychology, 16,* 29–44.

Angold, A. (2003). Adolescent depression, cortisol and DHEA. *Psychological Medicine, 33,* 573–581.

Angold, A., Costello, E.J., Erkanli, A., & Worthman, C.M. (1999). Pubertal changes in hormone levels and depression in girls. *Psychological Medicine, 29,* 1043–1053.

Angold, A., Costello, E.J., & Worthman, C.M. (1998). Puberty and depression: The roles of age, pubertal status and pubertal timing. *Psychological Medicine, 28,* 51–61.

Angold, A. & Rutter, M. (1992). Effects of age and pubertal status on depression in a large clinical sample. *Development and Psychopathology, 4,* 5–28.

Bao, W.-N., Whitbeck, L.B., & Hoyt, D.R. (2000). Abuse, support, and depression among homeless and runaway adolescents. *Journal of Health and Social Behavior, 41,* 408–420.

Beck, A.T. (1963). Thinking and depression: 1. Idiosyncratic content and cognitive distortions. *Archives of General Psychiatry, 9,* 324–333.

Beck, A.T. (1964). Thinking and depression: 2. Theory and therapy. *Archives of General Psychiatry, 10,* 561–571.

Beck, A.T. (1967). *Depression: Causes and treatment.* Philadelphia: University of Pennsylvania Press.

Beck, A.T. (1976). *Cognitive therapy and the emotional disorders.* New York: International University Press.

Beck, A.T. (1983). Cognitive therapy of depression: New perspectives. In P.J. Clayton & J.E. Barrett (Eds.), *Treatment of depression: Old controversies and new approaches* (pp. 265–290). New York: Raven.

Beck, A.T. (2005). The current state of cognitive therapy: A 40–year retrospective. *Archives of General Psychiatry, 62,* 953–959.

Beck, A.T., Rush, A.J., Shaw, B.F., & Emery, G. (1979). *Cognitive therapy of depression.* New York: Guilford.

Beevers, C.G., Gibb, B.E., McGeary, J.E., & Miller, I.W. (2006). Serotonin transporter genetic variation and biased attention for emotional word stimuli among psychiatric inpatients. *Journal of Abnormal Psychology, 116,* 208–212.

Beidel, D.C., & Turner, S.M. (1997). At risk for anxiety: psychopathology in the offspring of anxious parents. *Journal of the American Academy of Child and Adolescent Psychiatry, 36,* 918–924.

Birmaher, B., Dahl, R.E., Williamson, D.E., Perel, J.M., Brent, D.A., Axelson, D.A., et al. (2000). Growth hormone secretion in children and adolescents at high risk for major depressive disorder. *Archives of General Psychiatry, 57,* 867–872.

Bland, R.C., Newman, S.C., & Orn, H. (1986). Recurrent and nonrecurrent depression: A family study. *Archives of General Psychiatry, 43*, 1085–1089.

Blechman, E.A., McEnroe, M.J., Carella, E.T., & Audette, D.P. (1986). Childhood competence and depression. *Journal of Abnormal Psychology, 95*, 223–227.

Blyth, D.A., Simmons, R.G., & Carlton-Ford, S. (1983). The adjustment of early adolescents to school transitions. *Journal of Early Adolescence, 3*, 105–120.

Bond, L., Carlin, J.B., Thomas, L., Rubin, K., & Patton, G. (2001). Does bullying cause emotional problems? A prospective study of young teenagers. *British Medical Journal, 323*, 480–484.

Brown, J., Cohen, P., Johnson, J.G., & Smailes, E.M. (1999). Childhood abuse and neglect: Specificity of effects on adolescent and young adult depression and suicidality. *Journal of the American Academy of Child and Adolescent Psychiatry, 38*, 1490–1496.

Bruce, A.E., Cole, D.A., Dallaire, D.H., Jacquez, F.M., Pineda, A.Q., & LaGrange, B. (2006). Relations of parenting and negative life events to cognitive diatheses for children of depression. *Journal of Abnormal Child Psychology, 34*, 321–333

Burhans, K.K. & Dweck, C.S. (1995). Helplessness in early childhood: The role of contingent worth. *Child Development, 66*, 1719–1738.

Burt, C.E., Cohen, L.H., & Bjorck, J.P. (1988). Perceived family environment as a moderator of young adolescents' life stress adjustment. *American Journal of Community Psychology, 16*, 101–122.

Cairney, J. (1998). Gender differences in the prevalence of depression among Canadian adolescents. *Canadian Journal of Public Health, 89*, 181–182.

Caspi, A., Sugden, K., Moffitt, T.E., Taylor, A., Craig, I.W., Harrington, H.L., et al. (2003). Influence of life stress on depression: Moderation by a polymorphism in the 5-HTT gene. *Science, 301*, 386–389.

Cicchetti, D., Rogosch, F.A., Toth, S.L., & Spanola, M. (1997). Affect, cognition, and the emergence of self-knowledge in the toddler offspring of depressed mothers. *Journal of Experimental Child Psychology, 67*, 338–362.

Clark, D.A., Beck, A.T., & Alford, B.A. (1999). *Scientific foundations of cognitive theory and therapy of depression*. Philadelphia: Wiley.

Clark, L.A., Watson, D., & Mineka, S. (1994). Temperament, personality, and the mood and anxiety disorders. *Journal of Abnormal Psychology, 103*, 103–116.

Cohen, L.H., Burt, C.E., & Bjorck, J.P. (1987). Life stress and adjustment: Effects of life events experienced by young adolescents and their parents. *Developmental Psychology, 23*, 583–592.

Cole, D.A., Nolen-Hoeksema, S., Girgus, J., & Paul, G. (2006). Stress exposure and stress generation in child and adolescent depression: A latent trait-state-error approach to longitudinal analyses. *Journal of Abnormal Psychology, 115*, 40–51.

Compas, B.E. (1987). Stress and life events during childhood and adolescence. *Clinical Psychology Review, 7*, 275–302.

Compas, B.E., Davis, G.E., Forsythe, C.J., & Wagner, B.M. (1987). Assessment of major and daily stressful events during adolescence: The Adolescent Perceived Events Scale. *Journal of Consulting and Clinical Psychology, 55*, 534–541.

Compas, B.E., Grant, K.E., & Ey, S. (1994). Psychosocial stress and child and adolescent depression: Can we be more specific? In W.M. Reynolds & H.F. Johnston (Eds.), *Handbook of depression in children and adolescents* (pp. 509–523). New York: Plenum Press.

Compas, B.E., & Wagner, B.M. (1991). Psychological stress during adolescence: Intrapersonal and interpersonal processes. In M.E. Colten & S. Gore (Eds.), *Adolescent stress: Causes and consequences* (pp. 67–86). New York: Aldine de Gruyter.

Costello, E.J., Erkanli, A., & Angold, A. (2006). Is there an epidemic of child or adolescent depression? *Journal of Child Psychology and Psychiatry, 47*, 1263–1271.

Dahl, R.E., Birmaher, B., Williamson, D.E., Dorn, L., Perel, J., Kaufman, J., et al. (2000). Low growth hormone response to growth hormone-releasing hormone in child depression. *Biological Psychiatry, 48*, 981–988.

Daley, S.E., Hammen, C., & Rao, U. (2000). Predictors of first onset and recurrence of major depression in young women during the 5 years following high school graduation. *Journal of Abnormal Psychology, 109*, 525–533.

Daniels, D. & Moos, R.H. (1990). Assessing life stressors and social resources among adolescents: Applications to depressed youth. *Journal of Adolescent Research, 5*, 268–289.

Davidson, R.J. (1998). Anterior electrophysiological asymmetries, emotion, and depression: Conceptual and methodological conundrums. *Psychophysiology, 35*, 607–614.

Depue, R.A. & Collins, P.F. (1999). Neurobiology of the structure of personality: Dopamine, facilitation of incentive motivation, and extraversion. *Behavioral and Brain Sciences, 22*, 491–569.

Dierker, L.C., Merikangas, K.R., & Szatmari, P. (1998). Influence of parental concordance for psychiatric disorders on psychopathology in offspring. *Journal of the American Academy of Child and Adolescent Psychiatry, 38*, 280–288.

Dobson, K.S. & Dozois, D.J.A. (2004). The prevention of anxiety and depression: Promises and prospects. In D.J.A. Dozois & K.S. Dobson (Eds.), *The prevention of anxiety and depression: Theory, research, and practice* (pp. 283–295). Washington, DC: American Psychological Association.

Dornbusch, S.M., Mont-Reynaud, R., Ritter, P.L., Chen, Z., & Steinberg, L. (1991). Stressful events and their correlates among adolescents of diverse backgrounds. In M.E. Cohen & S. Gore (Eds.), *Adolescent stress: Causes and consequences* (pp. 111–130). New York: Aldine de Gruyter.

Downey, G. & Coyne, J.C. (1990). Children of depressed parents: An integrative review. *Psychological Bulletin, 108*, 50–76.

Dozois, D.J.A. (2007). Stability of negative self-structures: A longitudinal comparison of depressed, remitted, and nonpsychiatric controls. *Journal of Clinical Psychology, 63*, 319–338.

Dozois, D.J.A. & Dobson, K.S. (2001). A longitudinal investigation of information processing and cognitive organization in clinical depression: Stability of schematic interconnectedness. *Journal of Consulting and Clinical Psychology, 69*, 914–925.

Dozois, D.J.A. & Dobson, K.S. (2004). *The prevention of anxiety and depression: Theory, research, and practice.* Washington, DC: American Psychological Association.

DuBois, D.L., Felner, R.D., Brand, S., Adan, A.M., & Evans, E.G. (1992). A prospective study of life stress, social support, and adaptation in early adolescence. *Child Development, 63*, 542–557.

Duggal, S., Carlson, E.A., Sroufe, L.A., & Egeland, B. (2001). Depressive symptomatology in childhood and adolescence. *Development and Psychopathology, 13*, 143–164.

Dunn, V. & Goodyer, I.M. (2006). Longitudinal investigation into childhood and adolescence-onset depression: Psychiatric outcome in early adulthood. *British Journal of Psychiatry, 188*, 216–222.

Durbin, C.E., Klein, D.N., Hayden, E.P., Buckley, M.E., & Moerk, K.C. (2005). Temperamental emotionality in preschoolers and parental mood disorders. *Journal of Abnormal Psychology, 114*, 28–37.

Eberhart, N.K. & Hammen, C.L. (2006). Interpersonal predictors of onset of depression during the transition to adulthood. *Personal Relationships, 13*, 195–206.

Egeland, B. (1997). Mediators of the effects of child maltreatment on developmental adaptation in adolescence. In D. Cicchetti & S.L. Toth (Eds.), *Rochester Symposium on Developmental Psychopathology: Vol. 8. The effects of trauma on the developmental process* (pp. 403–434). Rochester, NY: University of Rochester Press.

Eley, T.C., Sugden, K., Corsico, A., Gregory, A.M., McGuffin, P., Plomin, R., et al. (2004). Gene-environment interaction analysis of serotonin system markers with adolescent depression. *Molecular Psychiatry, 9*, 908–915.

Essau, C.A. (2004). Primary prevention of depression. In D.J.A. Dozois & K.S. Dobson (Eds.), *The prevention of anxiety and depression: Theory, research, and practice* (pp. 185–204). Washington, DC: American Psychological Association.

Feldman, S.S., Rubenstein, J.L., & Rubin, C. (1988). Depressive affect and restraint in early adolescents: Relationship with family structure, family process and friendship support. *Journal of Early Adolescence, 8*, 279–296.

Fowles, D.C. (1994). A motivational theory of psychopathology. In W.D. Spaulding (Ed.), *Integrative views on motivation, cognition, and emotion. Nebraska symposium on motivation* (pp. 181–238). Lincoln, NE: University of Nebraska Press.

Fox, N.A., Nichols, K.E., Henderson, H.A., Rubin, K., Schmidt, L., Hamer, D., et al. (2005). Evidence for a gene–environment interaction in predicting behavioral inhibition in middle childhood. *Psychological Science, 16*, 921–926.

Garber, J. & Flynn, C. (2001a). Predictors of depressive cognitions in young adolescents. *Cognitive Therapy & Research, 25*, 353–376.

Garber, J. & Flynn, C. (2001b). Vulnerability to depression in childhood and adolescence. In R.E. Ingram & J.M. Price (Eds.), *Vulnerability to psychopathology: Risk across the lifespan* (pp. 175–225). New York: Guilford.

Garber, J. & Horowitz, J.L. (2002). Depression in children. In I.H. Gotlib & C.L. Hammen (Eds.), *Handbook of depression* (pp. 510–540). New York: Guilford.

Garber, J. & Martin, N.C. (2002). Negative cognitions in offspring of depressed parents: Mechanisms of risk. In S.H. Goodman & I.H. Gotlib (Eds.), *Children of depressed parents: Mechanisms of risk and implications for treatment* (pp. 121–153). Washington, DC: American Psychological Association.

Garber, J. & Robinson, N.S. (1997). Cognitive vulnerability in children at risk for depression. *Cognition and Emotion, 11*, 619–635.

Garber, J., Robinson, N.S., & Valentiner, D. (1997). The relation between parenting and adolescent depression: Self-worth as a mediator. *Journal of Adolescent Research, 12*, 12–33.

Garber, J., Weiss, B., & Shanley, N. (1993). Cognitions, depressive symptoms, and development in adolescents. *Journal of Abnormal Psychology, 102*, 47–57.

Ge, X., Conger, R.D., & Elder, G.H., Jr. (1996). Coming of age too early: Pubertal influences on girls' vulnerability to psychological distress. *Child Development, 67*, 3386–3400.

Ge, X., Conger, R.D., & Elder, G.H., Jr. (2001). Pubertal transition, stressful life events, and the emergence of gender differences in adolescent depressive symptoms. *Developmental Psychology, 37*, 404–417.

Ge, X., Lorenz, F.O., Conger, R.D., Elder, G.H., Jr., & Simons, R.L. (1994). Trajectories of stressful life events and depressive symptoms during adolescence. *Developmental Psychology, 30*, 467–483.

Golan, J., Rafferty, B., Gortner, E., & Dobson, K. (2005). Course profiles of early- and adult-onset depression. *Journal of Affective Disorders, 86*, 81–86.

Goldberg, D. (2006). The aetiology of depression. *Psychological Medicine, 36*, 1341–1347.

Goldston, D.B., Reboussin, B.A., & Daniel, S.S. (2006). Predictors of suicide attempts: State and trait components. *Journal of Abnormal Psychology, 115*, 842–849.

Goodman, S.H., Adamson, L.B., Riniti, J., & Cole, S. (1994). Mothers' expressed attitudes: Associations with maternal depression and children's self-esteem and psychopathology. *Journal of the American Academy of Child and Adolescent Psychiatry, 33*, 1265–1274

Goodman, S.H. & Gotlib, I.H. (1999). Risk for psychopathology in the children of depressed mothers: A developmental model for understanding mechanisms of transmission. *Psychological Review, 106*, 458–490.

Goodman, S.H. & Gotlib, I.H. (Eds.). (2002). *Children of depressed parents: Mechanisms of risk and implications for treatment.* Washington, DC: American Psychological Association.

Goodyer, I.M., Herbert, J., & Altham, P.M.E. (1998). Adrenal steroid secretion and major depression in 8- to 16-year-olds: III. Influence of cortisol/DHEA ratio at presentation on subsequent rates of disappointing life events and persistent major depression. *Psychological Medicine, 28*, 265–273.

Goodyer, I.M., Herbert, J., & Tamplin, A. (2003). Psychoendocrine antecedents of persistent first-episode major depression in adolescence: A community-based longitudinal enquiry. *Psychological Medicine, 33*, 601–610.

Goodyer, I.M., Herbert, J., Tamplin, A., & Altham, E (2000). Recent life events, cortisol, dehydroepiandosterone and the onset of major depression in high risk adolescents. *British Journal of Psychiatry, 177*, 499–504.

Goodyer, I.M., Herbert, J., Tamplin, A., Secher, S.M., & Pearson, J. (1997). Short-term outcome of major depression: II. Life events, family dysfunction, and friendship difficulties as predictors of persistent disorder. *Journal of the American Academy of Child and Adolescent Psychiatry, 36*, 474–480.

Goodyer, I.M., Wright, C., & Altham, P.M.E. (1989). Recent friends in anxious and depressed school age children. *Psychological Medicine, 19*, 165–174.

Gotlib, I.H., Lewinsohn, P.M., & Seeley, J.R. (1998a). Consequences of depression during adolescence: Marital status and marital functioning in early adulthood. *Journal of Abnormal Psychology, 107*, 686–690.

Gotlib, I.H., Ranganath, C., & Rosenfeld, J.P. (1998b). Frontal EEG alpha asymmetry, depression, and cognitive functioning. *Cognition and Emotion, 12*, 449–478.

Gottesman, I.I. & Gould, T.D. (2003). The endophenotype concept in psychiatry: Etymology and strategic intentions. *American Journal of Psychiatry, 160*, 636–645.

Granger, D.A., Weisz, J.R., & Kauneckis, D. (1994). Neuroendocrine reactivity, internalizing behavior problems, and control-related cognitions in clinic-referred children and adolescents. *Journal of Abnormal Psychology, 103*, 267–276.

Gray, J.A. (1972). The psychophysiological basis of introversion–extraversion: A modification of Eysenck's theory. In V.D. Nebylitsyn,& J.A. Gray (Eds.), *The biological bases of individual behaviour* (pp. 182–205). NY: Academic Press.

Gray, J.A. (1990). Brain systems that mediate both emotion and cognition. *Cognition and Emotion, 4*, 269–288.

Gray, J.A. (1994). Personality dimensions and emotion systems. In P. Ekman & R.J. Davidson (Eds.), *The nature of emotion: Fundamental questions* (pp. 329–331). NY: Oxford University Press.

Gubba, E.M., Netherton, C.M., & Herbert, J. (2000). Endangerment of the brain by glucocorticoids: Experimental and clinical evidence. *Journal of Neurocytology, 29*, 439–449.

Haaga, D.A.F., Dyck, M.J., & Ernst, D. (1991). Empirical status of the cognitive theory of depression. *Psychological Bulletin, 110*, 215–236.

Halligan, S.L., Murray, L., Martins, C., & Cooper, P.J. (2007). Maternal depression and psychiatric outcomes in adolescent offspring: A 13-year longitudinal study. *Journal of Affective Disorders, 97*, 145–154.

Hammen, C. (1991). The generation of stress in the course of unipolar depression. *Journal of Abnormal Psychology, 100*, 555–561.

Hammen, C. (1992). Life events and depression: The plot thickens. *American Journal of Community Psychology, 2*, 179–193.

Hammen, C. (2002). Context of stress in families of children with depressed parents. In S.H. Goodman & I.H. Gotlib (Eds.), *Children of depressed parents: Mechanisms of risk and implications for treatment* (pp. 175–199). Washington, DC: American Psychological Association.

Hammen, C., Burge, D., & Stansbury, K. (1990). Relationship of mother and child variables to child outcomes in a high risk sample: A causal modelling analysis. *Developmental Psychology, 26*, 24–30.

Hammen, C. & Rudolph, R.D. (1996). Childhood depression. In E.J. Mash & R.A. Barkley (Eds.), *Child psychopathology* (pp. 153–195). New York: Guilford.

Hammen, C. & Rudolph, R.D. (2003). Childhood mood disorders. In E.J. Mash & R.A. Barkley (Eds.), *Child psychopathology* (2nd ed., pp. 233–278). New York: Guilford.

Hankin, B.L. & Abela, J.R.Z. (2005). Depression from childhood through adolescence and adulthood: A developmental vulnerability and stress perspective. In B.L. Hankin & J.R.Z. Abela (Eds.), *Development of psychopathology: A vulnerability–stress perspective* (pp. 245–288). Thousand Oaks: Sage.

Hankin, B.L. & Abramson, L.Y. (2001). Development of gender differences in depression: An elaborated cognitive vulnerability–transactional stress theory. *Psychological Bulletin, 127*, 773–796.

Hankin, B.L., Abramson, L.Y., Miller, N., & Haeffel, G.J. (2004). Cognitive vulnerability–stress theories of depression: Examining affective specificity in the prediction of depression versus anxiety in three prospective studies. *Cognitive Therapy and Research, 28*, 309–345.

Hankin, B.L., Abramson, L.Y., Moffitt, T.E., Silva, P.A., McGee, R., & Angell, K.E. (1998). Development of depression from preadolescence to young adulthood: Emerging gender differences in a 10-year longitudinal study. *Journal of Abnormal Psychology, 107*, 128–140.

Hankin, B.L., Abramson, L.Y., & Siler, M. (2001). A prospective test of the hopelessness theory of depression in adolescence. *Cognitive Therapy and Research, 25*, 607–632.

Hankin, B.L., Fraley, C., & Abela, J.R.Z. (2005). Daily depression and cognitions about stress: Evidence for a trait-like depressogenic cognitive style and the prediction of depressive symptoms in a prospective daily diary study. *Journal of Personality and Social Psychology, 88*, 673–685.

Hankin, B.L., Mermelstein, R., & Roesch, L. (2007). Sex differences in adolescent depression: Stress exposure and reactivity models. *Child Development, 78*, 279–295.

Harrington, R., Rutter, M., Weissman, M., Fudge, H., Groothues, C., Bredenkamp, D., et al. (1997). Psychiatric disorders in the relatives of depressed probands: I. Comparisons of prepubertal, adolescent and early adult onset cases. *Journal of Affective Disorders, 42,* 9–22.

Hassler, G., Drevets, W.C., Manji, H.K., & Charney, D.S. (2004). Discovering endophenotypes for major depression. *Neuropsychopharmacology, 29,* 1765–1781.

Hauser, S.T., Vieyra, M.A.B., Jacobson, A.M., & Wertlieb, D. (1985). Vulnerability and resilience in adolescence: Views from the family. *Journal of Early Adolescence, 5,* 81–100.

Hayden, E.P., Klein, D.N., & Durbin, C.E. (2005). Parent reports and laboratory assessments of child temperament: A comparison of their associations with risk for depression and externalizing disorders. *Journal of Psychopathology and Behavioral Assessment, 27,* 89–100.

Hayden, E.P., Klein, D.N., Durbin, C.E., & Olino, T.M. (2006). Positive emotionality and age 3 predicts cognitive styles in 7-year-old children. *Development and Psychopathology, 18,* 409–423.

Hayward, C. & Sanborn, K. (2002). Puberty and the emergence of gender differences in psychopathology. *Journal of Adolescent Health, 30,* 49–58.

Hecht, H., van Calker, D., Berger, M., & von Zerssen, D. (1998). Personality in patients with affective disorders and their relatives. *Journal of Affective Disorders, 51,* 33–43.

Hedlund, S. & Rude, S.S. (1995). Evidence of latent depressive schemas in formerly depressed individuals. *Journal of Abnormal Psychology, 104,* 517–525.

Henriques, J.B. & Davidson, R.J. (1991). Left frontal hypoactivation in depression. *Journal of Abnormal Psychology, 100,* 535–545.

Hilsman, R. & Garber, J. (1995). A test of the cognitive diathesis–stress model of depression in children: Academic stressors, attributional style, perceived competence, and control. *Journal of Personality and Social Psychology, 69,* 370–380.

Hodges, E.V.E. & Perry, D. G. (1999). Personal and interpersonal antecedents and consequences of victimization by peers. *Journal of Personality and Social Psychology, 76,* 677–685.

Holahan, C.J., Valentiner, D.P., & Moos, R.H. (1994). Parental support and psychological adjustment during the transition to young adulthood in a college sample. *Journal of Family Psychology, 8,* 215–223.

Ingram, R.E. (2001). Developing perspectives on the cognitive-developmental origins of depression: Back is the future. *Cognitive Therapy and Research, 25,* 497–504.

Ingram, R.E., Bernet, C.Z., & McLaughlin, S.C. (1994). Attentional allocation processes in individuals at risk for depression. *Cognitive Therapy and Research, 18,* 317–332.

Ingram, R.E., Miranda, J., & Segal, Z. (2006). Cognitive vulnerability to depression. In L.B. Alloy & J.H. Riskind (Eds.), *Cognitive vulnerability to emotional disorders* (pp. 63–91). Mahwah, NJ: Erlbaum

Ingram, R.E., Miranda, J., & Segal, Z.V. (1998). *Cognitive vulnerability to depression.* New York: Guilford.

Ingram, R.E. & Ritter, J. (2000). Vulnerability to depression: Cognitive reactivity and parental bonding in high-risk individuals. *Journal of Abnormal Psychology, 109,* 588–596.

Ingram, R.E. & Snyder, C.R. (2006). Blending the good with the bad: Integrating positive psychology and cognitive psychotherapy. *Journal of Cognitive Psychotherapy: An International Quarterly, 20,* 117–122.

Jackson, S.W. (1986). *Melancholia and depression: From Hippocratic times to modern times.* New Haven, CT: Yale University Press.

Jaffee, S.R. & Price, T.S. (2007). Gene-environment correlations: A review of the evidence and implications for prevention of mental illness. *Molecular Psychiatry, 12,* 432–442.

James, I.A., Reichelt, F.K., Freeston, M.H., & Barton, S.B. (2007). Schemas as memories: Implications for treatment. *Journal of Cognitive Psychotherapy: An International Quarterly, 21,* 51–57.

Jang, K.L., McCrae, R.R., Angleitner, A., Riemann, R., & Livesley, W.J. (1998). Heritability of facet-level traits in a cross-cultural twin sample: Support for a hierarchical model of personality. *Journal of Personality and Social Psychology, 74,* 1556–1565.

Joiner, T.E., Jr., Metalsky, G.I., Lew, A., & Klocek, J. (1999). Testing the causal mediation component of Beck's theory of depression: Evidence for specific mediation. *Cognitive Therapy and Research, 23,* 401–412.

Jones, I., Kent, L., & Craddock, N. (2002). Genetics of affective disorders. In P. McGuffin, M.J., Owen, & I.I., Gottesman (Eds.), *Psychiatric genetics and genomics* (pp. 211–245). New York: Oxford University Press.

Joorman, J. & Gotlib, I.H. (2007). Selective attention to emotional faces following recovery from depression. *Journal of Abnormal Psychology, 116,* 80–85.

Joorman, J., Talbot, L., & Gotlib, I.H. (2007). Biased processing of emotional information in girls at risk for depression. *Journal of Abnormal Psychology, 116,* 135–143.

Just, N., Abramson, L.Y., & Alloy, L.B. (2001). Remitted depression studies as tests of the cognitive vulnerability hypotheses of depression onset: A critique and conceptual analysis. *Clinical Psychology Review, 21,* 63–83.

Kanner, A.D., Feldman, S.S., Weinberger, D.A., & Ford, M.E. (1987). Uplifts, hassles, and adaptational outcomes in early adolescence. *Journal of Early Adolescence, 7,* 371–394.

Kaplan, S.J., Pelcovitz, D., Salzinger, S., Weiner, M., Mandel, F.S., Lesser, M.L., et al., (1998). Adolescent physical abuse: Risk for adolescent psychiatric disorders. *American Journal of Psychiatry, 155,* 954–959.

Kaufman, J., Martin, A., King, R.A., & Charney, D. (2001). Are child-, adolescent-, and adult-onset depression one and the same disorder? *Biological Psychiatry, 49,* 980–1001.

Kaufman, J., Yang, B.-Z., Douglas-Palumberi, H., Grasso, D., Lipschitz, D., Houshyar, S., et al. (2006). Brain-derived neurotrophic factor-5-HTTLPR gene interactions and environmental modifiers of depression in children. *Biological Psychiatry, 59,* 673–680.

Kendler, K.S., Gardner, C.O., & Prescott, C.A. (2003). Personality and the experience of environmental adversity. *Psychological Medicine, 33,* 1193–1202.

Kendler, K.S. & Karkowski-Shuman, L. (1997). Stressful life events and genetic liability to major depression: Genetic control of exposure to the environment? *Psychological Medicine, 27,* 539–547.

Keyes, C.L.M. (2007). Promoting and protecting mental health as flourishing: A complementary strategy for improving national mental health. *American Psychologist, 62,* 95–108.

Klein, D.N., Durbin, C.E., Shankman, S.A., & Santiago, N.J. (2002a). Depression and personality. In I.H. Gotlib & C.L. Hammen (Eds.), *Handbook of depression* (pp. 115–140). New York: Guilford.

Klein, D.N., Lewinsohn, P.M., Rohde, P., Seeley, J.R., & Durbin, C.E. (2002b). Clinical features of major depressive disorder in adolescents and their relatives: Impact on familial aggregation, implications for phenotype definition, and specificity of transmission. *Journal of Abnormal Psychology, 111,* 98–106.

Klomek, A.B., Marrocco, F., Kleinman, M., Schonfeld, I.S., & Gould, M.S. (2007). Bullying, depression, and suicidality in adolescents. *Journal of the American Academy of Child and Adolescent Psychiatry, 46*, 40–49.

Kochanska, G. (1991). Patterns of inhibition to the unfamiliar in children of normal and affectively ill mothers. *Child Development, 62*, 250–263.

Kupfer, D.J., Frank, E., Carpenter, L.J., & Neiswanger, K. (1989). Family history in recurrent depression. *Journal of Affective Disorders, 17*, 113–119.

Kwon, S.-M. & Oei, T.P.S. (1992). Differential causal roles of dysfunctional attitudes and automatic thoughts in depression. *Cognitive Therapy and Research, 16*, 309–328.

Lakdawalla, Z., Hankin, B.L., & Mermelstein, R. (2007). Cognitive theories of depression in children and adolescents: A conceptual and quantitative review. *Clinical Child and Family Psychology, 10*, 1–24.

Larson, R. & Ham, M. (1993). Stress and 'storm and stress' in early adolescence: The relationship of negative events with dysphoric affect. *Developmental Psychology, 29,* 130–140.

Lau, J.Y.F. & Eley, T.C. (2006). Changes in genetic and environmental influences on depressive symptoms across adolescence and young adulthood. *British Journal of Psychiatry, 189*, 422–427.

Lau, S. & Kwok, L.-K. (2000). Relationship of family environment to adolescents' depression and self-concept. *Social Behavior and Personality, 28*, 41–50.

Leschied, A.W., Chiodo, D., Whitehead, P.C., & Hurley, D. (2005). The relationship between maternal depression and child outcomes in a child welfare sample: Implications for treatment and policy. *Child and Family Social Work, 10,* 281–291.

Lewinsohn, P.M., Joiner, T.E., & Rohde, P. (2001). Evaluation of cognitive diathesis–stress models in predicting major depressive disorder in adolescents. *Journal of Abnormal Psychology, 110*, 203–215.

Lewinsohn, P.M., Rohde, P., & Seeley, J.R. (1998). Major depressive disorder in older adolescents: Prevalence, risk factors, and clinical implications. *Clinical Psychology Review, 18*, 765–794.

Licitra-Kleckler, D.M. & Waas, G.A. (1993). Perceived social support among high-stress adolescents: The role of peers and family. *Journal of Adolescent Research, 8*, 381–402.

Lonigan, C.J., Phillips, B.M., & Hooe, E.S. (2003). Relations of positive and negative affectivity to anxiety and depression in children: Evidence from a latent variable longitudinal study. *Journal of Consulting and Clinical Psychology, 71*, 465–481.

Malcarne, V.L., Hamilton, N.A., Ingram, R.E., & Taylor, L. (2000). Correlates of distress in children at risk for affective disorder: Exploring predictors in the offspring of depressed and nondepresssed mothers. *Journal of Affective Disorders, 59*, 243–251.

Mathews, A. & MacLeod, C. (2005). Cognitive vulnerability to emotional disorders. *Annual Review of Clinical Psychology, 1*, 167–195.

McGuffin, P., Katz, R., & Bebbington, P. (1987). Hazard, heredity and depression: A family study. *Journal of Psychiatric Research, 21*, 365–375.

Meehl, P.E. (1975). Hedonic capacity: Some conjectures. *Bulletin of the Menninger Clinic, 39*, 295–307.

Miranda, J. & Persons, J.B. (1988). Dysfunctional attitudes are mood-state dependent. *Journal of Abnormal Psychology, 97*, 76–79.

Monroe, S.M., Rohde, P., Seeley, J.R., & Lewinsohn, P.M. (1999). Life events and depression in adolescence: Relationship loss as a prospective risk factor for first onset of major depressive disorder. *Journal of Abnormal Psychology, 108*, 606–614.

Munafò, M.R., Clark, T.G., Moore, L.R., Payne, E., Walton, R., & Flint, J. (2003). Genetic polymorphisms and personality in healthy adults: A systematic review and meta-analysis. *Molecular Psychiatry, 8,* 471–484.

Murray, L., Woolgar, M., Cooper, P., & Hipwell, A. (2001). Cognitive vulnerability to depression in 5-year-old children of depressed mothers. *Journal of Child Psychology and Psychiatry, 42,* 891–899.

Nestler, E.J. & Carlezon, W.A., Jr. (2006). The mesolimbic dopamine reward circuit in depression. *Biological Psychiatry, 59,* 1151–1159.

Nolan, S.A., Flynn, C., & Garber, J. (2003). Prospective relations between rejection and depression in young adolescents. *Journal of Personality and Social Psychology, 85,* 745–755.

Pandey, G.N., Dwivedi, Y., Rizavi, H.S., Ren, Z., Pandey, S.C., Pesold, C., et al. (2002). Higher expression of serotonin 5-HT-sub(2A) receptors in the postmortem brains of teenage suicide victims. *American Journal of Psychiatry, 159,* 419–429.

Patterson, G.R. & Stoolmiller, M. (1991). Replications of a dual failure model for boys' depressed mood. *Journal of Consulting and Clinical Psychology, 59,* 491–498.

Peciña, S., Cagniard, B., Berridge, K.C., Aldridge, J.W., & Zhuang, X. (2003). Hyperdopaminergic mutant mice have higher 'wanting' but not 'liking' for sweet rewards. *Journal of Neuroscience, 23,* 9395–9402.

Petersen, A.C., Sarigiani, P.A., & Kennedy, R.E. (1991). Adolescent depression: Why more girls? *Journal of Youth and Adolescence, 20,* 247–271.

Pizzagalli, D.A., Nitschke, J.B., Oakes, T.R., Hendrick, A.M., Horras, K.A., Larson, C.L., et al. (2002). Brain electrical tomography in depression: The importance of symptom severity, anxiety and melancholic features. *Biological Psychiatry, 52,* 73–85.

Reid, S.A., Duke, L.M., & Allen, J.J.B. (1998). Resting frontal electroencephalographic asymmetry in depression: Inconsistencies suggest the need to identify mediating factors. *Psychophysiology, 35,* 389–404.

Reinecke, M. & DuBois, D. (2001). Socio-environmental and cognitive risk and resources: Relations to mood and suicidality among inpatient adolescents. *Journal of Cognitive Psychotherapy, 15,* 195–222.

Rice, F., Harold, G.T., Shelton, K.H., & Thapar, A. (2006). Family conflict interacts with genetic liability in predicting childhood and adolescent depression. *Journal of the American Academy of Child and Adolescent Psychiatry, 45,* 841–848.

Roberts, R.E., Alegria, M., Roberts, C.R., & Chen, I.G. (2005). Concordance of reports of mental health functioning by adolescents and their caregivers: A comparison of European, African and Latino Americans. *Journal of Nervous and Mental Disease, 193,* 528–534.

Robinson, N.S., Garber, J., & Hilsman, R. (1995). Cognitions and stress: Direct and moderating effects on depressive versus externalizing symptoms during the junior high school transition. *Journal of Abnormal Psychology, 104,* 453–463.

Rudolph, K., & Hammen, C. (1999). Age and gender as determinants of stress exposure, generation, and reactions in youngsters: A transactional perspective. *Child Development, 70,* 660–677.

Rudolph, K.D., Hammen, C., & Burge, D. (1994). Interpersonality functioning and depressive symptoms in childhood: Addressing the issues of specificity and comorbidity. *Journal of Abnormal Child Psychology, 22,* 355–371.

Rudolph, K., Hammen, C., Burge, D., Lindberg, N., Herzberg, D., & Daley, S.E. (2000). Toward an interpersonal life-stress model of depression: The developmental context of stress generation. *Development and Psychopathology, 12,* 215–234.

Rutter, M., Dunn, J., Plomin, R., Simonoff, E., Pickles, A., Maughan, B., et al. (1997). Integrating nature and nurture: Implications of person-environment correlations and inter-actions for developmental psychopathology. *Development and Psychopathology, 9*, 335–364.

Safford, S.M., Alloy, L.B., Abramson, L.Y., & Crossfield, A.G. (2007). Negative cognitive style as a predictor of negative life events in depression-prone individuals: A test of the stress generation hypothesis. *Journal of Affective Disorders, 99*, 147–154.

Scher, C.D., Ingram, R.E., & Segal, Z.V. (2005). Cognitive reactivity and vulnerability: Empirical evaluation of construct activation and cognitive diatheses in unipolar depression. *Clinical Psychology Review, 25*, 487–510.

Segal, Z.V., Gemar, M., & Williams, S. (1999). Differential cognitive response to a mood chal-lenge following successful cognitive therapy or pharmacotherapy for unipolar depression. *Journal of Abnormal Psychology, 108*, 3–10.

Segal, Z.V., Kennedy, S., Gemar, M., Hood, K., Pedersen, R., & Buis, T. (2006). Cognitive reac-tivity to sad mood provocation and the prediction of depressive relapse. *Archives of General Psychiatry, 63*, 749–755.

Seligman, M.E.P., Schulman, P., & Tyron, A.M. (2007). Group prevention of depression and anxiety symptoms. *Behaviour Research and Therapy, 45*, 1111–1126.

Shea, A., Walsh, C., MacMillan, H., & Steiner, M. (2005). Child maltreatment and HPA axis dysregulation: Relationship to major depressive disorder and post traumatic stress disorder in females. *Psychoneuroendocrinology, 30*, 162–178.

Shih, J.H., Eberhart, N.K., Hammen, C.L., & Brennan, P.A. (2006). Differential exposure and reactivity to interpersonal stress predict sex differences in adolescent depression. *Journal of Clinical Child and Adolescent Psychology, 35*, 103–115.

Siddique, C.M., & D'Arcy, C. (1984). Adolescence, stress, and psychological well-being. *Journal of Youth and Adolescence, 13*, 459–473.

Silberg, J., & Rutter, M. (2002). Nature–nurture interplay in the risks associated with parental depression. In S.H. Goodman & I.H. Gotlib (Eds.), *Children of depressed parents: Mechanisms of risk and implications for treatment* (pp. 13–36). Washington, DC: American Psychological Association.

Simmons, R.G., Burgeson, R., Carlton-Ford, S., & Blyth, D.A. (1987). The impact of cumula-tive change in early adolescence. *Child Development, 58,* 1220–1234.

Smiley, P. & Dweck, C.S. (1994). Individual differences in achievement goals among young children. *Child Development, 65*, 1723–1743.

Solomon, A., Haaga, D.A.F., Brody, C., Kirk, L., & Friedman, D.G. (1998). Priming irrational beliefs in recovered-depressed people. *Journal of Abnormal Psychology, 107*, 440–449.

Spirito, A. & Esposito-Smythers, C. (2006). Attempted and completed suicide in adolescence. *Annual Review of Clinical Psychology, 2*, 237–266.

Stark, K.D., Schimidt, K.L., & Joiner, T.E., Jr. (1996). Cognitive triad: Relationship to depres-sive symptoms, parents' cognitive triad, and perceived parental messages. *Journal of Abnormal Child Psychology, 24,* 615–631.

Stice, E., Ragan, J., & Randall, P. (2004). Prospective relations between social support and depression: Differential direction of effects for parent and peer support? *Journal of Abnormal Psychology, 113*, 155–159.

Sullivan, P.F., Neale, M.C., & Kendler, K.S. (2000). Genetic epidemiology of major depression: Review and meta-analysis. *American Journal of Psychiatry, 157*, 1552–1562.

Swickert, R.J., Rosentreter, C.J., Hittner, J.B., & Mushrush, J.E. (2002). Extraversion, social support processes, and stress. *Personality and Individual Differences, 32*, 877–891.

Taylor, L. & Ingram, R.E. (1999). Cognitive reactivity and depressotypic information processing in children of depressed mothers. *Journal of Abnormal Psychology, 108,* 202–210.

Taylor, S.E. & Brown, J.D. (1988). Illusion and well-being: A social psychological perspective on mental health. *Psychological Bulletin, 103,* 193–210.

Teasdale, J.D. & Dent, J. (1987). Cognitive vulnerability to depression: An investigation of two hypotheses. *British Journal of Clinical Psychology, 26,* 113–126.

Thapar, A. & McGuffin, P. (1994). A twin study of depressive symptoms in childhood. *British Journal of Psychiatry, 165,* 259–265.

Thase, M.E., Jindal, R., & Howland, R.H. (2002). Biological aspects of depression. In I.H. Gotlib & C.L. Hammen (Eds.), *Handbook of depression* (pp. 192–218). New York: Guilford.

Thibodeau, R., Jorgensen, R. S., & Kim, S. (2006). Depression, anxiety, and resting frontal EEG asymmetry: A meta-analytic review. *Journal of Abnormal Psychology, 115,* 715–729.

Timbremont, B. & Braet, C. (2004). Cognitive vulnerability in remitted depressed children and adolescents. *Behaviour Research and Therapy, 42,* 423–437.

Tyano, S., Zalsman, G., Ofek, H., Blum, I., Apter, A., Wolovik, L., et al. (2006). Plasma serotonin levels and suicidal behavior in adolescents. *European Neuropsychopharmacology, 16,* 49–57.

Valle, M.F., Huebner, E.S., & Suldo, S.M. (2006). An analysis of hope as a psychological strength. *Journal of School Psychology, 44,* 393–406.

Vazsonyi, A.T. & Belliston, L.M. (2006). The cultural and developmental significance of parenting processes in adolescent anxiety and depressive symptoms. *Journal of Youth and Adolescence, 35,* 491–505.

Wagner, B.M., Cohen, P., & Brook, J.S. (1996). Parent/adolescent relationships: Moderators of the effects of stressful life events. *Journal of Adolescent Research, 11,* 347–374.

Weiss, J.M. & Kilts, C.D. (1998). Animal models of depression and schizophrenia. In A.F. Schatzberg & C.B. Nemeroff (Eds.), *Textbook of psychopharmacology* (2nd ed., pp. 89–131). Washington, DC: American Psychiatric Press.

Weissman, M.M., Warner, V., Wickramaratne, P., Moreau, D., & Olfson, M. (1997). Offspring of depressed parents: Ten years later. *Archives of General Psychiatry, 54,* 932–940.

Willner, P. (1995). Dopaminergic mechanisms in depression and mania. In F.E. Bloom & D.J. Kupfer (Eds.), *Psychopharmacology: The fourth generation of progress* (pp. 921–931). New York: Raven Press.

Wolfradt, U., Hempel, S., & Miles, J.N.V. (2003). Perceived parenting styles, depersonalization, anxiety and coping behavior in adolescents. *Personality and Individual Differences, 34,* 521–532.

Youngstrom, E., Loeber, R., & Stouthamer-Loeber, M. (2000). Patterns and correlates of agreement between parent, teacher, and male adolescent ratings of externalizing and internalizing problems. *Journal of Consulting and Clinical Psychology, 68,* 1038–1050.

Zammit, S. & Owen, M.J. (2006). Stressful life events, 5-HTT genotype and risk of depression. *British Journal of Psychiatry, 188,* 199–201.

Zimmerman, M.A., Ramirez-Valles, J., Zapert, K.M., & Maton, K.I. (2000). A longitudinal study of stress-buffering effects for urban African–American male adolescent problem behaviors and mental health. *Journal of Community Psychology, 28,* 17–33.

Zubenko, G.S., Maher, B.S., Hughes, H.B., Zubenko, W.N., Stiffler, J.S., Kaplan, B.B., et al. (2003). Genome-wide linkage survey for genetic loci that influence the development of depressive disorders in families with recurrent, early-onset, major depression. *American Journal of Medical Genetics, 123B,* 1–18.

Chapter 3

Empirically supported treatments for adolescent depression

Thomas H. Ollendick & Matthew A. Jarrett

Although the movement to develop empirically supported treatments has revolutionized the field of mental health, this movement is of relatively recent origin (Chambless & Ollendick, 2001). To appreciate the reasons for this movement, it is important to consider the historical backdrop for psychotherapy research. In his now in(famous) review of the effects of adult psychotherapy, Eysenck (1952) boldly asserted that psychotherapy practices utilized in the 1950s were no more effective than the passage of time (i.e., spontaneous remission). Levitt (1957, 1963) subsequently reviewed the child psychotherapy literature and offered a similar conclusion. Although these reviews were unsettling for clinicians and researchers alike, they served as a wake-up call to the mental health professions (Kazdin, 2000). Since the time of these reviews, advances in the study of developmental psychopathology, psychiatric diagnostic nomenclature, assessment and treatment practices, and longitudinal experimental designs have resulted in well over 1500 studies (Durlak et al., 1995; Kazdin, 2000; Ollendick et al., 2006) and four major meta-analyses examining the effects of child psychotherapy (Casey & Berman, 1985; Kazdin et al., 1990; Weisz et al., 1987, 1995b). These meta-analyses have provided strong empirical evidence that child and adolescent psychotherapy works for children and their families (Weersing & Weisz, 2002). More specifically, systematic reviews of the literature now show that therapy for children and adolescents outperforms wait-list and attention-placebo conditions. In addition, it is becoming abundantly clear that some forms of psychotherapy work better than others, a finding that has allowed the fields of clinical child psychology and child psychiatry to move beyond the question of whether psychotherapy works for children and adolescents to identifying the efficacy of *specific* treatments for children who present with *specific* behavioural, emotional, and social problems. These are exciting times for the field of child and adolescent psychotherapy, and the various chapters in this volume attest to what we know and what we have yet to learn in treating depression in adolescence.

The current chapter reviews past work used to identify empirically supported psychosocial treatments for children and adolescents and raises a series of critical issues relevant to this movement. First, it should be noted that this movement is embedded within a larger movement known as 'evidence-based medicine' or 'evidence-based practice' (Sackett et al., 1997, 2000). Evidence-based practice at its core is an approach to knowledge and a strategy for improving performance outcomes

(Ollendick & King, 2004; Ollendick et al., 2006). Although it is not wedded to any one theoretical position, it does require treatments to be based on objective and scientifically credible evidence that is obtained largely through randomized clinical trials (RCTs). In a RCT, children with a specific presenting problem are randomly assigned to a treatment condition or a control condition, such as a wait-list or attention-placebo condition, and the effects of these conditions are compared. Although there are limitations to such a design (Westen et al., 2004), it appears to be the best strategy currently available for rigorously evaluating the effects of treatment (i.e., controlling for extraneous variables through randomization) and ruling out biases and expectations (on the part of the child, the child's parents, and the therapist) that can result in misleading findings. Although the RCT is the gold standard for evaluating treatment conditions, information or opinions obtained from observational studies, logical intuition, personal experiences, and the testimony of experts can also serve as evidence for treatment efficacy. Although such evidence is valuable, it represents a less credible and acceptable form of evidence from a scientific standpoint (i.e., it occupies a lower rung on the ladder of evidentiary support). At the same time, it is these initial clinical observations and 'clinical hunches' that frequently lead to the development of new and innovative treatments that can eventually be more rigorously evaluated in RCTs. It is clear that evidence-based treatments do not simply emerge all at once or from a vacuum, but often have their own developmental trajectory, a consideration that is reflected in the varying levels of evidence identified in the evidence-based practice approach.

Although the approach to develop, identify, disseminate, and use empirically supported psychosocial treatments (initially referred to as empirically 'validated' treatments; see Chambless, 1996; Chambless & Hollon, 1998) seems both scientifically and ethically desirable (if not necessary), this movement has been highly controversial in the field of mental health. On the surface, it hardly seemed possible that anyone could or would object to the initial report developed by the Society of Clinical Psychology (Division 12) of the American Psychological Association in 1995 or that the movement associated with it would be so hotly contested. Surely, identifying, developing, and disseminating treatments that 'work' and possess empirical support should be encouraged, not discouraged, especially by a profession that is committed to the welfare of those whom it serves.

Unfortunately, this task force report was not only controversial; moreover, and unfortunately, it served to foster a divide within the mental health professions (Ollendick & King, 2000, 2004; Ollendick et al., 2006). In this chapter, we attempt to not only present the core of this approach to evaluating empirically supported treatments but also to address myths about the nature and use of empirically supported treatments (i.e., dangers of manualization, loss of therapist creativity). We believe that in order to create a more unified field, it will be important for advocates of empirically supported treatments to not only communicate the approach to others but to address the concerns of those who oppose this movement. In the first part of this chapter, we will define empirically supported treatments. We will then subsequently illustrate and discuss some of the lingering and contentious issues associated with empirically supported treatments and their development and promulgation. Finally, we conclude the chapter by offering recommendations for future research and practice with a particular focus on evidence-based treatments for adolescent depression. Other chapters in this volume will provide a more in-depth review on the efficacy of specific treatments for adolescent depression.

Defining empirically supported treatments

Although the movement to evaluate the efficacy of psychosocial treatments occurred prior to 1995, the first report to address the evidence-based practice movement was issued at that time. This report on empirically validated treatments, issued by the Society of Clinical Psychology Task Force on Promotion and Dissemination of Psychological Procedures, was developed by clinicians and researchers from a number of theoretical orientations, including psychodynamic, interpersonal, cognitive–behavioural, and systemic points of view. This diversity in membership was crucial in identifying and promulgating *all* psychotherapies of proven worth, not just those emanating from a particular school of thought. This diversity was valuable in generating alternative ways of thinking about treatment evaluation, but it also made defining empirically validated treatments a difficult task. One point that was emphasized in the report was that no treatment is ever fully validated as there are always important questions to ask about any treatment (e.g., the essential components of treatments, client characteristics that predict or moderate treatment outcome, and the mechanisms or mediators that account for behaviour change). In turn, the committee chose to substitute the more felicitous term 'empirically supported' for the term 'empirically validated.'

According to the 1995 report, three categories were established for empirically supported treatments: (1) well-established treatments, (2) probably efficacious treatments, and (3) experimental treatments (see Table 3.1). The primary distinction between *well-established* and *probably efficacious* treatments is that a well-established treatment must prove to be superior to a psychological placebo, pill, or another treatment, whereas a probably efficacious treatment must prove to be superior only to a wait-list or no treatment control condition. In addition, well-established treatments require evidence from at least two different investigatory teams, whereas the effects of a probably efficacious treatment only require evidence from one investigatory team. For both types of empirically supported treatments, client characteristics should be well-specified (e.g., age, sex, ethnicity, diagnosis), and the clinical trials should be conducted with treatment manuals. Furthermore, outcomes of treatment should be demonstrated in 'good' group design studies or a series of controlled single-case design studies. 'Good' designs were those in which it was reasonable to conclude that the benefits observed were due to the effects of treatment and not due to chance or confounding factors such as the passage of time, the effects of psychological assessment, or the presence of different types of clients in the various treatment conditions (Chambless & Hollon, 1998; also see Kazdin, 1998; Kendall et al., 1999 for a fuller discussion of research design issues). Treatment efficacy should also ideally be demonstrated in randomized clinical trials (RCTs) or carefully controlled single-case experiments and their group analogues. Finally, *experimental* treatments are those treatments not yet shown to be at least probably efficacious. This category was intended to capture treatments

Table 3.1 Criteria for empirically validated treatments

I. Well-established treatments

    A. At least two good between-group design experiments demonstrating efficacy in one or more of the following ways:

        1. Superior to pill or psychological placebo or to another treatment

        2. Equivalent to an already established treatment in experiments with adequate statistical power (about 30 per group)

    or

    B. A large series of single case design experiments ($n > 9$) demonstrating efficacy. These experiments must have

        1. Used good experimental designs, and

        2. Compared the intervention to another treatment in A.1.

Further criteria for both A and B

    C. Experiments must be conducted with treatment manuals

    D. Characteristics of the client samples must be clearly specified

    E. Effects must have been demonstrated by at least two different investigators or investigatory teams

II. Probably efficacious treatments

    A. Two experiments showing the treatment is more effective than a waiting-list control group

    or

    B. One or more experiments meeting the Well-Established Treatment Criteria A, C, D, but not E

    C. A small series of single case design experiments ($n > 3$) otherwise meeting Well-Established Treatment Criteria B, C, and D

frequently used in clinical practice but not yet fully evaluated *or* newly developed ones not yet put to the test of scientific scrutiny. It should be noted that the development of new treatments was strongly encouraged in the report. In addition, treatments can 'move' from one category to another depending on the empirical support available for that treatment *over time*. For example, an experimental treatment might move into probably efficacious or well-established status after further scientific evaluation. As noted earlier, the categorical system was intended to be a dynamic one, so that new and innovative treatments could build evidentiary support over time.

Empirically supported treatments: issues of concern

In an earlier paper, Ollendick (1999) identified three major concerns associated with the empirically supported treatment movement: (a) some treatments have been shown to be more effective than others and, as a result, the 'Dodo Bird' effect (i.e., all treatments are equivalent) was no longer tenable and some practices might be preferred over others, (b) use of treatment manuals might lead to mechanical, inflexible interventions that result in a loss of creativity and innovation in the therapy process, and (c) treatments shown to be effective in clinical research settings might not generalize or transport to 'real-life' clinical practice settings. Although these concerns are reasonable ones, we hope to address them in order to shed light on whether they necessarily compromise the empirically supported treatment movement. These concerns will be addressed in detail in the following sections.

Differential Effectiveness of Psychosocial Treatments. In our prior and recent reviews of the literature (Ollendick & King, 1998, 2000, 2004; Ollendick et al., 2006), we have reported a rather alarming set of findings. Namely, it is now clear that many treatments that are currently in use in clinical practice have not been systematically evaluated (with the exception of behavioural and cognitive–behavioural treatments) and therefore do not qualify as well-established or even probably efficacious treatments. For example, across problem areas such as depression, phobias, anxiety, ADHD, oppositional behaviours, and conduct problems, *no* randomized controlled trials using 'good' experimental designs have been identified for psychodynamic psychotherapies or family systems therapies (with the exception of oppositional behaviour wherein psychodynamic and family systems interventions have been shown to be *less* efficacious than behavioural based ones; see Brestan & Eyberg, 1998). In addition, interpersonal psychotherapy (Mufson et al., 1994, 1999; Rossello & Bernal, 1999) has only been established as efficacious in the treatment of depression in adolescents, but not for other disorders in adolescence. Given that many of these treatments have not been evaluated, we simply do not know whether or not they are effective.

Although a number of treatments have not been evaluated, there is considerable evidence for the efficacy of behavioural and cognitive–behavioural treatment procedures in the treatment of diverse child psychopathologies. These treatments have not only been found to be effective, but they have also been found to fare better than other interventions in meta-analytic studies (see Weisz et al., 1987, 1995b, for reviews that indicate the superiority of behavioural over 'non-behavioural' treatments). Although these findings are exciting for advocates of behavioural and cognitive–behavioural therapies, the results are less exciting for practitioners of other psychotherapies. Moreover, behavioural and cognitive–behavioural therapists should proceed with caution, since there is a limited evidentiary base for the efficacy of even these treatments. For example, in the child and adolescent area, we have been able to identify only one well-established treatment for the anxiety disorders (cognitive behaviour therapy), two well-established treatments for specific phobias (participant modeling, reinforced practice), two well-established treatments for ADHD (behavioural parent training, operant classroom management), and two well-established treatments for oppositional and conduct problems (Patterson's social learning parent training program, Webster-Stratton's videotape modeling parent training). Specific to adolescent depression, we have found limited support for cognitive–behavioural treatments and interpersonal psychotherapy, but then only as probably efficacious (Seligman et al., 2004).

Although the evidence is limited, these treatments still serve as a good start in the movement towards evidence-based practice. It is clear that additional treatments will need to be developed and evaluated, but how should clinical practice proceed until that time? What is the current status of 'treatment as usual' in clinical practice settings and should such treatments continue to be used until more empirical support is available? These questions are crucial if we are to move into an age of evidence-based practice. Weisz et al. (1998) examined these questions in a re-analysis of their 1995 meta-analytic study. The authors selected treatment studies of clinic-referred children who were treated in service-oriented clinics or clinical agencies by practicing clinicians. Over a period 50 years, nine studies were identified that compared 'treatment as usual' to a control condition in a clinical setting. Effect sizes associated with these nine studies ranged from −0.40 to +0.29, with a mean effect size of 0.01, an effect size well below the average effect size (+0.70) obtained in their meta-analyses of 'research'-based treatments. An effect size of 0.01 indicates that the treated children were no better off than the untreated children following treatment, a finding that is disquieting if not alarming.

Unfortunately, findings regarding treatment as usual are not limited to the clinical studies reviewed by Weisz et al. (1998). Bickman and colleagues have reported similar outcomes in their examination of a comprehensive mental health services program for children (Bickman, 1996; Bickman et al., 1995). In what became known as the Fort Bragg Project, the United States Army spent over $80 million to provide an organized continuum of mental health care to children and their families and to test its cost-effectiveness relative to a more conventional and less comprehensive intervention (treatment as usual) in a matched comparison site. The findings showed good evidence for better access to treatment and higher levels of client satisfaction in the experimental condition, but the program failed to demonstrate clinical and functional outcomes superior to those in the comparison site. Overall, this study resulted in more interventions at a greater cost, but more positive outcomes were not associated with greater intensity of treatment and costs. Moreover, neither treatment produced gains that approached those found in clinical trials reported by Weisz et al. (1995b) in their meta-analytic review. It is clear that expensive and intensive treatments do not always result in greater outcomes.

Furthermore, in a school setting, Weiss et al. (1999) evaluated the effectiveness of child psychotherapy as typically delivered ('treatment as usual') in that setting using a RCT design. A total of 160 children who presented with problems of anxiety, depression, aggression, and attention were randomly assigned to treatment and control conditions. Children were enrolled in normal elementary and middle schools and their mean age was 10.3 years. Treatment was provided by mental health professionals hired through regular clinic practices (six were masters' level clinicians and one was a doctoral level clinical psychologist). Overall, the therapists reported favouring psychodynamic-humanistic approaches over cognitive and behavioural ones. The treatment itself was open-ended (i.e., not guided by manuals) and delivered over an extended 2-year period on an 'as needed' and individualized basis. The results of the trial provided little support for the effectiveness of 'treatment as usual' in this setting (overall effect size of −0.08), indicating that the treatment was no better than the academic tutoring comparison control condition.

Overall, then, results from these studies and others show the importance of developing, validating, and transporting effective treatments to clinical and school settings.

'Treatment as usual' does not appear to be very effective treatment when it is compared to non-therapy alternatives (e.g., tutoring) or to no treatment at all. Interestingly, these results seem to mirror the findings of Levitt (1957, 1963) reported over fifty years ago in which treatment was found to be no more effective than the passage of time. If we are to move into an age of evidence-based practice and bring legitimacy to treatment outcome research, we must take these findings seriously, as they have important implications for the future of child and adolescent mental health treatment. Of even greater concern may be the often understudied area of iatrogenic effects of treatment, a field of study showing that our profession may at times do more harm than good (Lilienfeld, 2007).

Finally, we must consider the ethics of continuing to provide either ineffective or harmful treatments to children and their families (recall that the effect sizes for the nine clinic-based studies reviewed by Weisz et al. ranged from −0.40 to +0.29 and that the effect size reported by Weiss et al. was −0.08). As psychologists, the identification, promulgation, and use of empirically supported treatments are consistent with the ethical standard that psychologists 'should rely on scientifically and professionally derived knowledge when making scientific or professional judgments' (Canter et al., 1994, p. 36). Yet, as noted in a lively debate on this issue (Eiffert et al., 1998; Persons, 1998; Zvolensky & Eiffert, 1998, 1999), the identification and use of empirically supported treatments represent a two-edged sword. On the one hand, it might seem unethical to use a treatment that has not been empirically supported; on the other hand, given that few empirically supported treatments have been developed, it might be unethical to restrict practice to problem areas and disorders for which treatment efficacy has been established (Ollendick & Davis, 2004). What should a clinician do when children and their families present with problems for which empirically supported treatments have not yet been developed? Although there is not an obvious answer to this question, we agree with the conclusions reached earlier by Kinscherff (1999) in an article entitled 'Empirically supported treatments: What to do until the data arrive (or now that they have)?' Kinscherff suggests that 'clinicians should develop a formulation of the case and select the best approaches for helping a client from among the procedures in which the clinician is competent. Clinicians should remain informed about advances in treatment, including empirically supported treatments, and maintain their own clinical skills by learning new procedures and strengthening their skills in areas in which they are already accomplished. Because there are limitations to how many treatments any one clinician can master, a key professional competence is knowing when to refer for a treatment approach that may be more effective for the client' (p. 4). Overall, this approach emphasizes the importance of knowing one's limitations, the importance of continuing education, and the need to refer when the appropriate treatment is outside of one's competencies.

In those situations in which a referral is not possible (e.g., rural settings, few practitioners), or when the evidentiary support is lacking, Chorpita and his colleagues have proposed an 'evidence-based' decision making model, a model that was recently implemented in the Hawaii Child and Adolescent Mental Health Division (Chorpita & Donkervoet, 2005; Daleiden & Chorpita, 2005). Under this model, the therapist is encouraged to use individual case-specific evidence to guide clinical choices that need to be made for treatment. Routine measurement of clinical progress has the potential to provide empirical support for the clinical choices made when evidence from RCTs is not available (e.g., Hayes et al., 1999; Ollendick & Hersen, 1984). This model allows for services to continue in the face of minimal supportive evidence, but requires that clinical and functional improvements are evident *for that individual case*. Only preliminary evaluation of this alternative model is available at this time (Daleiden, 2004), but it appears to offer promise and accountability when it is not possible to use or implement evidence-based treatments.

Manualization of psychosocial treatments

The recommendation that well-established and probably efficacious treatments use a treatment manual was identified by Ollendick (1999) as the second major source of controversy in the empirically supported treatment movement. As noted by Chambless (1996), the inclusion of a treatment manual leads to greater standardization and an operational definition of the treatment. The treatment manual provides a description of the treatment that makes it possible to determine whether the treatment was actually delivered as intended (i.e., the treatment possesses 'integrity'). Second, the use of a manual allows other mental health professionals and researchers to know the actual components of treatments that were supported in the efficacy trial. This manualization of therapy is especially important to clarify the many types or variants of therapy. For example, given the many types of cognitive–behaviour therapy or psychodynamic therapy, it is largely meaningless to claim that a study found that cognitive–behaviour therapy or psychodynamic therapy was efficacious. What type of psychodynamic therapy was used in this study? What form of cognitive–behaviour therapy was used in that study? As Chambless (1996, p. 6) noted, 'brand names are not the critical identifiers. The manuals are.'

In response to this controversy about the use of manuals, Chorpita et al. (2005) proposed an alternative model that emphasized underlying *principles* of change rather than *procedures* of change. In their critique of procedural manuals, three primary concerns were raised. First, the requirement that a treatment is defined by the procedures outlined in the manual (and not by the principles underlying the procedures) implies that revisions to a manual require empirical justification to begin afresh every time a manual is changed or altered in some way. For example, although the Coping Cat (Kendall et al., 1990) has been subjected to several good randomized clinical trials for the treatment of childhood anxiety disorders, the currently available Coping Cat manual (Kendall, 2002) is an updated and revised version of the original manual. Strict adherence to the manualization principle would indicate that the latter manual is not empirically supported in its present form, a conclusion that seems counter to good clinical practice (i.e., treatment manuals change based on experience obtained while using them). Relaxing the strict interpretation of 'manualization' might allow for small revisions to benefit from prior empirical support, but, of course, then the issue becomes one of defining a boundary. How much change is too much? Is the manual basically the same or has it been altered appreciably?

The second concern raised by Chorpita et al. (2005) involves the unavailability of manuals for several problem areas. For example, there are currently no empirically supported treatment manuals for adolescent panic disorder (although a treatment approach based on the work with adults with panic disorder has been proposed and evaluated by Ollendick (1995a) and Mattis and Ollendick (2002), with single-case but not RCT support). Under a strict interpretation of the Division 12 guidelines, any treatment for adolescent panic might be as good as any other one (because none has received strong empirical support). Again, this is a conclusion that would be unfortunate, especially given the strong support for cognitive–behavioural interventions with adults with panic disorder and the promising support for adolescents (see Barlow et al., 2002; Mattis & Ollendick, 2002). Treatments based on the underlying principles in the adult and single-case studies would seem to be fruitful to apply, and to be evaluated systematically before using other interventions with little or no support.

Third, Chorpita and colleagues raised the issue of what to do when more than one manual exists for a given disorder and how clinicians should go about selecting one of them for use. For example, for childhood and adolescent depression, there are at least two promising treatment manuals (Kaslow & Thompson, 1998, Seligman et al., 2004), including those based on cognitive–behavioural and interpersonal approaches. How does a therapist determine which one or ones to use? There are few extant guidelines for how one selects one of the available treatments.

As noted, the model proposed to address these three concerns involves a methodology for the identification and selection of 'common elements' or underlying principles of evidence-based protocols. Chorpita et al. (2005) demonstrated that 'practice elements' (e.g., 'time out,' 'exposure,' 'cognitive restructuring') could be reliably coded and then empirically 'factored' into groupings representing particular approaches. Each factor could yield a practice element profile, which denotes the relative frequency of the occurrence of different practice elements for a particular problem. For example, the practice element profile for childhood anxiety showed that exposure was universally present in the evidence-based protocols coded, and other practice elements such as psychoeducation, relaxation, and self-monitoring were highly common. Similarly, common elements for the treatment of adolescent depression appear to include behavioural activation, cognitive restructuring, and address of interpersonal issues (Seligman et al., 2004). Such a 'common elements' approach represents an alternative to the strict definition of manuals at the level of individual manuals, allowing the grouping of manuals empirically determined to be similar in content. In that manner, the model addresses the three concerns reviewed above, in that the similarity of revised manuals can be empirically defined (e.g., the revised Coping Cat would share the support of the original), unavailability of manuals can be addressed through the construction of a profile averaging across similar problem areas (e.g., a cognitive–behavioural protocol for childhood anxiety would be recommended for panic disorder), and the presence of more than one manual could be addressed by creating a master profile, which represents the aggregate frequency of approaches (e.g., a clinician could select the manual that is most similar to the depression profile or could develop a new approach including the elements outlined in the profile). Although this model offers some promising alternatives, its use as an intervention strategy awaits additional empirical investigation.

The model proposed by Chorpita et al. (2005) arose in the context of considerable controversy regarding the use of 'procedural' manuals, as noted above. In recent years, a flood of commentaries—some commendatory, others derogatory—have filled the pages of several major journals, including the *American Psychologist, Australian Psychologist, Journal of Clinical Psychology, Journal of Consulting and Clinical Psychology, Clinical Psychology: Science and Practice, Clinical Psychology Review, and Psychotherapy*. Some authors have viewed manuals as 'promoting a cookbook mentality' (Smith, 1995), 'paint by numbers' (Silverman, 1996), 'more of a straightjacket than a set of guidelines' (Goldfried & Wolfe, 1996), 'somewhat analogous to cookie cutters' (Strupp & Anderson, 1997), and a 'hangman of life' (Lambert, 1998). Others have viewed them in more positive terms (e.g., Chambless & Hollon, 1998; Craighead & Craighead, 1998; Heimberg, 1998; Kendall, 1998; King & Ollendick, 1998; Ollendick, 1995b, 1999; Strosahl, 1998; Wilson, 1996a, b, 1998). Wilson (1998, p. 363), for example, suggested that 'the use of standardized, manual-based treatments in clinical practice represents a new and evolving development with far-reaching implications for the field of psychotherapy.'

In its simplest form, a treatment manual can be defined as a set of guidelines that instruct or inform the user as to 'how to do' a certain treatment and, ideally, specify the principles that underlie that treatment (Ollendick, 1999). They both specify and standardize the treatment at the same time. Although some opponents of manual-based treatment support the evidence-based practice movement, they express other concerns, including the notion that treatments evaluated in research settings will not generalize to 'real-life' clinical settings or that manual-based treatments will offer little opportunity for flexibility or clinical judgment. Seligman (1995, p. 967), for example, indicated that unlike the manual-based treatment of controlled, laboratory research—in which 'a small number of techniques, all within one modality' are delivered in fixed order for a fixed duration—clinical practice is, by necessity, self-correcting. 'If one technique is not working, another technique—or even modality—is usually tried.' As noted by Wilson (1998), this characterization or depiction of manual-based treatment is simply wrong. A variety of treatments have been 'manualized', including those embedded in psychodynamic (e.g., Strupp & Binder, 1984), interpersonal (e.g., Klerman et al., 1984), behavioural (Patterson & Gullion, 1968) and cognitive–behavioural theory (e.g., Beck et al., 1979); moreover, these manuals allow for flexible use and, for the most part, are responsive to progress or regress in treatment.

It should be recalled that the movement to manualize treatment practices existed long before the Task Force issued its report in 1995. Almost 30 years earlier, Patterson and Gullion (1968) published their now-classic book 'Living with Children: New Methods for Parents and Teachers', a 'how to' parent and teacher that has been the foundation for many behavioural treatment programs of oppositional, defiant, and conduct problem children. Not surprisingly, treatment based on this 'manual' was one of the first treatments designated as 'evidence-based'. Once again, prior to the task force report, Luborsky and DuRubeis (1984) commented upon the potential use of treatment manuals in a paper entitled 'The use of psychotherapy treatment manuals: A small revolution in psychotherapy research style.' Similarly, Lambert and Ogles (1988) indicated that manuals were not new; rather, they noted, manuals have been used to train therapists and define treatments since the 1960s. It seems to us that the 1995 Task Force Report simply reaffirmed a movement that had been present for some years and that had been adopted by the mental health field for studies designed to explore the efficacy of various psychotherapies.

At the same time, probably the most contentious issue may be that the Task Force Report asserted that psychotherapies described and operationalized by manuals should not only be identified, but they should also be promulgated and disseminated to clinical training programs, practicing mental health professionals, the public, and to third party payors (i.e., insurance companies, health maintenance organizations). Many clinicians were concerned that such actions were premature and that they would prohibit or, in the least, constrain the practice of those psychotherapies that had not yet been manualized or shown to be effective. They also were concerned that the development of new psychotherapies would be limited, if not stifled totally. Although these are possible outcomes of the evidenced-based treatment movement, they need not be an inevitable outcome. In fact, it seems to us that these developments can serve to stimulate additional treatments by systematically examining the parameters of effective treatments as well as the therapeutic mechanisms of change (see Kendall [1998] and Wilson [1998] for examples), a position that we fully support.

What is the current status of this movement toward manualization in the treatment of children and adolescents? First, it should be clear that the studies summarized in our reviews of empirically supported treatments for children either used manuals or the procedures were described in sufficient detail as to not require manuals (as originally suggested by the Task Force Report [1995] and by Chambless [1996]). As we noted earlier, manuals are simply guidelines that describe treatment procedures and therapeutic strategies, and in some instances, provide an underlying theory of change on which the procedures or techniques are based. Kendall and his colleagues (Kendall, 1998; Kendall & Chu, 2000; Kendall et al., 1998) have addressed misperceptions surrounding use of treatment manuals and have identified six (mis)perceptions that plague manual-based treatments: How flexible are they? Do they replace clinical judgment? Do manuals detract from the creative process of therapy? Does a treatment manual reify therapy in a fixed and stagnant fashion, and thereby stifle improvement and change? Are manual-based treatments effective with patients who present with multiple diagnoses or clinical problems? And, are manuals primarily designed for use in research programs, with little or no use or application in service-providing clinics? Although clear answers to these questions are not available at this time, careful research is desperately needed to explore these (mis)perceptions. In addition, Kendall and his colleagues provide evidence from their own work with children who have anxiety disorders that at least some of these issues or questions may be not be problematic. For example, flexibility of treatment implementation is an issue that many critics have raised; accordingly, it should be investigated empirically to determine if the degree to which a manual is implemented flexibly affects treatment outcome.

In a study by Kendall and Chu (2000), the degree to which flexibility affected treatment outcome was explored. In their study, Kendall and Chu defined flexibility as a construct that measures the therapist's adaptive stance to the *specific* situation at hand while adhering *generally* to the instructions and suggestions in the manual. Ratings on the degree to which the manual was implemented in a flexible manner were obtained from 18 different therapists who had implemented the Coping Cat cognitive–behavioural, manual-based treatment for anxious children (Kendall, 2002). Flexibility ratings were obtained retrospectively on a 13-item questionnaire, with each item rated on a 1- to 7-point scale as to the extent of flexibility used in implementing treatment (e.g., 'The manual suggests that clinicians spend 40–45 minutes of the session teaching the outlined skills to the child and 10–15 minutes of the session playing games. How flexible with this were you?' And, 'During therapy sessions, how flexible were you in discussing issues not related to anxiety or directly related to the child's primary diagnoses?'). Results of the study revealed that therapists reported being flexible in their implementation of the treatment plan (both in general and with specific strategies). Second, and perhaps more unexpectedly, the indices of flexibility were *not* related to whether the children were co-morbid with other disorders *or* treatment outcome. The important point here is that flexibility, however defined, is amenable to careful and systematic inquiry. Kendall (1998) asserts that other issues raised by the manualization of treatment are also amenable to empirical investigation and they need not remain in the area of 'heated' speculation.

A second example may help to illustrate how issues such as flexibility might be addressed empirically. In studies conducted primarily with adults, manual-based treatments have been 'individualized' in a flexible manner by matching certain characteristics or profiles of the individuals being treated to specific elements or components of previously established effective treatments. These efforts have been labelled 'prescriptive matching' by Acierno et al. (1994). At the core of this approach is the assumption that an idiographic approach to treatment is more effective in producing positive treatment outcomes than a nomothetic approach (e.g., not all patients who receive a diagnosis of major depression are *really* the same—the homogeneity myth put forth some years ago by Kiesler, 1966). For example, in one of these studies, Jacobson et al. (1989) designed individually tailored marital therapy treatment plans, where the number of sessions and the specific modules selected in each case were determined by the couple's specific needs and presenting problems. Individualized treatments were compared to a standard cognitive–behavioural treatment program with each treatment being manualized. Although couples treated with individually tailored protocols could not be distinguished from those receiving standardized protocols at post-treatment, a greater proportion of couples receiving standardized treatment showed decrements in marital satisfaction at 6-month follow-up, whereas a majority of those in the individually tailored program maintained their treatment gains. These findings suggest individually tailored programs may help to reduce treatment relapse.

Similar beneficial findings have been obtained in the treatment of adults with depression (Nelson-Gray et al., 1990). In this study, Nelson-Gray et al. assigned adult depressed patients to treatment protocols (e.g., cognitive treatment, social skills treatment) that were either matched or mismatched to presenting problems (e.g., irrational cognitions, social skills problems). Those in the matched conditions fared better than those in the mismatched condition upon completion of treatment. Similarly, Ost et al. (1981) examined the efficacy of social skills training and applied relaxation in the treatment of adults with social phobia who were categorized as either 'behavioural' or 'physiological' responders. Physiological responders benefited most clearly from the applied relaxation training, whereas behavioural responders showed the most benefit from the social skills program. It should be noted, though, that not all studies with individualized treatments have produced such positive results. For example, Schulte et al. (1992) found that standardized treatment, contrary to expectations, proved more successful than either matched or mismatched treatments in an investigation of adults with agoraphobia. Mersch et al. (1989) also failed to demonstrate the value of categorizing adults with social phobia into those with primarily cognitive or behavioural deficiencies and assigning them to matched or mismatched treatments. Matched treatments were not found to be superior to mismatched ones.

In the child arena, Eisen and Silverman (1993, 1998) provided preliminary support for the value of prescriptive matching in the treatment of fearful and anxious children. In the first study, the efficacy of cognitive therapy, relaxation training, and their combination was examined with four overanxious children, 6–15 years of age, using a multiple baseline design across subjects. The children received both relaxation training and cognitive therapy (counterbalanced), followed by a combined treatment that incorporated elements of both treatments. Results suggested that interventions were most effective when they matched the specific problems of the children. That is, children with primary symptoms of worry responded more favourably to cognitive therapy, whereas children with primary symptoms of somatic complaints responded best to relaxation treatment. Similar findings were obtained in the second study (Eisen & Silverman, 1998) with four children between 8 and 12 years of age who were diagnosed with overanxious disorder. The interventions that were prescribed on the basis of a match between the treatment and the response class (cognitive therapy for cognitive symptoms, relaxation therapy for somatic symptoms) produced the greatest changes and resulted in enhanced treatment effectiveness. These findings must be considered preliminary because of limitations associated with single case designs; to our knowledge, no controlled group design studies have been conducted examining these issues. Nonetheless, these studies and those conducted with adults show yet another possible way of individualizing treatment and exploring flexibility in the use of empirically supported treatment manuals.

In a related vein, Chorpita et al. (2004) demonstrated the successful application of a 'modular' intervention for childhood anxiety that allowed for systematic adaptation of the protocol to client characteristics. The modular approach involved defining each practice technique as an independent module that could be integrated with other techniques through a flowchart that served to guide module selection. In that investigation, seven youth with anxiety disorders were successfully treated using a multiple baseline design. Data on patterns of use indicated that the protocol administration was highly individualized. For example, although all children participated in techniques such as psychoeducation, exposure, and maintenance exercises, only 29% participated in differential reinforcement strategies and 43% participated in formal cognitive exercises. Moreover, 29% received only the four core components of the manual (self-monitoring, psychoeducation, exposure, and maintenance). The sessions delivered ranged from 5 to 17, and occurred in durations ranging from 7 to 30 weeks (Chorpita et al., 2004). Thus, treatment was highly individualized and found to be effective.

One final comment on manualization seems important. Recently, some have reminded us that manuals are only a part of defining the proper treatment operations.

For example, Henggeler and Schoenwald (2002) argued that practitioner behaviour needs to be examined within a social ecological framework: 'Practitioners are embedded in quality assurance systems (e.g., manuals, supervision), which are embedded within organizations, which are embedded within community contexts' (p. 419). These authors demonstrate that the successful implementation of an intervention requires all of these dimensions to work in combination. Thus, although a manual can be defined as the specific treatment operations, the proper implementation of these operations is not guaranteed simply because a manual is present.

If the spirit of the manual requirement is accepted (i.e., it is important to assure proper implementation), then perhaps the specification of these other dimensions bears additional consideration as well. For example, one could detail the supervision protocol used for many of the current evidence-based treatments, as each manual was surely tested within a richly supported supervision model relative to community-based usual care. The requirement that the manual only details the clinical operations and not the supervision or quality assurance operations might falsely imply the primacy of the treatment over its delivery context. We know of no research demonstrating that treatment alone (or supervision alone) universally accounts for successful clinical outcomes.

Issues with efficacy and effectiveness: the transportability of treatments

The third major concern about the empirically supported or evidence-based treatment movement is embedded in the difference between *efficacy* studies and *effectiveness* studies (Hibbs, 1998; Hoagwood et al., 1995; Ollendick, 1999). Efficacy studies demonstrate that the benefits obtained from a treatment administered in a fairly standard way (with a treatment manual) are due to the treatment and not due to chance factors or other factors that threaten the internal validity of the demonstration of efficacy. These studies are conducted under tightly controlled conditions, typically in laboratory or university settings. Most of these studies consist of RCTs and clearly specify the sample characteristics in accordance with the definition of 'good' experimental designs. In recent years, concern has been raised about the exportability of these 'laboratory-based' treatments to the real world of clinical practice. Some argue that the 'subjects' in randomized clinical trials do not represent real-life 'clients' or that the 'experimenters' in these trials do not represent 'clinical therapists' in practice settings. Moreover, it has been argued that the settings themselves are significantly different, ranging from tightly controlled laboratory conditions to ill-defined and highly variable conditions in practice settings. Weisz et al. (1995a) have referred to practice settings as the 'real test' or the 'proving ground' of interventions. This distinction reminds us of the importance of building a strong bridge between science and practice, a bridge recommended over 50 years ago in the Boulder model of clinical training. Building this bridge is admittedly not easy, and a gap between efficacy and effectiveness studies remains.

Nonetheless, it is clear that effectiveness studies that demonstrate the external validity of psychotherapies are very important; moreover, they need to be conducted in a way that allows us to conclude that the treatments are responsible for the changes observed in our clients, not chance or other extraneous factors. In this search for effectiveness, it will be important to emphasize both internal and external validity, as both should be viewed as equally important (Ollendick & King, 2000). Of course, not all treatments shown to be efficacious in clinical trials research will necessarily be shown to be effective in clinical settings. Reasons for such failure may include problems in implementing the treatment procedures in less-controlled clinical settings and the 'acceptability' of the efficacious treatments to clients and therapists in those settings. In the final analysis, whether the effects found in RCTs and conducted in research-based settings generalize to 'real-world' clinical settings is an empirical question that awaits additional research (see Kendall & Southam-Gerow (1995) and Persons & Silberschatz (1998) for further discussion of these issues).

The issues surrounding transportability and efficacy versus effectiveness studies are numerous (e.g., training of therapists, supervision of therapists, homogeneous/heterogeneous samples, development of manuals, adherence to manuals, competence in executing manual-based treatment, and the acceptability of manual-based treatments to clinicians and clients, among others). Weisz et al. (1998) have identified a set of characteristics associated with child psychotherapy outcome research that distinguishes efficacy from effectiveness research. Weisz et al. characterize 'research' therapy as serving a relatively homogeneous group of children who exhibit less severe forms of child psychopathology and who present with single-focus problems. Moreover, they suggest that such studies are conducted in research laboratories or school settings with clinicians who are 'really' researchers, who are carefully trained and supervised, and who have 'light' client loads. Finally, such studies typically use manualized treatments of a behavioural or cognitive–behavioural nature. In contrast, 'clinic' therapy is characterized by heterogeneous groups of children who are frequently referred for treatment and who have a large and diverse range of clinical problems. Treatment in such settings is delivered in a clinic, school, or hospital setting by 'real' therapists who have 'heavy' caseloads, little pre-therapy training, and who are not carefully supervised or monitored. Finally, treatment manuals are rarely used and the primary form of treatment is non-behavioural.

Clearly, a number of differences are evident. Although such distinctions are important, they also tend to be broad generalizations that may or may not be true for various studies conducted in laboratory *or* clinical settings. Moreover, they may serve to accentuate differences in types of studies rather than to define areas of rapprochement and, inadvertently, create a chasm, rather than a bridge, between laboratory and clinic research. We shall illustrate how these distinctions become blurred by describing three studies: (a) a 'research' therapy study conducted by Kendall et al. (1997), (b) a 'clinic' therapy study conducted by Weiss et al. (1999), and (c) a study examining the transportability of effective treatment into a practice setting (Tynan et al., 1999).

In the Kendall et al. (1997) study, the efficacy of a cognitive–behavioural treatment for anxious children was compared to a wait-list condition. Efficacy of treatment was determined at post-treatment and at 1-year follow-up. Using a RCT, the researchers developed a detailed but flexible manual, and the therapists were well-trained and supervised graduate clinicians who carried 'light' clinical loads. Treatment was conducted in a university-based clinic. Ninety-four children (aged 9–13 years) and their parents referred from multiple community sources (not volunteers or normal children in school settings) participated in the study. All participants received primary anxiety disorder diagnoses (attesting to the relative severity of their problems), and the majority were co-morbid with other disorders (affirming multiple problems in these children, including other anxiety disorders, affective disorders, and disruptive behaviour disorders). In short, a relatively heterogeneous sample of children with anxiety disorders was treated. Treatment was found to be highly effective both at post-treatment and 1-year follow-up. It is evident that this study utilized some of the characteristics associated with 'research' therapy but also some of the characteristics of 'clinic' therapy.

In the Weiss et al. (1999) study previously described, treatment as routinely practiced in an outpatient setting (a school setting) was evaluated by comparing it to an attention control placebo (academic tutoring). The seven therapists were hired through standard clinic practices (six were masters' level clinicians and one was a doctoral level clinical psychologist) and were allowed to select and use whatever interventions they believed were necessary (most selected and used psychodynamic–humanistic or cognitive strategies). No manuals were used. They received no additional clinical training as part of the clinical trial and were provided with a minimal amount of supervision. One hundred and sixty children were randomly assigned to one of the two 'experimental' conditions. Children were identified in the school setting and presented with problems of anxiety, depression, aggression, and inattention. Diagnostic data were not obtained; however, the identified children were thought to represent a heterogeneous sample of children with multiple and serious problems. As noted earlier, traditional therapy, as implemented in this study, was determined to be largely ineffective. It is evident that only some of the characteristics of 'clinic' therapy were applicable to this study and at least some of the characteristics of 'research' therapy were examined.

Finally, in the study undertaken by Tynan et al. (1999), the transportability of a well-established treatment for oppositional defiant disorder and ADHD in children between 5 and 11 years of age (behavioural parent management training and child social skills training) was examined in a 'real-life' clinical setting (a child psychiatry outpatient clinic). Therapy was conducted in a group format. All children who were referred for ADHD or oppositional defiant disorder were assigned to the groups as the first line of treatment. Parents and children were treated in separate groups. Diagnostic interviews determined that most children met diagnostic criteria for disruptive behaviour disorders and a majority was co-morbid with other disorders. Problems were judged by the clinicians to be serious. Treatment was manualized and therapists in this clinical setting were carefully trained and supervised by the primary author. No control condition was used and no follow-up data were reported. Nonetheless, the treatment was reported to be highly efficacious at post-treatment (effect size of 0.89 from pre-treatment to post-treatment). Although several methodological problems exist with this 'uncontrolled' clinical trial, it nicely illustrates the potential to extend findings from laboratory settings to clinical settings. This study also illustrates characteristics of 'research' therapy and 'clinic' therapy. To which is it more similar? These three studies illustrate that demarcations between efficacy and effectiveness studies are not always clear. Perhaps more importantly, they illustrate the types of studies that need to be conducted that will bridge the gap between research and clinic settings.

Recently, Chorpita (2003) has noted that the efficacy–effectiveness distinction involves at least four different levels of consideration. With true efficacy research, the point is to determine the relation between therapeutic practices or strategies and outcomes (e.g., Chambless & Hollon, 1998; Chambless & Ollendick, 2001). With such research, 'upstream' elements are typically controlled (i.e., children and families are carefully screened and selected, therapists are highly trained, and supervision is intensive and often provided by a national expert). Under conditions that maximize these upstream elements, we have considerable confidence that fidelity to a particular protocol matched to a certain problem is related to positive results.

The second type of research, which would be considered effectiveness research by many and has been termed 'transportability research' by Schoenwald and Hoagwood (2001), speaks of whether a particular intervention might be promising for delivery in a true clinical practice setting. Essentially, transportability research allows for inferences about the performance of a protocol under a wider range of client conditions that closely approximate client conditions in a practice setting, but at the same time still maximizing therapist and supervisor performance in a contrived laboratory setting. This approach would allow us to say, for example, that 'interpersonal psychotherapy is a promising approach for real world cases of depression in youth.'

A third type of approach to be considered involves the use of system employees (e.g., school counsellors, private practitioners) as therapists. Schoenwald and Hoagwood (2001) termed this approach 'dissemination' research, in that it relates to the performance of a protocol once deployed into a system. This research is likely what is most commonly implied when one encounters the term 'effectiveness', and it allows for inferences about the performance of the intervention under highly naturalistic conditions (e.g., Henggeler et al., 1998). Nevertheless, in such research the supervision is still provided by the investigator team, and thus questions remain about whether the same practice standards would be maintained after the investigator team withdrew from the system.

The final question regarding system independence can only be addressed directly by 'system evaluation' research, in which the system to be evaluated and the investigative team are fully independent. This strategy would allow the final inference to be made: whether treatment operations can lead to positive outcomes when a system stands entirely on its own. Although studies of entire systems exist (Bickman, 1996; Bickman et al., 2000; Burns et al., 1996), they do not truly represent evidence-based system evaluation research, because they have not used evidence-based interventions in one of the experimental conditions, but rather have compared different arrangements of 'treatments as usual'. Consequently, the outcomes of these studies primarily show differences in practice patterns (e.g., access to system, dropout rates) but are unsupportive with respect to differential outcomes at the level of the child (Bickman, 1999).

This absence of favourable child outcomes noted earlier in treatment as usual practices such as the Fort Bragg Demonstration and other similar investigations is perhaps due to the fact that such 'systems' studies have not controlled and specified the 'downstream' elements involving specific therapeutic practices. Thus, there is no guarantee that strategies at the higher level (e.g., care coordination, quality assurance) will not be neutralized or compromised by poor strategies at the lower level (cf. Weisz et al., 1997). Ultimately, the understanding of what works in system contexts awaits not only new research, but new paradigms of research, in which treatments and systems are simultaneously manipulated.

Conclusions

We have discussed salient issues associated with empirically supported treatments and concluded that some treatments are more effective than others, that manualization need not be a stumbling block to providing effective therapy in both research and clinic settings, and that the transportability of treatments from the laboratory setting to the practice setting is feasible (although still being tested). We have also noted that tensions remain about each of these issues, and we have illustrated various avenues of possible rapprochement.

Somewhat unexpectedly, however, our present review of empirically supported psychosocial treatments reveals that our armamentarium is relatively 'light' and that much more work remains to be done. We really do not have very many psychosocial treatments that possess well-established status in research settings let alone clinical settings; however, this is an exciting time as we continue to develop interventions to close the gap between laboratory and clinic practice. Adolescents and their families presenting at our clinics deserve our concerted attention to further the true synthesis of these approaches and to transform our laboratory findings into rich and clinically sensitive practices.

Although subsequent chapters will examine the empirical support of treatments for adolescent depression, we would like to conclude our chapter with a brief discussion of potential avenues for future studies in the treatment of adolescent depression. As noted earlier in this chapter, we now know that specific treatments work better for children and adolescents with specific behavioural, emotional, and social problems. Although studies to date suggest that factors that may moderate treatment outcome (e.g., comorbidity) may not be as important as originally thought, additional empirical evidence is needed before concluding that moderators such as comorbidity are not important in treatment outcome studies (Ollendick et al., 2008).

In the area of adolescent depression research, cognitive–behavioural therapy and interpersonal psychotherapy have been shown to be largely effective in the treatment of adolescent depression, qualifying as probably efficacious interventions. At the same time, a number of questions remain in determining which treatment works best for whom. One promising avenue for future research in adolescent depression treatment outcome research is an examination of the mediators and moderators of treatment outcome (Weersing et al., 2009). Another promising line of research involves the use of longitudinal designs—designs that will be particularly important in capturing the effects of treatment that may appear later in time. The recently completed multi-site Treatment of Adolescent Depression Study (TADS) illustrates the value of both moderational research and longitudinal studies. TADS has allowed for the first large-scale evaluation of cognitive–behavioural, medication (fluoxetine), and combined treatments for adolescent depression. Although studies conducted immediately following treatment pointed to the probable benefits of pharmacological and combined treatments over cognitive–behavioural ones for adolescent depression, recent analyses have shown that cognitive–behavioural therapy alone fared better at 36 week follow-up than either pharmacological or combined treatments at these longer follow-up intervals (J. Curry, Personal communication, July 20, 2007; Curry et al., 2006; TADS, 2004). Future studies will be needed to better understand the moderators and mediators of treatment outcome as well the role of time in capturing both short-term and long-term treatment effects. Promising results are being detected at this time.

References

Acierno, R., Hersen, M., Van Hasselt, V.B., & Ammerman, R.T. (1994). Remedying the Achilles heel of behavior research and therapy: Prescriptive matching of intervention and psychopathology. *Journal of Behavior Therapy and Experimental Psychiatry, 25,* 179–188.

Barlow, D.H., Gorman, J.M., Shear, M.K., & Woods, S.W. (2000). Cognitive–behavioral therapy, imipramine, or their combination for panic disorder: A randomized controlled trial. *Journal of the American Medical Association, 283,* 2529–2536.

Beck, A.T., Rush, A.J., Shaw, B.F., & Emery, G. (1979). *Cognitive therapy of depression.* New York: Guilford.

Bickman, L. (1996). A continuum of care: More is not always better. *American Psychologist, 51,* 689–701.

Bickman, L. (1999). Practice makes perfect and other myths about mental health services. *American Psychologist, 54,* 965–977.

Bickman, L., Guthrie, P.R., Foster, E.M., Lambert, E.W., Summerfelt, W.T., Breda, C.S. et al. (1995). *Evaluating managed mental health services: The Fort Bragg experiment.* New York: Plenum Press.

Bickman, L., Lambert, E.W., Andrade, A.R., & Penaloza, R.V. (2000). The Fort Bragg continuum of care for children and adolescents: Mental health outcomes over 5 years. *Journal of Consulting and Clinical Psychology, 68,* 710–716.

Brestan, E.V. & Eyberg, S. M. (1998). Effective psychosocial treatments of conduct-disordered children and adolescents: 29 years, 82 studies, and 5,272 kids. *Journal of Clinical Child Psychology, 27,* 179–188.

Burns, B.J., Farmer, E.M.Z., Angold, A., Costello, E.J., & Behar, L. (1996). A randomized trial of case management for youths with serious emotional disturbance. *Journal of Clinical Child Psychology, 25,* 476–486.

Canter, M.B., Bennett, B.E., Jones, S.E., & Nagy, T.F. (1994). *Ethics for psychologists: A commentary on the APA ethics code.* Washington, DC: American Psychological Association.

Casey, R.J. & Berman, J.S. (1985). The outcome of psychotherapy with children. *Psychological Bulletin, 98,* 388–400.

Chambless, D.L. (1996). In defense of dissemination of empirically supported psychological interventions. *Clinical Psychology: Science and Practice, 3,* 230–235.

Chambless, D.L. & Hollon, S.D. (1998). Defining empirically supported therapies. *Journal of Consulting and Clinical Psychology, 66,* 7–18.

Chambless, D.L. & Ollendick, T.H. (2001). Empirically supported psychological interventions: Controversies and evidence. *Annual Review of Psychology, 52,* 685–716.

Chorpita, B.F. (2003). The frontier of evidence-based practice. In A. E. Kazdin & J. R. Weisz (Eds.), *Evidence-based psychotherapies for children and adolescents* (pp. 42–59). New York: Oxford.

Chorpita, B.F., Daleiden, E.L., & Weisz, J.R. (2005). Identifying and selecting the common elements of evidence based interventions: A distillation and matching model. *Mental Health Services Research, 7,* 5–20.

Chorpita, B.F. & Donkervoet, C.M. (2005). Implementation of the Felix Consent Decree in Hawaii: The impact of policy and practice development efforts on service delivery. In R.G. Steele &

M.C. Roberts (Eds.), *Handbook of mental health services for children, adolescents, and families* (pp. 317–332). New York: Kluwer.

Chorpita, B.F., Taylor, A.A., Francis, S.E., Moffitt, C.E., & Austin, A.A. (2004). Efficacy of modular cognitive behavior therapy for childhood anxiety disorders. *Behavior Therapy, 35,* 263–287.

Craighead, W.E. & Craighead, L.W. (1998). Manual-based treatments: Suggestions for improving their clinical utility and acceptability. *Clinical Psychology: Science and Practice, 5,* 403–407.

Curry, J., Rohde, P., Simons, A., Silva, S., Vitiello, B., Kratochvil, C., et al. (2006). Predictors and moderators of acute outcome in the treatment for adolescents with depression study (TADS). *Journal of the American Academy of Child and Adolescent Psychiatry, 45,* 1427–1439.

Daleiden, E. (2004). Child status measurement: System performance improvements during Fiscal Years 2002–2004. Honolulu, HI: Hawaii Department of Health Child and Adolescent Mental Health Division. Available via Internet at http://www.hawaii.gov/health/ mentalhealth/camhd/resources/rpteval/ge/library/pdf/er-ge/ge010.pdf

Daleiden, E.L. & Chorpita, B.F. (2005). From data to wisdom: Quality improvement strategies supporting large-scale implementation of evidence based services. *Child and Adolescent Psychiatric Clinics of North America, 14,* 329–349.

Durlak, J.A., Wells, A.M., Cotton, J.K., & Johnson, S. (1995). Analysis of selected methodological issues in child psychotherapy research. *Journal of Clinical Child Psychology, 24,* 141–148.

Eiffert, G.H., Schulte, D., Zvolensky, M.J., Lejuez, C.W., & Lau, A.W. (1998). Manualized behavior therapy: Merits and challenges. *Behavior Therapy, 28,* 499–509.

Eisen, A.R. & Silverman, W.K. (1993). Should I relax or change my thoughts? A preliminary examination of cognitive therapy, relaxation training, and their combination with overanxious children. *Journal of Cognitive Psychotherapy: An International Quarterly, 7,* 265–279.

Eisen, A.R. & Silverman, W.K. (1998). Prescriptive treatment for generalized anxiety disorder in children. *Behavior Therapy, 29,* 105–121.

Eysenck, H.J. (1952). The effects of psychotherapy: An evaluation. *Journal of Consulting Psychology, 16,* 319–324.

Goldfried, M.R., & Wolfe, B.E. (1996). Psychotherapy practice and research: Repairing a strained alliance. *American Psychologist, 51,* 1007–1016.

Hayes, S.C., Barlow, D.H., & Nelson-Gray, R.O. (1999). *The scientist practitioner: Research and accountability in the age of managed care (2nd Ed.).* Boston: Allyn and Bacon.

Heimberg, R.G. (1998). Manual-based treatment: An essential ingredient of clinical practice in the 21st century. *Clinical Psychology: Science and Practice, 5,* 387–390.

Henggeler, S.W. & Schoenwald, S.K. (2002). Treatment manuals: Necessary, but far from sufficient. *Clinical Psychology: Science and Practice, 9,* 419–420.

Henggeler, S.W., Schoenwald, S.K., Borduin, C.M., Rowland, M.D., & Cunningham, P.B. (1998). *Multisystemic treatment of antisocial behavior in children.* New York: Guilford Press.

Hibbs, E.D. (1998). Improving methodologies for the treatment of child and adolescent disorders. *Journal of Abnormal Child Psychology, 26,* 1–6.

Hoagwood, K., Hibbs, E., Brent, D., & Jensen, P. (1995). Introduction to the special section: Efficacy and effectiveness in studies of child and adolescent psychotherapy. *Journal of Consulting and Clinical Psychology, 63,* 683–687.

Jacobson, N.S., Schmaling, K.B., Holtzworth-Munroe, A., Katt, J.L., Wood, L.F., & Follette, V.M. (1989). Research-structured vs. clinically flexible versions of social learning-based marital therapy. *Behavior Research and Therapy, 27,* 173–180.

Kaslow, N.J. & Thompson, M.P. (1998). Applying the criteria for empirically supported treatments to studies of psychosocial interventions for child and adolescent depression. *Journal of Clinical Child Psychology, 27*, 146–155.

Kazdin, A.E. (1998). *Research design in clinical psychology* (3rd Ed.). Boston: Allyn & Bacon.

Kazdin, A.E. (2000). Developing a research agenda for child and adolescent psychotherapy. *Archives of General Psychiatry, 57*, 829–836.

Kazdin, A.E., Bass, D., Ayers, W.A., & Rodgers, A. (1990). Empirical and clinical focus of child and adolescent psychotherapy research. *Journal of Consulting and Clinical Psychology, 58*, 729–740.

Kendall, P.C. (1998). Directing misperceptions: Researching the issues facing manual-based treatments. *Clinical Psychology: Science and Practice, 5*, 396–399.

Kendall, P.C. (2002). *Coping Cat Therapist Manual.* Ardmore, PA: Workbook Publishing.

Kendall, P.C. & Chu, B.C. (2000). Retrospective self-reports of therapist flexibility in a manual-based treatment for youths with anxiety disorders. *Journal of Clinical Child Psychology, 29*, 209–220.

Kendall, P.C., Chu, B., Gifford, A., Hayes, C., & Nauta, M. (1998). Breathing life into a manual: Flexibility and creativity with manual-based treatments. *Cognitive and Behavioral Practice, 5*, 177–198.

Kendall, P.C., Flannery-Schroeder, E., Panichelli-Mindel, S.M., Southam-Gerow, M., Henin, A., & Warman, M. (1997). Therapy for youths with anxiety disorders: A second randomized clinical trial. *Journal of Consulting and clinical Psychology, 65*, 366–380.

Kendall, P.C., Flannery-Schroeder, E., & Ford, J.D. (1999). Therapy outcome research methods. In P.C. Kendall, J.N. Butcher, & G.N. Holmbeck (Eds.), *Handbook of research methods in clinical psychology* (2nd ed., pp. 330–363). New York: John Wiley & Sons, Inc.

Kendall, P.C., Kane, M., Howard, B., & Siqueland, L. (1990). *Cognitive–behavioral treatment of anxious children: Treatment manual.* Ardmore, PA: Workbook Publishing.

Kendall, P.C. & Southam-Gerow, M.A. (1995). Issues in the transportability of treatment: The case of anxiety disorders in youth. *Journal of Consulting and Clinical Psychology, 63*, 702–708.

Kiesler, D.J. (1966). Some myths of psychotherapy research and the search for a paradigm. *Psychological Bulletin, 65*, 110–136.

King, N.J., & Ollendick, T.H. (1998). Empirically validated treatments in clinical psychology. *Australian Psychologist, 33*, 89–95.

Klerman, G. L., Weissman, M. M., Rounsaville, B. J., & Chevron, E. (1984). *Interpersonal psychotherapy of depression.* New York: Academic Press.

Kinscherff, R. (1999). Empirically supported treatments: What to do until the data arrive (or now that they have)? *Clinical Child Psychology Newsletter, 14*, 4–6.

Lambert, M.J. (1998). Manual-based treatment and clinical practice: Hangman of life or promising development? *Clinical Psychology: Science and Practice, 5*, 391–395.

Lambert, M.J. & Ogles, B.M. (1988). Treatment manuals: Problems and promise. *Journal of Integrative and Eclectic Psychotherapy, 7*, 187–204.

Levitt, E.E. (1957). The results of psychotherapy with children: An evaluation. *Journal of Consulting and Clinical Psychology, 21*, 189–196.

Levitt, E.E. (1963). Psychotherapy with children: A further evaluation. *Behavior Research and Therapy, 60*, 326–329.

Lilienfeld, S.O. (2007). Psychological treatments that cause harm. *Perspectives on Psychological Science, 2,* 53–70.

Luborsky, L. & DuRubeis, R. (1984). The use of psychotherapy treatment manuals: A small revolution in psychotherapy research style. *Clinical Psychology Review, 4*, 5–14.

Mattis, S.G. & Ollendick, T.H. (2002). *Panic disorder and anxiety in adolescence*. Oxford: BPS Blackwell.

Mersch, P.P.A., Emmelkamp, P.M.G., Bogels, S.M., & van der Sleen, J. (1989). Social phobia: Individual response patterns and the effects of behavioral and cognitive interventions. *Behavior Research and Therapy, 27*, 421–434.

Mufson, L., Moreau, D., Weissman, M.M., Wickramaratne, P., Martin, J., & Samoilov, A. (1994). Modification of interpersonal psychotherapy with depressed adolescents (IPT-A): Phase I and II studies. *Journal of the American Academy of Child and Adolescent Psychiatry, 33*, 695–705.

Mufson, L. Weissman, M.M., Moreau, D., & Garfinkel, R. (1999). Efficacy of interpersonal psychotherapy for depressed adolescents. *Archives of General Psychiatry, 56*, 573–579.

Nelson-Gray, R.O., Herbert, J.D., Herbert, D.L., Sigmon, S.T., & Brannon, S.E. (1990). Effectiveness of matched, mismatched, and package treatments of depression. *Journal of Behavior Therapy and Experimental Psychiatry, 20*, 281–294.

Ollendick, T.H. (1995a). Cognitive-behavior treatment of panic disorder with agoraphobia in adolescents: A multiple baseline analysis. *Behavior Therapy, 26*, 517–531.

Ollendick, T.H. (1995b). AABT and empirically validated treatments. *The Behavior Therapist, 18*, 81–82.

Ollendick, T.H. (1999). Empirically supported treatments: Promises and pitfalls. *The Clinical Psychologist, 52*, 1–3.

Ollendick, T.H. & Davis, T.E., III. (2004). Empirically supported treatments for children and adolescents: Where to from here? *Clinical Psychology: Science and Practice, 11*, 289–294.

Ollendick, T.H. & Hersen, M. (1984). *Child behavioral assessment: Principles and procedures*. New York: Pergamon Press.

Ollendick, T.H., Jarrett, M.A., Grills-Taquechel, A.E., Hovey, L.D., & Wolff, J. (2008). Comorbidity as a predictor and moderator of treatment outcome in youth with anxiety, affective, AD/HD, and oppositional/conduct disorders. *Clinical Psychology Review, 28*, 1447–1471.

Ollendick, T.H. & King, N.J. (1998). Empirically supported treatments for children with phobic and anxiety disorders: Current status. *Journal of Clinical Child Psychology, 27*, 156–167.

Ollendick, T.H. & King, N.J. (2000). Empirically supported treatments for children and adolescents. In P.C. Kendall (Ed.), *Child and adolescent therapy: Cognitive behavioral procedures* (2nd Ed., pp. 386–425). New York: Guilford Publications.

Ollendick, T.H. & King, N.J. (2004). Empirically supported treatments for children and adolescents: Advances toward evidence-based practice. In P.M. Barrett & T.H. Ollendick (Eds.), *Handbook of interventions that work with children and adolescents: Prevention and treatment* (pp. 1–26). Chichester: John Wiley & Sons, Ltd.

Ollendick, T.H., King, N.J., & Chorpita, B.F. (2006). Empirically supported treatments for children and adolescents. In P.C. Kendall (Ed.), *Child and adolescent therapy: Cognitive–behavioral procedures* (3rd ed., pp. 492–520). New York: Guilford Press.

Ost, L.G., Jerremalm, A., & Johansson, J. (1981). Individual response patterns and the effects of different behavioral methods in the treatment of claustrophobia. *Behavior Research and Therapy, 20*, 445–560.

Patterson, G.R. & Gullion, M.E. (1968). *Living with children: New methods for parents and teachers*. Champaign, IL: Research Press.

Persons, J.B. (1998). Paean to data. *The Behavior Therapist, 21*, 123.

Persons, J.B., & Silberschatz, G. (1998). Are results of randomized controlled trials useful to psychotherapists? *Journal of Consulting and Clinical Psychology, 66*, 126–135.

Rossello, J. & Bernal, G. (1999). The efficacy of cognitive–behavioral and interpersonal treatments for depression in Puerto Rican adolescents. *Journal of Consulting and Clinical Psychology, 67*, 734–745.

Sackett, D., Richardson, W., Rosenberg, W., & Haynes, B. (1997). *Evidence-based medicine.* London: Churchill Livingston.

Sackett, D., Richardson, W., Rosenberg, W., & Haynes, B. (2000). *Evidence-based medicine* (2nd Ed.). London: Churchill Livingston.

Schoenwald, S.K. & Hoagwood, K. (2001). Effectiveness, transportability, and dissemination of interventions: What matters when? *Psychiatric Services, 52*, 1190–1197.

Schulte, D., Kunzel, R., Pepping, G., & Schulte-Bahrenberg, T. (1992). Tailor-made versus standardized therapy of phobic patients. *Advances in Behavior Research and Therapy, 14*, 67–92.

Seligman, M.E.P. (1995). The effectiveness of psychotherapy. *American Psychologist, 50*, 965–974.

Seligman, L.D., Goza, A.B., & Ollendick, T.H. (2004). Treatment of depression in children and adolescents. In P.M. Barrett & T.H. Ollendick (Eds.), *Handbook of interventions that work with children and adolescents* (pp. 301–328). Chicester, UK: Wiley.

Silverman, W.H. (1996). Cookbooks, manuals, and paint-by-numbers: Psychotherapy in the 90s. *Psychotherapy, 33*, 207–215.

Smith, E.W.L. (1995). A passionate, rational response to the 'manualization' of psychotherapy. *Psychotherapy Bulletin, 30*, 36–40.

Strosahl, K. (1998). The dissemination of manual-based psychotherapies in managed care: Promises, problems, and prospects. *Clinical Psychology: Science and Practice, 5*, 382–386.

Strupp, H.H., & Anderson, T. (1997). On the limitations of therapy manuals. *Clinical Psychology: Science and Practice, 4*, 76–82.

Strupp, H.H., & Binder, J.L. (1984). *Psychotherapy in a new key: A guide to time-limited dynamic psychotherapy.* New York: Basic Books.

Task Force on Promotion and Dissemination (1995). Training in and dissemination of empirically validated treatments. Report and recommendations. *The Clinical Psychologist, 48*, 3 23.

Treatment for Adolescents with Depression Study (TADS) Team (2004). Fluoxetine, cognitive-behavior therapy, and their combination for adolescents with depression. *Journal of the American Medical Association, 292*, 807–820.

Tynan, W.D., Schuman, W., & Lampert, N. (1999). Concurrent parent and child therapy groups for externalizing disorders: From the laboratory to the world of managed care. *Cognitive and Behavioral Practice, 6*, 3–9.

Weersing, V.R., Rozenamn, M., & Gonzalez, A. (2009). Core components of therapy in youth: Do we know what to disseminate? *Behavior Modification, 33*, 24–47.

Weersing, V.R., & Weisz, J.R. (2002). Community clinic treatment of depressed youth: Benchmarking usual care against CBT clinical trials. *Journal of Consulting and Clinical Psychology, 70*, 299–310.

Weiss, B., Catron, T., Harris, V., & Phung, T.M. (1999). The effectiveness of traditional child psychotherapy. *Journal of Consulting and Clinical Psychology, 67*, 82–94.

Weisz, J.R., Donenberg, G.R., Han, S.S., & Weiss, B. (1995a). Bridging the gap between laboratory and clinic in child and adolescent psychotherapy. *Journal of Consulting and Clinical Psychology, 63*, 688–701.

Weisz, J.R., Han, S.S., & Valeri, S.M. (1997). More of what? Issues raised by the Fort Bragg Study. *American Psychologist, 52*, 541–545.

Weisz, J.R., Huey, S.J., & Weersing, V.R. (1998). Psychotherapy outcome research with children and adolescents: The state of the art. In T.H. Ollendick & R.J. Prinz (Eds.), *Advances in Clinical Child Psychology* (Vol. 20, pp. 49–91). New York: Plenum Publishing.

Weisz, J.R., Weiss, B., Alicke, M.D., & Klotz, M.L. (1987). Effectiveness of psychotherapy with children and adolescents: A meta-analysis for clinicians. *Journal of Consulting and Clinical Psychology, 55*, 542–549.

Weisz, J.R., Weiss, B., Han, S.S., Granger, D.G., & Morton, T. (1995b). Effects of psychotherapy with children and adolescents revisited: A meta-analysis of treatment outcome studies. *Psychological Bulletin, 117*, 450–468.

Westen, D., Novotny, C.M., & Thompson-Brenner, H. (2004). The empirical status of empirically supported psychotherapies: Assumptions, findings, and reporting in controlled clinical trials. *Psychological Bulletin, 130*, 631–663.

Wilson, G.T. (1996a). Manual-based treatments: The clinical application of research findings. *Behavior Research and Therapy, 34*, 295–314.

Wilson, G.T. (1996b). Empirically validated treatments: Reality and resistance. *Clinical Psychology: Science and Practice, 3*, 241–244.

Wilson, G.T. (1998). Manual-based treatment and clinical practice. *Clinical Psychology: Science and Practice, 5*, 363–375.

Zvolensky, M.J. & Eiffert, G.H. (1998). Standardized treatments: Potential ethical issues for behavior therapists? *The Behavior Therapist, 21*, 1–3.

Zvolensky, M.J. & Eiffert, G.H. (1999). Potential ethical issues revisited: A reply to Persons. *The Behavior Therapist, 22*, 40.

Part 2

Cognitive–behavioral therapy

Chapter 4

Challenges in school-based, universal approaches to the prevention of depression in adolescents

Susan H. Spence

Concern about depression in young people has resulted in a recent surge in interest in the development of programs to prevent the onset of this disorder. The majority of such interventions draw upon treatment methods such as cognitive–behaviour therapy or interpersonal psychotherapy, based on the assumption that approaches that have been shown to be effective in treating depression will also be effective in preventing its onset. Most preventive interventions for depression recognize the role of adverse life events at home or school, such as parental conflict, separation or divorce, parental mental health problems, illness, unemployment, bullying by peers, or academic failure, in the aetiology of the disorder. However, rather than attempting to change the environment in which the young person lives, preventive approaches have focussed on enhancing individual skills that are thought to produce resilience against the negative effects of adverse life situations. Similarly, while most approaches recognize the importance of a biological or genetic predisposition to the development of mental health problems, there has been little attempt to directly modify such characteristics. Rather, most approaches to prevention of depression assume that enhancing individual cognitive and behavioural skills, such as social skills, coping skills, self-regulation, optimistic and adaptive cognitive style, and problem solving skills, will influence the development of depression, either through a direct association or by reducing the adverse effects of a biological predisposition or negative life events upon depression (Abramson et al., 1999; Clarke et al., 1999; Lewinsohn et al., 1990; Stark et al., 1991; Vostanis & Harrington, 1994).

Two broad approaches to prevention of psychological disorders have been developed; the first involving universal intervention, delivered to children in general, usually in a school setting, and the second taking a targeted approach with those at increased risk of developing the disorder because they have been exposed to some risk factor or because they already show elevated, but non-clinical signs of depression. For example, young people selected for targeted depression prevention programs have included those with a parent with an affective disorder, with a pessimistic cognitive style, and/or having experienced abuse, family conflict, parental divorce, or death of a parent. There are relative advantages and disadvantages of universal versus targeted approaches (Offord et al., 1998). The proponents of universal interventions note the advantage of avoiding potential labelling effects associated with being selected as being 'at-risk'. Also, they suggest that by reaching a broad range of children, it is possible to help those with a wide spectrum of risk-factors, rather than being limited to those with specific characteristics. The universal prevention model assumes that the intervention will produce a small effect on risk and protective factors across a large number of individuals in a population, thereby preventing a significant number of clinical cases from developing (Rose, 1992).

In contrast, targeted programs usually involve individual, family, or small group interventions, with a focus on the specific issues facing that group of young people. Supporters of targeted approaches suggest that universal approaches waste a good deal of effort (and therefore money) by working with the majority of children who are not at risk of developing the disorder. They suggest that targeted approaches enable a higher 'dosage' and greater capacity to focus on the specific needs of individual children than is possible with universal prevention.

This chapter focuses specifically upon universal approaches to prevention of depression, the majority of which have been conducted in schools. It examines the evidence relating to the outcomes of school-based universal prevention for depression, explores the issues involved in implementation of such interventions, and discusses the types of approaches that we might need to consider in order to make a more significant impact in the prevention of this disorder.

Outcome studies

There have now been several randomized controlled trials that have investigated the effects of school-based, universal programs for the prevention of depression among adolescents. The majority has focussed on teenagers in the 12–15 year age group. Generally, the results have been disappointing and the methodological designs of most studies have been weak (Merry et al., 2004a; Spence & Shortt, 2007). Of the published, randomized controlled trials that compared intervention with no-intervention, several failed to find significant effects upon depression either in the short-term or at follow-up (Bond et al., 2004; Cardemil et al., 2002; Clarke et al., 1993; Gillham et al., 2007; Pattison & Lynd Stevenson, 2001; Sheffield et al., 2006). Of those studies that reported positive effects upon depression immediately after intervention (Cardemil et al., 2002; Chaplin et al., 2006; Pössel et al., 2004; Spence et al., 2003), the benefits were not maintained in one study (Spence et al., 2003) and Chaplin et al. (2006) did not conduct a follow-up. Only two studies (Cardemil et al., 2002; Pössel et al., 2004) found effects at post-intervention that were also maintained at follow-up (6 months and 3 months respectively). Interestingly, Gillham et al. (2007) reported positive effects upon the prevention of depressive symptoms in two of their three schools over a three-year follow-up. Quayle et al. (2001) found no benefits immediately after intervention, but significant effects upon depression at 6 month follow-up. Of those that compared preventive intervention with a placebo, one failed to find a significant benefit for intervention (Pattison & Lynd Stevenson, 2001), one reported a very small positive effect (Merry et al., 2004b) and one found intervention to reduce depression symptoms to a significantly greater extent than placebo in two schools, but placebo to be superior to intervention in the third school (Gillham et al., 2007).

There have also been several studies that used quasi experimental, rather than randomized controlled designs, again with mixed results. For example, Shochet et al. (2001), using a cohort design, reported positive effects for a school-based universal intervention compared to no intervention for one of two measures of depression. However, the same intervention was not found to produce significant changes in a subsequent evaluation (Harnett & Dadds, 2004).

Taken together, the evidence suggests that we should proceed with caution. Spence and Shortt (2007) concluded that there is, as yet, insufficient evidence regarding efficacy and effectiveness to justify the widespread dissemination of universal, school-based interventions for the prevention of depression in children and adolescents. We also need to be mindful of the methodological limitations of most of the outcome studies in this area, such as inadequate sample sizes, reliance on self-report data, absence of diagnostic interview data and 'blind' evaluation, and insufficient long-term follow-up. Furthermore, most studies failed to report data regarding program attendance and compliance by students and failed to conduct fidelity checks of implementation by teachers/clinicians. Participation and retention rates were also poor in most studies, raising issues about generalization of findings to real world situations.

The *beyondblue* schools research initiative

In response to the relatively weak results from universal approaches to the prevention of depression in young people, the *beyondblue* schools research initiative was established to develop, implement, and evaluate a multi-component school-based intervention that aimed to overcome the perceived weaknesses of previous interventions. In contrast to previous interventions, the program involved a 3-year period including a classroom-based curriculum, a whole school climate change component, and pathways system that aimed to increase mental health literacy, help-seeking, and access to help and support.

The content of the intervention was driven by a conceptual framework that emphasized the importance of factors within the individual and their environment that provided resilience against the impact of adverse life and stressful events (Garmezy, 1991; Rutter, 1987). Although the importance of biological and temperament factors in the development of depression is acknowledged, the study focussed upon building protective factors within the individual (e.g., optimistic thinking style, coping and interpersonal skills, and help seeking behaviour), and the school environment (e.g., positive peer and teacher relationships, safety, student participation, and access to professional help). The intervention consisted of four main strategies, including (i) building individual protective skills through a classroom program, (ii) building a supportive school environment, (iii) building pathways to support and professional assistance, and (iv) enhancing community involvement with the school. The program materials are available from the *beyondblue* website http://www.beyondblue.org.au/index.aspx?link_id=4.64.

Building individual protective skills: The classroom program

To enhance individual protective skills, a 3-year curriculum was developed that was delivered by teachers on a whole-class basis. It focused on teaching those cognitive and behavioural skills that have been proposed in the literature to reduce the risk of depression. Each year for 3 years, the students participated in 10 classes of 30–45 min duration, over one school term, starting in year 8 when the students were 11–13 years old. The curriculum was implemented by teachers, using small-group exercises, discussions, role-plays, deep-learning tasks, quizzes, and videotaped examples and dramatized stories to illustrate target skills. Each year, teachers completed a 1-day training session prior to implementation. In developing the content of the curriculum, we aimed to ensure that

- The skills taught had high face validity (acceptable and relevant) to staff and students
- The content, materials and teaching methods were developmentally appropriate
- Skills were taught in a hierarchical manner, ensuring that skills are well established before moving on to the next skill
- There were opportunities to practice skills in class, with guidelines for practice between sessions, in a variety of different, real-world contexts
- Tasks were designed that provided students with feedback from their practice attempts, and that high probability of leading to successful outcomes
- Role-plays were tailored to include real-life cues to increase the chance that skills would be used in real situations
- Examples and videotaped demonstrations illustrated use of skills by models with whom the students could identify
- The content was respectful of differences in culture, gender, sexuality, abilities, and life circumstances of the students.

The curriculum, outlined in Table 4.1, focused on 8 key domains, including emotional literacy and regulation, stress reduction, social skills, life problem solving skills, cognitive skills (to enhance rational and constructive thinking styles), building social supports and connectedness, participation in pleasant events, and awareness of mental health literacy and help-seeking.

Building a supportive school environment

The Supportive Environment component of the program involved a whole-school change approach that aimed to enhance safety, promote positive social relationships between and within students and staff, and encourage students to participate in the social, recreational, sporting, and decision-making aspects of school life. Together, these elements aimed to enhance students' sense of connectedness and belonging in school. Each school established a *school action team*, consisting of between 3–9 school staff (such as guidance officers, school counsellors, deputy principals or principals, pastors, year coordinators, or heads of departments) and a member of the research team (*the facilitator*). Each school action team took part in 2 days of training relating to the goals and strategies of the supportive environments program.

Table 4.1 Cognitive and behavioural skills taught within the curriculum

Domain	Target skills
1. Emotional literacy and regulation	Recognizing emotions in self and others distinguishing thoughts and feelings; Recognizing link between thoughts and feelings; Managing negative emotions; Increasing positive mood.
2. Stress reduction and emotional regulation	Identifying stress and the physical, emotional, psychological, and behavioural responses to stress; Techniques for managing stress to cope with challenging situations—relaxation, thought challenging, self-soothing; Time management and planning skills; Coping applied to relationship issues.
3. Social skills	Developing and maintaining relationships—conversation and listening skills; Assertive skills and negotiation; Conflict resolution skills; Perspective taking skills;
4. Life problem solving skills	Identifying challenging situations; Positive problem orientation; Steps and skills of interpersonal problem solving; Predicting consequences, evaluating options, selecting responses.
5. Cognitive skills—building rational and constructive thinking styles	Links between thoughts and feelings; Role of self-talk; Self-reflection; Identifying automatic thoughts; Challenging automatic thoughts and unhelpful beliefs; Realistic thinking and realistic expectations; Enhancing the six senses—positive sense of self/world/future/belonging/control/meaning; Importance of sense of humour; Setting goals.
6. Building social supports and connectedness	Identifying sources of support and social connections; Types of relationships, types of support; The value of relationships and value of belonging (family, friends, sporting groups, cultures); Building support networks; Evaluating the usefulness of sources of support.
7. Participation in pleasant events	Importance of participation in pleasant activities, laughter, and humour; Identifying personal pleasant events; Programming for pleasant events.
8. Awareness of mental health issues and help seeking	Awareness of concept of resiliency; Understanding health and well-being (including emotional well-being); Knowing how and when to access help for mental health issues; Skills to identify and access available health resources and services within school and community; Skills for seeking help for self and others; Evaluating the usefulness of sources of support.

The action team began by conducting an audit of the school's current structures, policies, programs, and practices relating to the promotion of student well-being, which were then compared with a set of principles of effective practice. The Action Team was also provided with information from student surveys (summarized and de-identified) relating to student perceptions of social support, participation, level and types of victimization, acceptance and belonging, and help seeking behaviour. De-identified summary data was also provided regarding staff perceptions of the school climate. Taken together, the information allowed the Action Team to identify the school's strengths and weaknesses relating to promotion of student emotional well-being. Each school team then developed an *action plan* for whole-school change. This plan specified the goals, objectives, strategies, required resources, timeframe, and person responsible for each planned action. Actions were developed for the classroom level, the whole school, and for school-community linkages. A resource book was developed that provided guidelines regarding whole-school change approaches to enhancing promotion of student emotional well-being, participation, and student support.

The supportive environment intervention took place over 3 years during which time the facilitator met with the school action team monthly, supported by weekly telephone contact. The Action teams reviewed progress in implementation and outcomes of their action plans at 6-month and annual intervals. Seminars were held at which Action Teams from different schools met to review progress and share information about activities. The exact content of the action plans varied according to the identified needs of each school, with some examples being illustrated in Table 4.2.

Building pathways to support and professional assistance

Large-scale mental health surveys of young people have shown that the majority does not receive any form of professional help for problems of depression (Sawyer et al., 2000). This may reflect a lack of knowledge on the part of teenagers and their families, friends, and teachers about the symptoms of depression and where to go to get help. It could also reflect fears of stigma associated with seeking help for a mental health problem. Given the long-term adverse consequences of depression referred to earlier in this chapter, there is a strong case for early identification and treatment of young people who do develop depression. The Pathways component of the *beyondblue* schools research initiative aims to facilitate young people's access to support and professional services both at school and within the community. It also attempts to increase the capacity of school staff to identify students who are in need of help and to increase their knowledge about the type and sources of help. Each school identifies a network of connections for appropriate pathways for help and builds partnerships between families, school staff, students, education support/welfare personnel, and community-based health professionals.

As part of the Pathways component, school staff and students are provided with resources that outline information about mental health issues, help and support services, and methods of referral. These resources include leaflets, posters, CD rom, and web-site material relevant to the local area. All school staffs attend a half-day training session to discuss their roles and responsibilities in relation to mental health

Table 4.2 Examples of whole-school change strategies to build supportive environments

---

Increasing opportunities to build positive relationships
- Increasing group and team work within class
- Using 'home-class' teachers and a 'home-group' structure
- Reducing the number of teachers working with each class
- Structuring the physical environment to encourage interaction and communication between students and teachers (e.g., set up of tables/desks)
- Reviewing curriculum to increase opportunities for interaction and communication
- Staff professional development activities in communication skills and classroom management
- Mentoring/coaching/buddy programs (within and across age groups)
- Peer mediation/peer support programs
- Enhancing activities of 'house' groups

Increasing student safety and reducing conflict
- Increasing the use of positive behaviour management approaches (use of praise, attention, rewards), rather than punitive.
- Creating a constructive, encouraging, and participative classroom environment
- Increasing supervision at free time periods, particularly in high-risk areas
- Establishing confidential reporting systems for dealing with bullying
- Developing and publicizing school policies and practices regarding bullying in line with international best practice

Increase recognition and rewards
- Active recognition of student efforts and achievements and showcasing student work and successes
- Encouraging and recognizing successes relative to each individual's abilities with opportunities for all students to succeed at their own level
- Providing feedback (re: academic and behavioural performance) in a constructive rather than critical manner

Increasing opportunities for student and family participation in school
- Inviting student input to planning of class activities
- Involving students in the development of classroom policies and practices to enhance safety, confidentiality, respect, and communication
- Enhancing parent and community participation in school activities, including decision making
- Increasing opportunities to participate in school activities and decision making through student councils and student representatives
- Enhancing communication content in school newsletters
- Actively seeking feedback from parents and caregivers (surveys and focus groups)
- Creating a welcoming atmosphere for parents and visitors to the school

Increasing Mental Health Literacy and Facilitating Help Seeking
- Increasing the number of student counselling and support staff
- Establishing a school mental health charter that recognizes and respects the needs and rights of students and teachers
- Training all staff in awareness of mental health issues
- Establishing confidential systems to facilitate student help-seeking behaviours
- Increasing information about support services within the school and the wider community staff, and creating easy access pathways

promotion, prevention and early intervention, and referral processes. In addition, students contribute to the development of the school's resource materials, as an activity within the curriculum (outlined above). As part of the Pathways component teachers and students in all schools work together to develop a mental health charter that emphasizes the vision, purpose, values/principles, rights, responsibilities, actions, and roles of all school members in relation to mental health of the school community. Schools also develop interagency protocols for ensuring students, staff, and families can access the education, health, and other community services in a timely manner.

Enhancing community involvement in the school

The fourth and final element of the intervention involved the implementation of a *Community Forum* towards the end of the first year, or early in the second year. The forums were designed to increase mental health literacy about depression and to reduce the stigma associated with mental health problems within the school and local community. Each forum provided information about the nature and prevalence of mental health issues among school students, risk, and protective factors, and help seeking strategies for students, family members, and friends. The events were held as joint initiatives between each school and its local community, and involved students, teachers, parents, service providers, and community organizations (such as Rotary and sporting clubs). They took various forms and were generally organized around themes, such as musical, dance, or drama productions, with students playing a significant role in planning the content.

Outcomes

The outcomes of the intervention are being assessed over a 5-year period, to determine the longer term impact, and it is expected that effects will be strongest in the final two years after the whole-school change process has had time to be fully implemented. The evaluation examines not only mental health outcomes (in terms of depression, anxiety and emotional well-being), but it also assesses the impact of the intervention upon the skills and competencies that it aims to develop. Thus, it examines the impact upon social skills, problem solving and coping skills, cognitive style, and interpersonal relationships. In addition, it explores whether the intervention is associated with changes in school environment factors, such as quality of supportive relationships, levels of bullying and safety, opportunities for participation, and sense of belonging from the perspectives of both students and staff. The evaluation compares outcomes for 25 intervention schools with 25 matched comparison schools that were initially randomized to either intervention or control conditions. Students and staff provide annual assessments over the 3 years of the intervention, and for the two subsequent years until the students leave school.

The preliminary results for the first 3 years of implementation were reported by Sawyer et al. (2007) and raise issues about whether the intervention will indeed be effective in producing a preventive effect upon depression. The results over this 3-year period revealed no significant differences between intervention and control groups on indicators of depression, anxiety, emotional well-being, or conduct problems. Furthermore, there were no significant differences between intervention and control groups on the mediating factors that were targeted in the program, such as problem solving, optimistic thinking, social relationships, social skills, and students' sense of belonging and participation in school.

Although it is still feasible that positive effects will become evident over the further two-year follow-up period, we need to consider why the intervention did not produce significant benefits over the first 3 years. The implementation of the 3-year curriculum would have been expected to at least produce some preventive effects upon depressive symptoms.

Is it premature to conclude the universal approaches to prevention of depression are ineffective?

We need to consider possible reasons for what appear to be relatively poor outcomes from universal, school-based interventions that are designed to prevent the development of depression. One possibility is that the universal approaches that have been used so far are based on incorrect assumptions and that no matter how well we implement them we will not prevent the development of depression. An alternative explanation is that the assumptions behind the interventions are correct but researchers have not implemented them well enough to produce significant effects on depression; thus, more careful implementation could produce the desired results. A third possibility is that the interventions were actually effective in preventing the development of depression, but methodological designs were flawed and were not sufficiently strong to detect the positive effects. Each of these possibilities needs to be explored.

Possibility 1. The approach is correct but the implementation is inadequate

One of the key questions relates to the degree to which the interventions have been implemented in the manner intended. In the *beyondblue* schools project, the classroom program was implemented by teachers after 2-days of training. We need to consider whether teachers administered the program correctly, in line with the protocols. Ideally, we should have used independent observers to assess quality of implementation, but we did not have the resources to do this and rely on teachers' own recordings of session implementation. It may be possible to use these data to determine whether preventive effects are evident for schools in which teachers implemented the program with greater fidelity. Similarly, we have collected data regarding that quality of implementation of the supportive environments and pathways elements of the intervention and it will be possible over the next two years to determine whether this factor is associated with future levels of depression among the students. One of the major challenges for prevention programs in the real world is to ensure high levels of fidelity of implementation. This becomes increasingly difficult with large scale studies, and those implemented by teachers rather than research project staff, as the project team has less control over the implementation process.

A further question relates to the degree to which the teaching staff in the *beyondblue* study had the skills and knowledge to implement a CBT-based curriculum effectively. Although the curriculum materials were highly structured, and teachers attended two days of training, it is possible that a greater level of expertise in CBT is required.

This issue requires further investigation in future studies, but the limited research to date does not suggest that effects are greater when preventive interventions are implemented by clinicians rather than teachers (Shatté, 1996).

A further factor that we need to consider relates to the degree to which students paid attention and participated in the classroom activities. We do not have a measure of attendance and student compliance in the program, but future research should consider these issues.

Possibility 2: The research designs have been inadequate

There are several methodological issues that could explain the failure to find positive outcomes. First, in most studies students are only able to take part in the evaluation if they and their parents have given written, informed consent. For example, in the *beyondblue* study, informed consent was limited to 63% of grade 8 students and it may be that there is something different about these students compared to those who did not return consent forms. Perhaps those most at risk, and who may have benefited most from the program, were not included in the evaluation. Similarly, over the years of the study 20% of students dropped out of the evaluation, and again it is possible that students who are most likely to benefit from the intervention may be those who leave the school or who are not contactable. Potential sample bias associated with consent and drop-out rates is a common issue in this type of research. Inadequacy in the psychometric properties of the measures used to assess depression, in terms of internal consistency and test-retest reliability, is a further issue that needs to be considered. It is possible that unreliability in questionnaires and diagnostic interviews may reduce the capacity to detect significant changes in depressive symptoms.

Possibility 3: The approach is not valid

There are many questions that arise in relation to the validity of universal, school-based approaches to prevention of depression. For example, is it valid to assume that we can produce changes in 'at risk' individuals using a universal approach, or is a more intensive, individually tailored intervention required? Are we tackling the correct risk and protective factors? Is an approach based on enhancing cognitive–behavioural skills appropriate and sufficient, even when combined with a supportive school environment? What is the best age to intervene? Is it too late to intervene in adolescence?

There is very little evidence that universal preventive programs for depression are effective in changing mediating or moderating factors, such as thinking style or coping skills. If the variables that are targeted by the intervention are not changing, then it is not surprising that minimal effects are found upon depression. A genuine test of whether it is possible to prevent depression by changing mediating or moderating factors requires that we can demonstrate that we are able to change those variables effectively. Evidence from treatment outcome studies of CBT for depression suggests that it is indeed possible to produce changes in social–cognitive and coping skills and that these changes are associated with reductions in depression (Oei et al., 2006). However, it is unclear whether it is reasonable to expect similar changes to occur in a universal sample where most individuals do not exhibit deficits in the targeted skills. It is also possible that the strength of universal interventions may not be sufficient to produce lasting improvements in cognitive and coping skills in those with significant deficits in these areas. Those with significant skills deficit may require more intensive, small group experiences, implemented by highly trained mental health professionals.

A further question that arises is whether it is feasible in a universal intervention to tackle all of the many different risk and protective factors associated with depression. There are a myriad of factors that influence children's risk of developing depression and each of these explains only a very small percent of variance (Kovacs, 2006). In any given classroom there will be a proportion of young people who are at elevated risk of developing depression, but the nature of these factors will vary considerably across individuals. For some the risk may reflect family circumstances, such as living with a parent with a mental illness, parental conflict, separation or divorce, unemployment, poor parenting practices, abuse, or neglect. For others the risk may relate to a biological or genetic predisposition, or to individual psychosocial characteristics, such as poor capacity in problem solving, social skills or emotional regulation, lack of social support, or relationship difficulties (including being bullied). Indeed, for some young people, the risk may relate to a complex interplay between various combinations and permutations of these environmental and individual risk factors. Programs that aim to enhance cognitive and behavioural skills, and to build a supportive school environment, may simply be insufficient to protect young people against the impact of such a complex matrix of risk factors. Also, rather than attempting to build protective factors, perhaps it is necessary to tackle the risk factors directly, where this is feasible. For example, effective interventions to enhance the quality of couple relationships to prevent marital breakup and couple conflict could be one way in which a risk factor for depression could be significantly reduced in the community. Similarly, positive parenting programs to optimize the quality of parenting practices could also reduce the prevalence of some key risk factors for depression.

Unfortunately, it is likely that families with the most risk factors will be those least likely to take part in couple relationship or parenting programs, meaning that there will always be a proportion of young people who are exposed to adverse family environments. Similarly, there will continue to be children who experience the death of a parent or close family member, significant illness, or trauma. Thus, we need an integrated approach that not only tackles risk factors at their source, but also includes interventions to enhance individual resiliency and build supportive social environments. Furthermore, there will continue to be a proportion of children for whom these preventive approaches are insufficient and for whom early detection and early referral for treatment is required.

Another possible criticism of current school-based approaches is that intervention is typically occurring too late in the trajectory towards the development of depression, and that effective prevention needs to commence in early childhood (Avenevoli & Merikangas, 2006). Such strategies could include home visiting programs, parent preparation classes, and teaching of social and problem-solving skills at kindergarten level (Spivack et al., 1976). In contrast, proponents of prevention in later adolescence suggest that, given limited resources, it is preferable to intervene just prior to the peak increase in the rate of onset of depression from ages 15 to 20 years (Fleming & Offord, 1990; Kessler et al., 2001). The age at which preventive interventions for depression are best targeted is debatable and currently we do not have evidence from which we can draw firm conclusions.

Summary and conclusions

At first sight, the results of school-based, universal approaches to prevention of depression seem rather discouraging. However, it would be premature to draw conclusions about their effectiveness or lack thereof. Given the strong case for prevention of depression, it is important that researchers and practitioners continue to seek to develop and evaluate new approaches. To produce significant and lasting effects in depression prevention, we may need to take a lifespan approach, and one that takes into account the wide range of individual and environmental factors that influence depression. We need a better understanding of causal variables and factors that influence trajectories in the development of depression at different ages (Garber, 2006; Kovacs, 2006). This information will inform the development of preventive interventions that take a lifespan approach, with different interventions being applicable at different ages, including adulthood. It must also be recognized that effective prevention of *all* new cases of depression is highly unlikely. Prevention therefore needs to be integrated within a multilevel framework involving universal and targeted interventions, plus early identification and intervention, and pathways to evidence-based treatment services for those who develop depressive disorders despite our best efforts.

One of the major challenges in depression prevention research will be the transition from small, highly controlled efficacy trials to the implementation of real-world, large-scale interventions. Even if we can identify a range of interventions that can produce small effects in highly controlled situations, it may be difficult to produce significant preventive effects in real-world contexts, where it is hard to ensure fidelity of implementation. Prevention of depression in the real world will require us to develop interventions that are not only effective in preventing depression, but are also sustainable. Sustainability requires that the intervention is relatively easy to implement with high fidelity, by staff without extensive training, at low cost, and that can be integrated into existing services and systems within the community. Clearly, we have a major challenge ahead.

References

Abramson, L.Y., Alloy, L., Hogan, M.E., Whitehouse, W.G., Donovan, W.G., Rose, D.T., et al. (1999). Cognitive vulnerability to depression: Theory and evidence. *Journal of Cognitive Psychotherapy, 13*, 5–20.

Avenevoli, S. & Merikangas, K.R. (2006). Implications of high-risk family studies for prevention of depression. *American Journal of Preventive Medicine, 31(6, Suppl 1)*, S126–S135.

Bond, L., Patton, G., Glover, S., Carlin, J.B., Butler, H., Thomas, L., et al. (2004). The Gatehouse Project: Can a multilevel school intervention affect emotional well-being and health risk behaviours? 10.1136/jech.2003.009449. *J Epidemiol Community Health, 58(12)*, 997–1003.

Cardemil, E.V., Reivich, K.J., & Seligman, M.E.P. (2002). The prevention of depressive symptoms in low-income minority middle school students. *Prevention and Treatment, 5, Article 8*, Retreived 15 August, 2000 http://www.journals.apa.org/prevention/volume2005/pre005500008a.html.

Chaplin, T.M., Gillham, J.E., Reivich, K., Elkon, A.G., Samuels, B., Freres, D.R., et al. (2006). Depression prevention for early adolescent girls: A pilot study of all girls versus co-ed groups. *Journal of Early Adolescence, 26(1)*, 110–126.

Clarke, G.N., Hawkins, W., Murphy, M., & Sheeber, L. (1993). School-based primary prevention of depressive symptomatology in adolescents: Findings from two studies. *Journal of Adolescent Research, 8(2)*, 183–204.

Clarke, G.N., Rohde, P., Lewinsohn, P.M., Hops, H., & Seeley, J.R. (1999). Efficacy of acute group treatment and booster sessions. *Journal of the American Academy of Child and Adolescent Psychiatry, 38(3)*, 272–279.

Fleming, J.E., & Offord, D.R. (1990). Epidemiology of childhood depressive disorders: A critical review. *Journal of the American Academy of Child and Adolescent Psychiatry, 29(4)*, 571–580.

Garber, J. (2006). Depression in children and adolescents: Linking risk research and prevention. *American Journal of Preventive Medicine, 31(6, Suppl 1)*, S104–S125.

Garmezy, N. (1991). Resiliency and vulnerability to adverse developmental outcomes associated with poverty. *American Behavioral Sciences, 34*, 416–430.

Gillham, J.E., Reivich, K.J., Freres, D.R., Chaplin, T.M., Shatte, A.J., Samuels, B., et al. (2007). School-based prevention of depressive symptoms: A randomized controlled study of the effectiveness and specificity of the penn resiliency program. *Journal of Consulting and Clinical Psychology, 75(1)*, 9–19.

Harnett, P.H., & Dadds, M.R. (2004). Training school personnel to implement a universal school-based prevention of depression program under real-world conditions. *Journal of School Psychology, 42(5)*, 343–357.

Kessler, R.C., Avenevoli, S., & Merikangas, K.R. (2001). Mood disorders in children and adolescents: An epidemiologic perspective. *Biological Psychiatry, 49(12)*, 1002–1014.

Kovacs, M. (2006). Next steps for research on child and adolescent depression prevention. *American Journal of Preventive Medicine, 31(6, Suppl 1)*, S184–S185.

Lewinsohn, P.M., Clarke, G.N., Hops, H., & Andrews, J.A. (1990). Cognitive–behavioral treatment for depressed adolescents. *Behavior Therapy, 21(4)*, 385–401.

Merry, S., McDowell, H., Hetrick, S., Bir, J., & Muller, N. (2004a). Psychological and/or educational interventions for the prevention of depression in children and adolescents (Cochrane Review). In *The Cochrane Library* (Vol. Issue 2). Chichester, UK: John Wiley & Sons, Ltd.

Merry, S., McDowell, H., Wild, C.J., Bir, J., & Cunliffe, R. (2004b). A randomized placebo-controlled trial of a school-based depression prevention program. *Journal of the American Academy of Child & Adolescent Psychiatry, 43(5)*, 538–547.

Oei, T.P.S., Bullbeck, K., & Campbell, J.M. (2006). Cognitive change process during group cognitive behaviour therapy for depression. *Journal of Affective Disorders, 92(2–3)*, 231–241.

Offord, D.R., Kraemer, H.C., Kazdin, A.-E., Jensen, P.S., & Harrington, R. (1998). Lowering the burden of suffering from child psychiatric disorder: Trade-offs among clinical, targeted, anduniversal interventions. *Journal of the American Academy of Child and Adolescent Psychiatry, 37(7)*, 686–694.

Pattison, C., & Lynd Stevenson, R.M. (2001). The prevention of depressive symptoms in children: The immediate and long-term outcomes of a school based program. *Behaviour Change, 18(2)*, 92–102.

Pössel, P., Horn, A.B., Groen, G., & Hautzinger, M. (2004). School-based prevention of depressive symptoms in adolescents: A 6-month follow-up. *Journal of the American Academy of Child & Adolescent Psychiatry, 43(8)*, 1003–1010.

Quayle, D., Dziurawiec, S., Roberts, C., Kane, R., & Ebsworthy, G. (2001). The effect of an optimism and lifeskills program on depressive symptoms in preadolescence. *Behavior Change, 18(4)*, 194–203.

Rose, G. (1992). *The strategy of preventative medicine.* Oxford: Oxford University Press.

Rutter, M. (1987). Psychosocial resilience and protective mechanisms. *American Journal of Orthopsychiatry, 57*, 316–331.

Sawyer, M.G., Arney, F.M., Baghurst, P.A., Clark, J.J., Graetz, B.W., Kosky, R.J., et al. (2000). *The Mental Health of Young People in Australia.* Canberra: Commonwealth Department of Health and Aged Care.

Shatté, A.J. (1996). *Prevention of depressive symptoms in adolescents: Issues of dissemination and mechanisms of change.* Unpublished PhD Thesis, University of Pennsylvania, Philadelphia.

Sheffield, J.K., Spence, S.H., Rapee, R.M., Kowalenko, N., Wignall, A., Davis, A., et al. (2006). Evaluation of universal, indicated, and combined cognitive–behavioral approaches to the prevention of depression among adolescents. *Journal of Consulting & Clinical Psychology, 74(1)*, 66–79.

Shochet, I.M., Dadds, M.R., Holland, D., Whitefield, K., Harnett, P.H., & Osgarby, S.M. (2001). The efficacy of a universal school-based program to prevent adolescent depression. *Journal of Clinical Child Psychology, 30(3)*, 303–315.

Spence, S.H., Sheffield, J.K., & Donovan, C.L. (2003). Preventing adolescent depression: An evaluation of the Problem Solving For Life program. *Journal of Consulting and Clinical Psychology, 71(1)*, 3–13.

Spence, S.H. & Shortt, A.L. (2007). Can we justify the widespread dissemination of universal, school-based interventions for the prevention of depression among children and adolescents? *Journal of Child Psychology and Psychiatry, 48(6)*, 526–542.

Spivack, G., Platt, J.J., & Shure, M.B. (1976). *The problem solving approach to adjustment.* San Francisco: Jossey Bass.

Stark, K.D., Rouse, L.W., & Livingston, R. (1991). Treatment of depression during childhood and adolescence: Cognitive–behavioural procedures for the individual and family. In P.C. Kendal (Ed.), *Child and adolescent therapy: Cognitive–behavioural procedures* (pp. 165–208). New York: Guilford Press.

Vostanis, P. & Harrington, R. (1994). Cognitive–behavioural treatment of depressive disorder in child psychiatric patients: Rationale and description of a treatment package. *European Child and Adolescent Psychiatry, 3(2)*, 111–123.

Chapter 5

Primary and secondary control enhancement training (PASCET): Applying the deployment-focused model of treatment development and testing

Sarah Kate Bearman & John R. Weisz

Over the past 5 decades, numerous treatment protocols have been developed to address youth mental health disorders; some estimates suggest that over 500 different named therapies are practiced with children and adolescents (Kazdin, 2002). Although quite a few of these protocols have been subjected to and supported by rigorous exam- ination—in the form of randomized clinical trials (RCTs)—the great majority are not a part of everyday practice in service settings, and thus not available to most treated youth. Moreover, for many of these protocols, we lack the evidence needed to assess their readiness for use in practice settings. To address this state of affairs, a deploy- ment-focused model (DFM) of treatment development and testing has been proposed (Weisz, 2004). In this paper, we describe the model and illustrate its application by focusing on the development of a specific program for youth depression, PASCET.

The PASCET (Primary and Secondary Control Enhancement Training) program for the treatment of child and adolescent depression is a cognitive–behavioural proto- col that has been under study for a decade. Because the research has followed the DFM, it provides an illustration of the prospects, and the challenges, of applying the model. In this chapter, we will provide an overview of youth depression, a description of the DFM, and an examination of PASCET's development within this context together with a summary of the evidence on its utility for the treatment of youth depression.

Youth depression is a major public health concern

A number of pivotal social, developmental, and emotional transitions occur as individuals progress through childhood and adolescence. Although most youth navi- gate these challenges successfully, a substantial literature suggests that many youngsters experience depressed mood and other symptoms of depressive disorders during these life phases. *Major depressive disorder* involves one or more episodes in which at least five depressive symptoms have been present for at least two weeks. One of these five must be either an increase in depressed or irritable mood, or greatly diminished interest or pleasure, known as *anhedonia*. The other symptoms may include significant changes in weight (loss or gain), sleep (insomnia or hypersomnia), or psychomotor activity (slowing or agitation), or increased fatigue, increased feelings of worthlessness or guilt, decreases in concentration or decisiveness, or recurrent thoughts of death or suicidal thoughts or actions. A second relevant condition, *dysthymic disorder*, entails sad or irritable mood most of the day, for more days than not, for at least one year with no symptom remission of longer than one month, and the presence, while depressed, of at least two of the following: poor appetite or overeating, insomnia or hypersomnia, low energy or fatigue, low self-esteem, poor concentration or decisiveness, and feelings of hopelessness. Although once considered a diagnosis only applicable to adults, today we know that youth depression is a relatively common and tremendously impairing condition.

Youth depression is among the most prevalent and impairing paediatric conditions. With adolescence comes a marked increase in rates of depression (Angold & Costello, 2001, 2006). Indeed, rates of depression increase from a relatively low 3% among pre-pubertal children to 9% in children aged 12–16 years old (Fleming & Offord, 1990; Garrison et al., 1992; Kaltiala-Heino et al., 2001; Lewinsohn et al., 1993), and rates of both depressive symptoms (Ge et al., 2001, 1994) and onset of depression (Hankin & Abramson, 2001) continue to rise dramatically from ages 15 to 18 for adolescent girls and boys. By age 18, nearly a fourth of all youth will have experienced a depressive disorder, making this one of the most prevalent forms of youth dysfunction (Clarke et al., 1993; Lewinsohn et al., 1993; Zalsman et al., 2006).

Youth epidemiologic studies reveal 12-month prevalence rates for major depressive disorder (MDD) exceeding 6%, and 12-month prevalence rates for dysthymic disorder (DD) exceeding 10% (Angold & Rutter, 1992; Cohen et al., 1993; Fleming & Offord, 1990; Lewinsohn et al., 1993, 1998). Point prevalence of adolescent MDD alone is estimated at 3–8% (Birmaher et al.,1996; Costello et al., 2006; Lewinsohn et al., 1993; Zalsman et al., 2006), but combined prevalence of MDD and DD has been reported at 14% in schools (Pfeffer et al., 1984), 30–40% in outpatient mental health clinics (Jensen & Weisz, 2002; Schiffman et al., 2006), and 49% in an educational diagnostic clinic (Weinberg et al., 1973).

The precipitous rise of depression in youth, in concert with the global impairment associated with depressive disorders, constitutes a major public health concern. Depression in childhood and adolescence predicts low academic achievement and school failure, substance abuse and dependence, unemployment, and early parenthood (Fergusson & Woodward, 2002). It is associated with high rates of psychiatric comorbidity (Birmaher et al., 1996) and a 30-fold increased risk of completed suicide (Stolberg et al., 2002)—the third leading cause of death among adolescents (Arias et al., 2003). Even subdiagnostic depression during youth persists over time and predicts onset of psychiatric disorders, inpatient hospitalization, substance abuse, academic problems, impaired social functioning, and suicidal ideation (Capaldi & Stoolmiller, 1999; Gotlib et al., 1998; Nolen-Hoeksema et al., 1992). It is also associated with significant physical health consequences, adding to the public health burden (Keenan-Miller et al., 2007). Moreover, depression in youth may continue to impair functioning even after recovery (Kovacs & Golston, 1991; Puig-Antich et al., 1993), suggesting that interventions that thwart the development of depressive disorders during this crucial period of development are imperative.

Despite the ubiquity of depression, the vast majority of depressed youth will never receive treatment (Lewinsohn et al., 1993; Newman et al., 1996). Equally troubling, research suggests that the treatment benefits for those few youth who do receive treatment may be relatively modest and short-lived (Weersing & Weisz, 2002). It follows that two priorities for mental health professionals must therefore be to (a) focus on transporting effective treatments into community settings where the majority of depressed youth receive treatment and (b) test the effectiveness of these treatments in real-world practice settings to ensure that there are robust benefits for afflicted youth. Although a number of treatments have been developed in academic settings to address youth depression, their migration into typical service settings has progressed slowly, and has often been fraught with difficulty as treatments developed under 'ideal conditions' fare less well when variables such as client characteristics, therapist training and supervision, and treatment fidelity are under less stringent control (Weisz et al., 2006). Despite a number of well-tested interventions, most of the interventions studied have not actually made their way into routine use in clinical practice settings or become part of the usual standard of care for practitioners. Indeed, even mature evidence-based treatments that have undergone rather extensive efficacy testing have, for the most part, not been subjected to 'effectiveness tests'—i.e., trials testing the treatments as provided to naturally referred individuals treated by practitioners in the settings and under the conditions of everyday practice.

Need for a new approach to treatment development: The deployment-focused model

In response to the concerns raised by research suggesting that some evidence-based treatments are not yet ready for use in service settings, Weisz and colleagues have suggested a *deployment-focused model (DFM) of treatment development and testing* (Weisz, 2004). The model is guided by three primary aims: (1) developing treatments that can be blended into everyday practice and work well with referred individuals treated in typical settings (clinics, schools) by practicing clinicians (2) generating evidence on treatment outcome in actual clinical practice, with a focus on the outcomes that stakeholders most need in order to assess the likely utility of the treatments for their settings; and (3) producing a body of evidence on the nature, necessary and sufficient components, boundary conditions (i.e., moderators), and change/causal processes (i.e., mediators) associated with treatment impact that will have a high level of external validity because it is derived from research in the practice context. In short, this model seeks to ensure that tests in practice settings occur, and to produce treatments that are designed *from the start* to work well in those settings. The model entails six steps of treatment development and testing, as shown in Figure 5.1.

Step 1: Theoretically and clinically guided construction of the treatment protocol

The initial step is development, refinement, pilot testing, and manualizing of the treatment protocol. Theory and evidence on the nature and treatment of the target

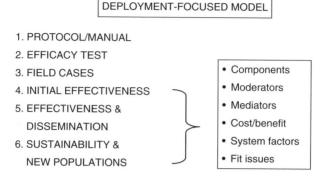

Figure 5.1 Steps in the deployment-focused model of treatment development and testing.

condition, the available clinical literature, and input from experienced clinicians are used to guide the design of treatment components. The goal is the production of a manual-guided treatment program that arises from both the theoretical and empirical literatures and that possesses a high level of adaptability across numerous clinical situations that are anticipated contexts for the intervention. The treatment protocol should grow out of a well-articulated model of the condition being treated, and of the hypothesized mechanism(s) by which change in that condition is brought about.

Step 2: Initial efficacy trial under controlled conditions, to establish potential for benefit

Next, an initial *efficacy* trial is used to assess whether the treatment (compared to a control group) can produce beneficial effects with youth treated under controlled laboratory conditions. The focus is the systematic study of symptomatic volunteers, not clinically referred cases, in order to avoid exposing severely disordered individuals to an untested intervention. Positive findings in this initial trial will provide evidence that the intervention has the potential to benefit the target population.

Step 3: Single-case applications in practice settings, with progressive adaptations to the protocol

Next, a series of single-case tests is conducted with referred individuals, treated within the kinds of service settings for which the treatment is ultimately intended. Ideally, the treatment is delivered by the practitioners who work within that service setting, and supervision is available both from a protocol supervisor (likely from the research team) who is expert in the treatment protocol to ensure faithfulness to the core treatment principles, plus a second supervisor who is an experienced clinic staff member—to monitor the appropriateness of the treatment for the family and the clinical setting. Importantly, modifications are made to the treatment protocol throughout the treatment to ensure goodness of fit, while also adhering to the model of change that guides the protocol. The process in Stage 3 guides decisions as to the *type* of manual best-suited to the clinical context, with choices ranging from highly structured, session-by-session instructions (see e.g., Clarke et al., 1990) to broad treatment principles with illustrations of how to apply them (see e.g., Henggeler et al., 1998).

Step 4: Initial effectiveness tests

The fourth step involves initial controlled effectiveness trials in which the treatment protocol—newly adapted to reflect the feedback from Step 3—is tested in a practice setting, with clinically referred youngsters who meet criteria for the target condition, and with treatment provided by practitioners who work in the setting. Outcomes for youths randomly assigned to the manualized treatment are compared to those randomized to receive the usual treatment procedures offered in the setting. Multiple effectiveness tests may be needed to permit investigators to move across steps of clinical representativeness (e.g., beginning with a focus on referred youths, then adding a focus on training practitioners to deliver the treatment, etc.). Comparison of the target intervention to usual care provides a test of whether the new intervention can improve upon the treatment youngsters would otherwise receive. More broadly, two paramount goals are represented in this effort to move from a series of individual cases and successive modifications in the protocol to more uniform applications of the protocol across clients and therapists. One goal is to provide initial evidence on whether introducing the target treatment improves outcomes relative to the interventions clients in the setting would have otherwise received. Another goal is to embark upon what is likely to be a lengthy journey of investigator education. That is, treatment developers will learn, as they attempt to complete a group-design treatment trial, a great deal about setting conditions, characteristics of referred youths and their families, therapist responses to training and supervision, and numerous other factors that need to be addressed in order to deploy the intervention effectively across groups of clinicians and youths in the practice context. Lessons learned in this process can inform the design of subsequent effectiveness tests.

Step 5: Tests of effectiveness, implementation, and transportability

In the next step, additional group-design effectiveness trials are carried out, with the target treatment provided to referred clients, in practice settings, by staff practitioners. As in Step 4, clients are randomly assigned to either the target treatment or usual care. Each of these tests builds on lessons learned in previous trials regarding ways to fit the treatment into the setting, ways to engage the kinds of clients who seek care there, ways to build therapist proficiency in the protocol, and ways to address a variety of problems that may arise with attempts to change current practices via dissemination of new procedures. The individual studies are intended to identify the most effective ways to implement the intervention within representative clinic practice conditions. The series of studies is intended to refine procedures for deploying the protocol to the point that it fits so well into the setting and works so well with referred clients that it can continue to be used effectively after the treatment researchers are gone. This brings us to Step 6.

Step 6: Tests of goodness-of-fit, benefit, and sustainability in practice contexts

The final step focuses on the fit of the treatment program to the practice context for which it is ultimately intended. The aim is to identify factors that predict (a) how likely it is that practitioners will use the treatment, (b) the level of treatment adherence demonstrated by those practitioners who do use the protocol, and (c) the degree to which use of the protocol improves youth outcomes. An overarching focus will be assessment of sustainability—i.e., continued use, with treatment integrity and youth outcomes maintained—over time in various practice settings.

Additional foci throughout Steps 4, 5, and 6: Components, moderators, mediators, cost-benefit, system factors, and fit issues

A great deal of additional learning can occur during Steps 4–6. As shown in Figure 5.1, a goal in these studies is to use variations in design and measurement to (a) ascertain the necessary and sufficient components of our complex treatment packages, (b) identify moderators of outcome that set boundaries around treatment impact, (c) assess whether proposed change processes in treatment do in fact mediate outcomes, (d) assess treatment costs in relation to benefits, (e) investigate which organizational factors in the systems and settings, where the treatments are used (e.g., community mental health clinics, inpatient psychiatric units, primary care clinics, schools, social service agencies), relate to how effectively the treatments are used, and (e) test variations in treatment procedures, packaging, training, and delivery designed to improve fit to various settings in which the treatment is deployed. The ultimate aim is to generate an assortment of information about the target treatment and the factors that enhance or mitigate its success.

PASCET as an exemplar of the deployment-focused model

The PASCET program for youth depression is an example of a treatment that has used the guidelines of the DFM from its inception and throughout its development and implementation. In the following section, the PASCET program will be described, and the corresponding DFM steps will be examined.

Step 1: Theoretically and clinically guided construction of the treatment protocol

Several major theories of depression posit that a perceived lack of control may be a root cause for the development of this disorder (Abramson et al., 1978; Bandura, 1977, 1986; Beck et al., 1979), potentially leading to feelings of helplessness, hopelessness, and low self-worth. The two-process model of control (Rothbaum et al., 1982;

Weisz et al., 1984) asserts that individuals pursue feelings of control via two distinct but complementary processes: Primary control consists of efforts to enhance reward or reduce negative consequences by attempting to modify objective conditions (e.g., one's grade in a class, or other people's opinions), in the service of making these conditions conform to one's wishes. Secondary control, on the other hand, consists of efforts to enhance reward or reduce negative consequences by attempting to modify oneself (e.g., one's hopes, expectations, or evaluation of an event) so as to achieve goodness-of-fit with the existing conditions. In short, primary control is an attempt to change the world to better suit one's needs, while secondary control is an attempt to change oneself to better suit the world.

The PASCET program evolved from the literature suggests that deficits in perceived control and coping were highly correlated with depression among children (Abramson et al., 1978; Weisz et al, 1993), and, in particular, from the theoretical two-process model of control described above (Rothbaum et al., 1982; Weisz et al., 1984). The PASCET program attempts to address youth depression by increasing depressed individuals' abilities to apply primary control strategies to distressing conditions that are modifiable, and to apply secondary control strategies to those conditions that are not easily altered. Most of the specific strategies included in the program were adapted from extant cognitive–behavioural treatments (Reynolds & Coats; 1986; Stark et al., 1987) and divided into 'ACT' skills (primary control) and 'THINK' skills (secondary control) aimed at bolstering perceptions of primary and secondary control (Table 5.1).

The inclusion of elements that have a solid foundation in cognitive–behavioural therapies in the development of PASCET is an attempt to respond to the evidence suggesting that these treatments may offer particularly robust effects for youth depression. A variety of CBT manuals and treatment programs exist and has been shown to reduce depressive symptoms among depressed youths (Clarke et al., 1999; Michael & Crowley, 2002; Lewinsohn et al., 1990; Reinecke et al., 1998), as well as for

Table 5.1 Coping skills emphasized in the PASCET program

ACT (Primary Control) SKILLS

- *Activities that solve problems*: Use systematic steps to find solutions to everyday problems.
- *Activities I enjoy*: Create a menu of pleasant activities and see how they change your mood!
- *Calming*: Learn and practice two methods of achieving relaxation and self-soothing.
- *Turn on my positive self*: Identify and practice showing a positive self to others!

THINK (Secondary Control) SKILLS

- *Think positive*: Identify and challenge thoughts that are unrealistically negative.
- *Help from a friend*: Call on others who can offer helpful views on troubling situations.
- *Identify the 'silver lining'*: Learn to find the hidden good things about difficult situations.
- *No replaying bad thoughts*: Use distraction to cut short rumination over bad experiences.
- *Keep thinking—Don't give up*: Plan multiple coping steps until you feel better!

high-risk or symptomatic youth (Clarke et al., 1995, 2001; Cardemil et al., 2002). Extant empirically supported programs that treat youth depression have primarily focused on reducing negative cognitions and negative attributions because dominant aetiologic models of depression implicate negative cognitions. Beck (1976) postulates that a negative view towards oneself, one's experiences, and the future; a negative schema that biases the selection, encoding, and evaluation of information; and a tendency to make cognitive errors (e.g., dichotomous thinking), increases risk for onset and persistence of depression. The reformulated learned helplessness model posits that a tendency to attribute negative events to internal, stable, and global causes, and positive events to external, unstable, and specific causes increases risk for depression (Abramson et al., 1978). Negative cognitions and attributional style predicted subsequent depression in youths (Hankin et al., 2001; Lewinsohn et al., 1994; Nolen-Hoeksema et al., 1986, 1992) and treatments for youth depression that focus on negative cognitions appear to be among the most thoroughly tested interventions (Brent et al., 1997; Chu & Harrison, 2007; Rehm et al., 1987).

Certain interventions have also included a behavioural activation component that involves increasing the frequency of pleasant activities. This focus is based on the behavioural theory of depression that posits that initial negative moods prompt a withdrawal from pleasant activities that serves to exacerbate and perpetuate depressed mood (Lewinsohn et al., 1979). Low rates of pleasant activities predicted subsequent depressive symptoms during adolescence (Clarke et al., 1992), and withdrawal from pleasurable activities appears to contribute to the maintenance of depressed mood in adults (Lewinsohn et al., 1988). Furthermore, treatments that focus on instigating active participation in reinforcing activities have been found to alleviate depression in adult samples (Addis & Jacobson, 1996; Jacobson et al., 1996).

Thus, PASCET represents a treatment that was guided both by a theoretical rationale and by the precedents of existing treatment elements, with a clearly articulated hypothesized mechanism of action (increases in primary and secondary control). Below, we describe characteristics of PASCET in greater detail, as it appears in its most current form.

Program overview

Consistent with the deployment-focused model, the PASCET protocol has been adapted in response to lessons learned at each stage of development and testing. In its current form, PASCET involves 18 individual youth sessions complemented by parent and school contact, with therapists directed through all steps with a treatment manual and an accompanying youth workbook. Youth (aged 8–15) take part in about 15 structured sessions, followed by about 3 individually tailored sessions involving (1) applications of the most personally relevant ('best fit') PASCET skills to important situations or stressors in the youth's life, (2) helping the youth plan his days in advance, building in activities that will maintain good mood throughout the day, and (3) planning for future applications of the PASCET skills after treatment has ended. The sessions include within-session exercises and take-home practice (i.e., homework) assignments, guided by an *ACT & THINK* Practice Book that each youth uses throughout the program and keeps afterward.

Individual youth sessions are complemented by contact with parents in three forms. (1) An individual parent session is held prior to the first meeting with the youth. During this parent session, the therapist explains the treatment program and solicits the parent's perspective on the youth's depression and his mood and behaviour at home. The therapist also explains the parent's role in treatment and discusses appropriate ways for the parent to effectively support treatment. (2) At the end of each individual session, a parent (or both, if available) joins the therapist and youth for 10–15 minutes, in which the main points of the day's session are briefly discussed (excluding information the youth does not want to have discussed) and the parent engages in an activity with the youth that demonstrates the skill(s) he or she learned that day. In this same meeting, the youth's practice assignment for the upcoming week is described, the parent is encouraged to assist him or her with this practice assignment, and a session handout is given to the parent. (3) As an optional feature, the therapist can make a home visit, to meet the youth's family and learn about the environment where the youth lives, and a school visit, to meet school staff who know the youth and to hear their perspective on the youth and his/her behaviour at school and with peers.

Initial youth session: Rapport building and setting goals

One of the most important jobs of the therapist is to build rapport with the youth, by being attentive to what he or she says. It may be helpful to refer back to things the youth has said, and use illustrations and examples during sessions that reflect his or her specific interests. Especially important is the following: The therapist must make the sessions fun, interesting, and active so that the youth always wants to come back for more. Of course, what is fun and interesting to a 9-year-old boy may not be fun or interesting to a 14-year-old girl. So, although the manual does suggest activities, the fun and interesting aspect cannot really be built into the manual very successfully. Instead, this becomes the job of the therapist—i.e., making the sessions enjoyable and engaging by designing clever, witty, and memorable ways to present and illustrate the main points of each session.

Identifying goals that are of importance to the youth is another essential way to establish rapport, and should begin at the initial session. Following a brief, psychoeducative discussion of depression and an exploration of how depression manifests for the youth, at least two treatment goals should be identified collaboratively by the youth and therapist. The therapist may need to rephrase the goal and guide the youth towards the identification of goals that are both meaningful and attainable. Throughout treatment, these goals should be linked to skills whenever possible, and progress towards these goals should be routinely assessed.

Individual youth formulation

Within the PASCET framework, the therapist's experience in individual youth sessions, parent sessions, home visit, and school visit is used to create, and continually revise and update, a formulation regarding the individual youth. The formulation should be a coherent, integrated description of the youth and his life situation, emphasizing the nature and behavioural expression of his depression, the coping strategies from the PASCET protocol that are most likely to be helpful to this particular youth, and how these coping strategies may best be applied given the conditions and constraints of this youngster's life. This therapist formulation is used, together with input from the youth and parent(s), to individualize the treatment for the youth's own stressors and problems. The therapist's formulation should include the following elements:

- Reason for referral
- Symptoms endorsed by the youth and parent during intake or pre-treatment assessment
- Problem areas (not covered by depression symptoms) endorsed during intake or pre-treatment assessment
- Core beliefs
- Behavioural indicators of the youth's depression
- Treatment goals
- Negative thoughts specific to problems/goals
- ACT and THINK skills that will likely work to reach treatment goals
- Potential obstacles to treatment
- Youth's strengths

A preliminary formulation should be written, for the first time, following the pre-treatment assessment, and refined after the initial session with the youth and initial individual parent session. An outline for developing the formulation is provided within the PASCET manual.

Identifying core beliefs

According to Beck (1983), individuals hold 'core beliefs' about themselves, the world, and the future. These core beliefs are cognitive structures that allow for efficient information processing, but the trade-off is the opportunity for the development of 'cognitive distortions' about the self, world, and future. Depressed youth perceive their environment in a way that is consistent with negative beliefs, which leads to the onset and maintenance of depressive symptoms. Without intervention, core beliefs are maintained through distorted cognitive processes, causing depressive symptoms to continue and worsen.

Common core beliefs that youth have are

- I am worthless
- I am flawed
- I am damaged
- I am unlovable
- I am helpless
- My future is hopeless.

Although the therapist will rarely 'know' what the youth's core beliefs are, hypotheses can be made using information from the parent, youth, and school reports, and by observing the youth's behaviour within sessions. For example, if the parent reports that the youth gives up easily and says things like 'what's the point in trying', 'this is not going to work', or 'I am just going to fail no matter how hard I try', the therapist may hypothesize that he has a 'helpless' core belief. If the parent reports that the youth becomes overly upset around social situations or says 'nobody loves me', the therapist may hypothesize an 'unlovable' core belief. The therapist should make hypotheses about the youth's core beliefs in the first conceptualization (following the individual parent session). Throughout treatment, the therapist and youth will 'catch' negative thoughts during treatment sessions, using a 'thought net'. These automatic thoughts, 'caught' during the treatment session, should be reviewed after each session to look for themes regarding the youth's core belief(s), and later in the treatment may be challenged collaboratively by the therapist and client. Hypotheses about core beliefs can be revised throughout treatment and included in later conceptualizations.

Individualizing the treatment to the youth's 'best fit' skills

In later sessions, there is an increasing emphasis on identifying the particular coping skills of the PASCET program that fit the individual youth's needs best, and seem most likely to be helpful in addressing the individual's depressive symptoms. In this process of tailoring and fitting, the therapist should rely on (a) the evolving formulation, and (b) information on how the youth has responded to the various components of the PASCET program (i.e., which parts he or she seemed to like and use effectively).

Skills emphasized in the PASCET program

PASCET uses the acronym 'ACT & THINK' to present the core coping skills included in the treatment program. The first set of skills, the 'ACT skills', emphasizes primary control, as conceptualized in the theoretical two-process model of control.

- *Activities that Solve Problems.* Depressed youth are more likely to display resignation in the face of perceived stressors; to counter this phenomenon, and to make big problems feel more solvable, we teach and practice STEPS ('Say what the problem is, Think of solutions, Examine each solution, Pick one and try it out, See if it worked'), applying the STEPS procedure to a problem within the session (in vivo), and then to a problem from the youth's own life that he identifies.

- *Activities that Boost Mood.* Depressed youth show a decrease in pleasant, naturally reinforcing events and activities, and this decrease is associated with the maintenance of depression among youth. To address this, the therapist works with the youth to create a menu of specific activities that are reliably mood-enhancing and relatively accessible. To help identify a large range of activities, youth are encouraged to identify activities that are enjoyable, can be shared with someone the youth likes, activities that use energy, and activities that help someone else. These activities are demonstrated within the session to show the profound impact even a few minutes of a highly reinforcing event has on the youth's mood.

- *Calming.* To address the tension, anxiety, and irritability that often accompany youth depression, two strategies for relaxation are taught and practiced. First, 'Complete Calming' uses progressive muscle relaxation via a ten-minute script or recording to help the youth gain control over the physiological effects of depression when time allows. Secondly, 'Quick Calming' uses imagery and diaphragmatic breathing to provide more immediate relaxation in public places.

- *Turn on my Positive Self.* To counter the unengaging social style that often accompanies youth depression, and to provide an additional measure of physiological control over depressed affect, the therapist and youth identify verbal and nonverbal behaviours that project a 'positive self' and a 'negative self' to others and do in vivo role plays of both styles to experience the impact each style has on mood. Take-home practice exercises allow the youth to further explore the impact that positive self-presentation has on her mood and the responses of others.

As the initial sessions focusing on the ACT skills are completed, the therapist and youth discuss the nature of difficult situations all individuals encounter, and how some of these situations cannot be objectively changed through direct actions. For these more intractable problems, the youth may only be able to change how he thinks about a situation, thereby mitigating the impact the situation has on his mood. This discussion introduces the second phase of treatment, focused on THINK skills:

- *Think Positive.* The focus of these sessions is to help the youth first identify and later revise automatic, maladaptive cognitions that are common among depressed youth. Numerous strategies (role-plays, experiential activities, therapist self-disclosure) are used to help the youth grasp the abstract concept that thinking influences feelings, and that she can exert control over her thoughts, by examining the evidence that supports or does not support the thoughts, and generating more realistic, helpful thoughts.

- *Help from a Friend.* Because depressed youth often engage in solitary rumination of negative events, this session focuses on generating a list of helpful people within the youth's life with whom he can 'think things over' in order to gain a different perspective of troubling solutions. A range of helpful people are identified, including adults, peers, and family members, and practice focuses partly on developing skills to appropriately ask for help.

- *Identify the 'Silver Lining'.* To counter the habit of negative selective abstraction, the therapist and youth practice identifying good things that arise as the direct result of situations that seem otherwise aversive.

- *No Replaying Bad Thoughts.* Rumination of past bad experiences or upcoming stressors has been shown to be associated with the onset and maintenance of youth depression; therefore, this session identifies and practices using highly distracting activities to effectively 'change the channel' when the youth is stuck engaging in unproductive rumination.

- *Keep On Using the ACT & THINK Skills.* To combat passivity and helplessness, and to encourage the pro-active use of PASCET skills for the prevention of future depressive episodes, therapists encourage perseverance in the face of failed first attempts to improve mood by teaching and practicing sequential coping—Plan A, B, and C—for problems the youth is likely to encounter. Additionally, the therapist and youth plan for the preventive use of PASCET skills as the youth's mood improves, with the overt message that the youth need not wait for his/her mood to diminish in order to use these skills.

The final few sessions focus on continuing to apply the most relevant coping skills to real-life stressors and the youth's treatment goals. In these sessions, the youth and therapist also create an end-of-treatment project. The project—which might be a poster, a booklet, or a video emphasizing the youngster's favourite skills—is a tangible product the youth can bring home at the end of treatment to remember the skills he learned, while at the same time reviewing and developing mastery of the preferred or most useful skills. The final session, #18, is a review and celebration of what the youth has accomplished.

Youth practice and use of the 'ACT & THINK' workbook

Many of the in-session activities and all the practice assignments are guided by the ACT & THINK Practice Book. At the beginning of the first individual youth session, this book is introduced, and then given to the youth to keep. The youth is expected to fill in pages relevant to each practice assignment during the weeks between sessions, and to bring the book back to the therapist's office for each session. The youth can earn up to two stamps or stickers each week—one for bringing the book to the session, and one for doing the practice assignment and filling in the relevant Practice Book pages. The stamps and stickers can be exchanged for rewards according to a schedule that is shown in the early pages of the Practice Book, and that is developed in collaboration with the parents.

Mood-boosters and teaching moments

A key aspect of the PASCET model is that youths will learn the skills best if they (a) practice them, and (b) experience them to be useful. We encourage therapists to watch for fluctuations in the youth's mood during the session and use these fluctuations as opportunities to help the youth experience how changing behaviour changes feelings. A youth's bad mood can actually turn into a 'teaching moment'. If he/she enters the session in a bad mood, or his/her mood declines during the session, the therapist may comment about this, and then ask the youth to rate his/her mood at that moment, using the 0–10 scale. The therapist may then suggest an appropriate activity designed to improve mood. Following the activity, the youth re-rates his/her mood, and the therapist can make the point that we can all find ways to improve our mood.

Step 2: Initial efficacy trial under controlled conditions, to establish potential for benefit

The original treatment trial of PASCET (Weisz et al., 1997) consisted of an eight-session intervention guided by a detailed therapist's manual, emphasizing two primary control skills (goal setting and increasing mood-enhancing activities) and three secondary control skills (identifying and modifying depressogenic cognitions, cognitive techniques for mood enhancement, and relaxation and positive imagery). It was initially tested among a sample of elementary aged children ($N = 48$, mean age = 9.6; 18% ethnic minority) with mild-to-moderate levels of depression as assessed via the self-report Children's Depression Inventory (CDI; Kovacs, 1992), the Children's Depression Rating Scale—Revised (CDRS-R; Poznanski & Mokros, 1996), and a standardized clinical interview. Children were randomly assigned to receive the abbreviated version of PASCET or a no-treatment control group. Children in the PASCET condition met weekly with two co-therapists in small groups (three to five children). The treatment was delivered by graduate students under the supervision of the treatment developer (JRW).

Outcomes were assessed post-treatment and at nine-month follow-up. Results indicated that children who received the eight-session PASCET program showed significantly greater reductions in depressive symptoms relative to children in the no-treatment control group at both assessment points. The clinical significance of group differences was further underscored by the fact that children treated with PASCET were more likely to shift from above the normal range for depressive symptoms to within the normal range on both the questionnaires at post-treatment (50% vs. 16%) and the questionnaires (62% vs. 31%) and the clinical interview at follow-up (69% vs. 24%).

In the context of the DFM, the paramount goal of the initial efficacy trial was to assess the potential for benefit of PASCET. Because the efficacy trial demonstrated potential benefit under rigorously controlled conditions, the next step suggested by the DFM—field cases—was deemed appropriate.

Step 3: Single-case applications in practice settings, with progressive adaptations to the protocol

Following the DFM approach, PASCET was progressively delivered in community mental health clinics, one of the primary settings in which it is ultimately intended. Advanced clinical trainees were supervised by both senior clinical staff and by the PASCET developer in field trials conducted to inform ways to adapt PASCET to increase effectiveness and utility in community practice. A number of changes resulted from these iterative field trials, including the following: (a) revising the format from the original group version to an individual format more typically utilized in community clinics, (b) the addition of a problem-solving skills and a positive self-presentation component, based on the clinical presentation of children treated in the field trials, (c) expanded parental involvement and optional home and school visits to address the complexity of the clinic youth's family and school situations, (d) increased treatment length to better individualize the treatment to each youth's real-life situations, and (e) improved organization of the therapist manual and youth practice book, in response to therapist feedback regarding usability.

Step 4: Initial effectiveness test

Consistent with the DFM, the next step in the development of PASCET was an initial effectiveness trial in which PASCET was delivered by clinicians in real-world practice settings under typical practice conditions, and compared to treatment offered at the same clinic by clinicians who did not receive training in PASCET. Fifty-seven youth (8–15 years old, $M = 11.77$, SD = 2.14) who met criteria for a DSM-IV depressive disorder (MDD, Dysthymia, Minor Depression), were randomly assigned to receive PASCET or Treatment as Usual (TAU), with therapy continuing until normal termination. Treatment occurred in seven Los Angeles-area community clinics and was administered by full-time practitioners. Therapists ($N = 26$ in CBT, 28 in TAU) represented diverse professional backgrounds (22% social workers, 14% doctoral-level psychologists, 56% masters level psychologists, 8% other masters level professionals) and experience, averaging 4.30 (SD = 1.70) years of training and 2.40 (SD = 3.50) years of additional professional experience. PASCET and TAU therapists did not differ significantly on any of these characteristics.

To provide a fair test of the relative effectiveness of usual care and PASCET used in an everyday clinical context, substantial efforts were made to ensure that this treatment trial used procedures that closely mimicked—and could fit smoothly into—everyday clinic procedures. Therefore, clinicians randomly assigned to the PASCET condition were provided only brief training in the PASCET model (a six-hour workshop commensurate with the professional trainings typically attended by therapists in community practice settings) and weekly group case supervision of 30 minutes per therapist. These procedures fit well within clinic productivity requirements, suggesting that they were realistic and potentially sustainable. Adherence ratings indicated that PASCET sessions contained the required elements from the treatment manual.

At termination, 75% of the sample had no remaining depressive disorder, but treatment groups did not differ significantly on symptom or diagnostic outcomes. However, compared to TAU, PASCET was significantly briefer (24 vs. 39 weeks). Guided by clinic administrators, the cost of treatment was estimated for each youth assigned to PASCET or TAU, and mean cost per case for TAU was significantly higher than for PASCET. Clients randomized to PASCET also received fewer adjunctive services during the study, including treatment from a second therapist, and school-based services; PASCET youths also showed significantly less use of psychotropic medications as a whole and depression-specific psychotropics in particular, when compared to the TAU group. Parents whose children received PASCET also rated therapeutic alliance as significantly stronger than parents of youths who received TAU.

It is important to consider that therapists using PASCET were using an unfamiliar approach guided by a manual they had not independently selected, whereas the TAU therapists used the treatment strategies that in which they were experienced and confident. Review of the PASCET videotapes suggested that although the clinicians showed reasonable treatment fidelity, the skilfulness with which the treatment was delivered varied widely. As noted by Fixsen et al. (2005), when a previously applied intervention is applied in a new context, null findings may reflect incomplete implementation in the new context rather than problems with the intervention per se. Overall, the findings show similar clinical outcomes for PASCET and TAU, but advantages for PASCET with regard to treatment duration, therapeutic alliance, reduced rates of other services (including medication), and cost. In the future, it will be useful to assess the impact of PASCET when delivered by community clinic therapists who have gained experience and familiarity with the protocol and can deliver it both faithfully and skilfully.

Step 5: Further tests of effectiveness and dissemination

Additional tests of PASCET with the goal of expanding its effectiveness and increasing its user-potential have been completed and are currently underway. Our research group is conducting a trial to test the effectiveness of a video-guided version of PASCET within public middle schools, compared to an enhanced treatment as usual condition. This study has two primary aims: to assess whether PASCET can be used to treat depression among young adolescents within the school setting and to examine the utility of the video-guided format. Thus far, PASCET-VG (Video-guided) has been implemented in ten public middle schools in California and Massachusetts, and 161 youth with elevated depressive symptoms, as assessed by the CDI and structured clinical interviews, were randomly assigned to receive either a 13-session group version of PASCET ($N = 86$) or a 13-session group treatment as usual, delivered by therapists working within the schools ($N = 77$). Because data collection is still active for this study, any report regarding the relative effectiveness of PASCET-VG is premature. Nonetheless, some lessons have already been learned over the course of the past five years of study implementation.

First, it is possible to identify treatment-appropriate youth within the school setting. Prior research has indicated that the majority of youth who receive any mental health services receive them in schools (Burns et al., 1995; Farmer et al., 2003), and that youth are more likely to engage in treatment when it is offered in school, rather than when services are offered within the community (Catron & Weiss, 1994). Furthermore, schools are the primary treatment provider for low-income and ethnic minority youth (Levy & Land, 1994), who face particular risk for depression (Roberts et al., 1997), yet are least likely to receive treatment in outpatient community clinics (Baruch, 2001). Thus, schools may be the ideal forum in which to focus efforts to better understand mental health services for youth. In the current study, we screened 1,237 6th and 7th grade students and identified 266 as high risk for depression and eligible for intervention (CDI score >12 or diagnosis of MDD, Dysthymia, or Minor Depression). Fifty-six percent of those received family consent to participate, and 166 participated in treatment with reasons for non-participation including scheduling conflicts, sufficient existing psychological services, or youth refusal.

Second, a video-guided group format works well within the context of the middle-school setting. Most schools offer a variety of therapeutic groups for students, thus reducing the stigma of participation in such a group. The video provides non-personal examples of same-aged actors experiencing difficulties common to youth (peer and parent conflict, academic difficulties, etc.), allowing for participating youth to participate without having to disclose personal information that may not be comfortable within the school setting. Finally, the use of the video and the structured, manualized treatment minimizes preparation time for treatment delivery, a necessary factor when considering the busy scheduled and limited resources of school-based clinicians.

Finally, there is tremendous interest and enthusiasm on the past of school clinicians and administrators to transport PASCET-VG into their schools. Following the active phase of the study at each school, training has traditionally been offered to interested school staff on the PASCET techniques. Attendance has been high at these training workshops, and school staff report the use of PASCET even after study staff are no longer working within the school—in numerous formats, including individual student meetings, group sessions, and in one case, as part of the health curriculum for seventh grade students.

Most recently, PASCET has been adapted in order to better match the conditions found in usual community care, where clients often present with numerous comorbid disorders, and where the use of multiple treatment manuals requires training and preparation that exceed the resources available to community clinicians (see, e.g., Weisz et al., 2006). The *Child Steps Clinic Treatment Project* (CTP) combines PASCET with well-tested treatments for childhood disruptive behaviour disorders and anxiety to form a modular treatment manual designed for flexible use. In the Modular Approach to Treatment for Children—Anxiety, Depression, and Conduct (MATCH-ADC), each treatment element of PASCET is presented as a single, stand alone 'module' that may be used as one session or extended to many sessions, and which may be used in tandem with other treatment elements from PASCET, or with elements used to address disruptive behaviour disorders or anxiety. Thus, when the treatment of depression is not sufficient, clinicians may seamlessly incorporate other well-established treatment elements, guided by a clinical decision flowchart that is informed by the evidence base for youth mental health treatment.

A large-scale, randomized effectiveness trial of MATCH-ADC with complex cases referred to community clinics is currently underway, with 175 children between the ages of 8–13 randomly assigned to receive treatment from clinicians trained in MATCH-ADC or alternately trained in the traditional, non-modular versions of PASCET and treatments for the other disorders. These conditions are also compared to a treatment-as-usual condition, and all clinicians at participating clinics are randomly assigned. The study is still underway, and thus results are not available. Nonetheless, The Child Steps CTP represents an important step towards tailoring treatments that have been tested in ideal settings for better fit to the practice contexts in which the majority of youth are treated.

Step 6: Tests of goodness-of-fit, benefit, and sustainability in practice contexts

In the decade since PASCET was developed and implemented in its first efficacy trial, it has moved through the first five stages of the proposed deployment-focused model of treatment development and testing, and has undergone adaptations and revisions throughout this process in response to scientific examination as well as feedback from clinicians, clinic and school stakeholders, and the youth and parents who have received treatment. In addition to the efforts of our own research group, PASCET has also been adopted by other intervention researchers, and varied somewhat in terms of intervention design, delivery format, and target population.

The Choosing Healthy Actions and Thoughts (CHAT) program. In one instance, PASCET has been adapted for use by the Hamilton-Wentworth District School Board (HWDSB) in Ontario, Canada. This school district has field-tested a parallel form of the video-guided PASCET program within a total of 19 grade seven classrooms over three separate trials. Under the rubric of CHAT (Choosing Healthy Actions and Thoughts), this adapted version is co-facilitated by a mental health professional and a grade seven teacher and is delivered during regular classroom time. The CHAT manual includes key references to the Ontario Curriculum so that teachers can easily relate how health, English, drama, and social-emotional learning expectations are met through this program. In all other respects, the CHAT program mirrors the original PASCET-VG intervention (e.g., use of video-guided format, skill areas, session structure, and activities). Here, PASCET is being used as a primary prevention intervention, and early results suggested that the program had positive effects on coping skills and mood (Polo et al., 2006). A larger, randomized clinical trial is currently underway to fully assess the preventive benefits of PASCET.

PASCET for medically ill depressed youth. As a means of testing its effectiveness among a unique population of interest, PASCET has been adapted for use with medically ill youth suffering from inflammatory bowel disease (IBD) and subsyndromal depression, because depression has been associated with IBD severity, and because for physically ill youth, depression is generally associated with less optimal medical outcomes, heightened functional impairment, and increased mortality (Szigethy et al., 2007). In the initial open trial of this PASCET adaptation, 11 adolescents (12–17 years) with inflammatory bowel disease and either major or minor depression underwent 12 sessions of PASCET-PI (Physical Illness) enhanced by social skills, physical illness narrative, and family psychoeducation components. Pre- to post-treatment assessment demonstrated changes in DSM-IV depression diagnoses and symptoms, physical health, global psychological functioning, and social functioning. Participants reported high satisfaction with the PASCET-PI intervention and no adverse events were reported (Szigethy et al., 2004). At 6 and 12-month follow-up, 10 of the 11 participants did not meet criteria for mood disorders. Improvements in depression, global functioning, and physical health perceptions at completion were maintained during the 12-month period, although additional therapy sessions (mean = 4.36; SD = 4.37) and psychopharmacology ($n = 5$) were required during the follow-up period (Szigethy et al., 2006).

Next, a randomized clinical trial tested the efficacy of PASCET-PI (Szigethy et al., 2007). In this study, youths with IBD (age 11–17, mean age = 14.99) were randomly assigned to receive a modified version of PASCET (PASCET-PI; Physical Illness, $N = 22$) or treatment as usual plus brief psychoeducation about depression (TAU, $N = 19$). Youth receiving PASCET-PI showed significantly greater improvement with regards to depressive symptoms as assessed by the CDI, global assessment of functioning, and perceived control, compared to the TAU group. Taken together, this series of studies suggest that PASCET may be an appropriate treatment to address depression among medically ill youth and can be effectively delivered within a hospital setting.

Caregiver–Child Relationship Enhancement Training. Another adaptation of PASCET has sought to increase the role of the caregiver in the intervention by more directly targeting parent-youth interactions. In the Caregiver–Child Relationship Enhancement Training (C-CRET) manual, developed by Eckshtain and Gaynor (2008), PASCET has been expanded to include skill-building of positive parenting practices, to complement the treatment of depressed youth. The caregiver/caregiver–child sessions focus on establishing a dedicated child–caregiver special time, noncontingent praise and contingent reinforcement of positive mood and behaviour, communication training and positive communication, and family problem solving. The treatment included 16 individual sessions and 7 caregiver sessions administered in the child's school to promote accessibility. Pre-, mid-, post-treatment, one-, and six-month follow-up assessments showed significant decreases in depressive symptoms as assessed by the CDI. Self-, caregiver-, and teacher-report of child psychosocial functioning, depressotypic cognitions, coping skills, caregiver–child relationships, and parenting stress also showed significant improvements. Benchmarking these results against those from the literature suggested that the treatment equalled CBT in other studies and appeared markedly superior to control conditions. Benchmarking the results against relevant pharmacotherapy studies revealed that the treatment compared favourably to pharmacotherapy and appeared to outperform a pill placebo.

Future directions for PASCET

In addition to the expanded use of PASCET among novel populations, it is also important to continue examining additional foci that have emerged in the previous DFM steps. For example, what are the necessary components of the treatment—and are some components more essential or potent than others? What are the treatment moderators that mitigate or bolster the impact of the treatment on youth depressive symptoms? And are the proposed treatment mediators—the enhancement of primary and secondary control, decreases in negative cognitive errors and increases in pleasant and reinforcing activities—acting as mechanisms of change for those youth who benefit from the PASCET treatment? Our current randomized clinical trial of the video-guided PASCET will yield a sample that is sufficiently large to attempt to answer some of these important questions.

It is also imperative that the final step of the DFM is not neglected: to explore the fit of the treatment program to the practice context in which it is ultimately intended, and identify factors that influence practitioners' willingness to use the treatment, the level of treatment adherence demonstrated by those practitioners, and the degree to which use of the protocol improves youth outcomes. An oft-noted weakness of children's mental health services research is the lack of consideration of how programs will be sustained once the funding agencies and research partners have departed (Atkins et al., 2003). Thus, future research will need to continue to investigate how well PASCET, in its various iterations, can be transported into community clinics, schools, and other practice settings, and whether it can be faithfully and effectively sustained once the scrutiny of funded research has lapsed.

Summary and conclusions

The PASCET program grew out of the theoretical model of primary and secondary control for depression, and was also informed by the cognitive–behavioural tradition of youth depression treatment with its focus on identifying and altering negative cognitions and increasing pleasant activities. Throughout the treatment sessions and via homework assignments, boys and girls learn and practice coping skills of two types: primary control skills for altering objective conditions in their lives, and secondary control skills for altering the subjective impact of stressors beyond their immediate control. Whenever possible, the sessions are lively and experiential, with an emphasis on helping youngsters experience the impact of the coping skills on mood in vivo. Over the course of the treatment, youths are encouraged to identify the 'best fit' skills that reliably work to enhance mood, and to practice applying these skills both sequentially in response to stressors and depressed mood, and preventively as a way of sustaining positive mood and engagement. Parents are likewise informed of these coping skills and provided examples of how to use them with their children.

Following the DFM, PASCET has been modified and enhanced over the past decade, expanding from a set of five skills to the current set of eight, shifting to incorporate both group and individual modalities, and examining the utility of different delivery methods, including a video-guided version and incorporation of PASCET into a modular protocol designed to address comorbidity. PASCET has been tested in community clinics, schools, and hospitals, and has been delivered by research staff as well as community practitioners. The age range has been broadened, and unique treatment populations have also been included, such as medically ill children. Via training and the outreach of research endeavours, PASCET has found its way into community child guidance clinics, outpatient child psychiatry clinics, academic classrooms, school-based clinics, and paediatric hospital settings.

The decade ahead holds additional challenges for the PASCET program, as we continue to balance the sometimes competing goals of stringent intervention research with the need for user-friendly treatments that can address the needs of real-world clinical cases and be delivered by practitioners outside the walls of academia. We have learned a good deal about the obstacles that face the task of bringing structured, manual-guided treatments into clinical practice settings, and even more about the potential benefit that such research–practice collaborations may offer to science, and practice, and to the youth and families who seek services.

References

Abramson, L.Y., Seligman, M.E., & Teasdale, J. (1978). Learned helplessness in humans: Critique and reformulation. *Journal of Abnormal Psychology, 87*, 49–74.

Addis, M.E. & Jacobson, N.S. (1996). Reasons for depression and the process and outcome of cognitive–behavioral psychotherapies. *Journal of Consulting and Clinical Psychology, 64*, 1317–1424.

Angold, A. & Costello, E.J. (2001). The epidemiology of depression in children and adolescents. In I.M. Goodyer (Ed.), *The depressed child and adolescent* (pp. 127–147). Cambridge, UK: Cambridge University Press.

Angold, A., & Costello, E.J. (2006). Puberty and depression. *Child and Adolescent Psychiatric Clinics of North America, 15*, 919–937.

Angold, A., & Rutter, M. (1992). Effects of age and pubertal status on depression in a large clinical sample. *Development and Psychopathology, 4*, 5–28.

Arias, E., MacDorman, M.F., Strobino, D.M., & Guyer, B. (2003). Annual summary of vital statistics—2002. *Pediatrics, 112*, 1215–1230.

Atkins, M.S., Graczyk, P.A., Frazier, S.L., & Abdul-Adil, J. (2003). Toward a new model for promoting urban children's mental health: Accessible, effective, and sustainable school-based mental health services. *School Psychology Review, 32*, 503–514.

Bandura, A. (1977). Self-efficacy: Toward a unifying theory of behavioral change. *Psychological Review, 84*, 191–215.

Bandura, A. (1986). Social foundations of thought and action: A social cognitive theory. New Jersey: Prentice-Hall.

Baruch, G. (2001). Mental health services in schools: The challenge of locating a psychotherapy service for troubled adolescent pupils in mainstream and special schools. *Journal of Adolescence, 24*, 549–570.

Beck, A.T. (1976). Cognitive therapy and the emotional disorders. Oxford: International Universities Press.

Beck, A.T. (1983). Cognitive therapy of depression: New perspectives. In P.J. Clayton & J.E. Barrett (Eds.), *Treatment of depression: Old controversies and new approaches* (pp. 265–290). New York: Raven Press.

Beck, A.T., Rush, A.J., Shaw, B.F., & Emery, G. (1979). *Cognitive therapy of depression.* New York: Guilford Press.

Birmaher, B., Ryan, N.D., Williamson, D.E., Brent, D.A., Kaufman, J., Dahl, R.E., et al. (1996). Childhood and adolescent depression: A review of the past 10 years. Part I. *Journal of the American Academy of Child and Adolescent Psychiatry, 35*, 1427–1439.

Brent, D.A., Holder, D., Kolko, D.J., Birmaher, B., Baugher, M., Roth, C. et al. (1997). A clinical psychotherapy trial for adolescent depression comparing cognitive, family, and supportive therapy. *Archives of General Psychiatry, 54*, 877–885.

Burns, B.J., Costello, E.J., Angold, A., Tweed, D., Stangl, D., Farmer, E., et al. (1995). Children's mental health service use across service sectors. *Health Affairs, 14*, 147–159.

Capaldi, D.M. & Stoolmiller, M. (1999). Co-occurrence of conduct problems and depressive symptoms in early adolescent boys: III. Prediction to young adulthood. *Developmental Psychopathology, 11*, 59–84.

Cardemil, E.V., Reivich, K.J., & Seligman, M.E.P. (2002). The prevention of depressive symptoms in low-income minority middle school students. *Prevention and Treatment, 5*, np.

Catron, T. & Weiss, B. (1994). The Vanderbilt school-based counseling program. *Journal of Emotional and Behavioral Disorders, 2*, 247–253.

Chu, B.C. & Harrison, T.L. (2007). Disorder-specific effects of CBT for anxious and depressed youth: A meta analysis of candidate mediators of change. *Clinical Child and Family Psychology Review, 10*, 1–35.

Clarke, G., Hawkins, W., Murphy, M., & Sheeber, L. (1993). School-based primary prevention of depressive symptomatology in adolescents: Findings from two studies. *Journal of Adolescent Research, 8*, 183–204.

Clarke, G.N., Hawkins, W., Murphy, M., Sheeber, L., Lewinsohn, P.M., & Seeley, J.R. (1995). Targeted prevention of unipolar depressive disorder in an at-risk sample of high school adolescents: A randomized trial of a group cognitive intervention. *Journal of the American Academy of Child and Adolescent Psychiatry, 34*, 312–321.

Clarke, G.N., Hornbrook, M., Lynch, F., Polen, M., Gale, J., Beardslee, W., et al. (2001). A randomized trial of a group cognitive intervention for preventing depression in adolescent offspring of depressed parents. *Archives of General Psychiatry, 58*, 1127–1134.

Clarke, G., Lewinsohn, P., & Hops, H. (1990). *Leader's manual for adolescent groups: Adolescent coping with depression course.* Eugene, OR: Castalia Publishing Company.

Clarke, G.N., Lewinsohn, P.M., Hops, H., Andrews, J.A., Seeley, J.R., & Williams, J.A. (1992). Cognitive–behavioral group treatment of adolescent depression: Prediction of change. *Behavior Therapy, 23*, 341–354.

Clarke, G.N., Rohde, P., Lewinsohn, P.M., Hops, H., & Seeley, J.R. (1999). Cognitive–behavioral treatment of adolescent depression: Efficacy of acute group treatment and booster sessions. *Journal of the American Academy of Child and Adolescent Psychiatry, 38*, 272–279.

Cohen, P., Cohen, J., Kasen, S., Velez, C.N., Hartmark, C., Johnson, J., et al. (1993). An epidemiological study of disorders in late childhood and adolescence: I. Age and gender specific prevalence. *Journal of Child Psychology and Psychiatry, 34,* 851–867.

Costello, E.J., Erkanli, A., & Angold, A. (2006). Is there an epidemic of child or adolescent depression? *Journal of Child Psychology and Psychiatry, 47,* 1263–1271.

Eckshtain, D. & Gaynor, S.T.(2008, November). Combined cognitive behavioral treatment plus caregiver sessions for childhood depression. In Sarah Kate Bearman (Chair), Bridging the Gap for Youth Depression: Using the Deployment-Focused Model (DFM) of Treatment Development and Testing in Children's Mental Health. Symposium accepted to the annual meeting of the Association for Behavioral and Cognitive Therapy, Orlando, FLA.

Farmer, E., Burns, B., Phillips, S., Angold, A., & Costello, E.J. (2003). Pathways into and through mental health services for children and adolescents. *Psychiatric Services, 54(1),* 60–66.

Fergusson, D.M. & Woodward, L.J. (2002). Mental health, educational, and social role outcomes of adolescents with depression. *Archives of General Psychiatry, 59,* 225–231.

Fixsen, D.L., Naoom, S.F., Blase, K.A., Friedman, R.M., & Wallace, F. (2005). *Implementation research: A synthesis of the literature* (No. Louis de la Parte Florida Mental Health Publication #231). Tampa: University of South Florida.

Fleming, J.E. & Offord, D. R. (1990). Epidemiology of childhood depressive disorders: A critical review. *Journal of the American Academy of Child and Adolescent Psychiatry, 29,* 571–580.

Garrison, C.Z., Addy, C.L., Jackson, K.L., McKeown, R.E., & Waller, J.L. (1992). Major depressive disorder and dysthymia in young adolescents. *American Journal of Epidemiology, 135,* 792–802.

Ge, X., Conger, R.D., & Elder, G.H. (2001). Pubertal transition, stressful life events, and the emergence of gender differences in adolescent depressive symptoms. *Developmental Psychology, 37,* 404–417.

Ge, X., Lorenz, F.O., Conger, R.D., Elder, G.H., & Simons, R.L. (1994). Trajectories of stressful life events and depressive symptoms during adolescence. *Developmental Psychology, 30,* 467.

Gotlib, I.H., Lewinsohn, P.M., & Seeley, J.R. (1998). Consequences of depression during adolescence: Marital status and marital functioning in early adulthood. *Journal of Abnormal Psychology, 107,* 686–690.

Hankin, B.L. & Abramson, L.Y. (2001). Development of gender differences in depression: An elaborated cognitive vulnerability–transactional stress theory. *Psychological Bulletin, 127,* 773–796.

Hankin, B.L., Abramson, L.Y., & Siler, M. (2001). A prospective test of the hopelessness theory of depression in adolescence. *Cognitive Therapy and Research, 25,* 607–632.

Henggeler, S.W., Schoenwald, S.K., Borduin, C.M., Rowland, M.D., & Cunningham, P.B. (1998). *Multisystemic treatment of antisocial behavior in children and adolescents.* New York: Guilford.

Jacobson, N., Dobson, K., Traux, P., Addis, M., Koerner, K., Gollan, J., et al. (1996). A component analysis of cognitive–behavioral treatment for depression. *Journal of Consulting and Clinical Psychology, 64,* 295–304.

Jensen, A.L., & Weisz, J.R. (2002). Assessing match and mismatch between practitioner-generated and standardized interview-generated diagnoses for clinic-referred children and adolescents. *Journal of Consulting and Clinical Psychology, 70,* 158–168.

Kaltiala-Heino, R., Rimpela, M., Rantanen, P., & Laippala, P. (2001). Adolescent depression: The role of discontinuities in life course and social support. *Journal of Affective Disorders, 64,* 155–166.

Kazdin, A.E. (2002). The state of child and adolescent psychotherapy research. *Child and Adolescent Mental Health, 7*, 53–59.

Keenan-Miller, D., Hammen, C.L., & Brennan, P.A. (2007). Health outcomes related to early adolescent depression. *Journal of Adolescent Health, 41*, 256–262.

Kovacs, M. (1992). *Children's Depression Inventory Manual.* North Tonawanda, NY: Multi-Health Systems.

Kovacs, M. & Golston, D. (1991). Cognitive and social cognitive development of depressed children and adolescents. *Journal of the American Academy of Child and Adolescent Psychiatry, 30*, 388–392.

Levy, A.J. & Land, H. (1994). School-based interventions with depressed minority adolescents. *Child & Adolescent Social Work Journal, 11*, 21–35.

Lewinsohn, P.M., Clarke, G.N., Hops, H., & Andrews, J. (1990). Cognitive–behavioral treatment for depressed adolescents. *Behavior Therapy, 21*, 385–401.

Lewinsohn, P.M., Hoberman, H.M., & Rosenbaum, M. (1988). A prospective study of risk factors for unipolar depression. *Journal of Abnormal Psychology, 97*, 251–264.

Lewinsohn, P.M., Hops, H., Roberts, R.E., Seeley, J.R., & Andrews, J.A. (1993). Adolescent psychopathology: I. Prevalence and incidence of depression and other DSM-III-R disorders in high school students. *Journal of Abnormal Psychology, 102*, 133–144.

Lewinsohn, P.M., Roberts, R.E., Seeley, J.R., Rohde, P., Gotlib, I.H., & Hops, H. (1994). Adolescent psychopathology: II. Psychosocial risk factors for depression. *Journal of Abnormal Psychology, 103*, 302–315.

Lewinsohn, P., Rohde, P., & Seeley, J. (1998). Major depressive disorder in older adolescents: Prevalence, risk factors, and clinical implications. *Clinical Psychology Review, 18*, 765–794.

Lewinsohn, P.M., Youngren, M.A., & Grosscup, S.J. (1979). Reinforcement and depression. In R.A. Dupue (Ed.), *The psychobiology of depressive disorders: Implications for the effects of stress* (pp. 291–316). New York: Academic Press.

Michael, K.D. & Crowley, S.L. (2002). How effective are treatments for child and adolescent depression? A meta-analytic review. *Clinical Psychology Review, 22*, 1–23.

Newman, D.L., Moffitt, T.E., Caspi, A., Magdol, L., Silva, P.A., & Stanton, W.R. (1996). Psychiatric disorder in a birth cohort of young adults: Prevalence, comorbidity, clinical significance, and new case incidence from ages 11 to 21. *Journal of Consulting and Clinical Psychology, 64*, 552–562.

Nolen-Hoeksema, S., Girgus, J.S., & Seligman, M.E. (1986). Learned helplessness in children: A longitudinal study of depression, achievement, and explanatory style. *Journal of Personality and Social Psychology, 51*, 435–442.

Nolen-Hoeksema, S., Girgus, J.S., & Seligman, M.E. (1992). Predictors and consequences of childhood depressive symptoms: A 5-year longitudinal study. *Journal of Abnormal Psychology, 101*, 405–422.

Pfeffer, C.R., Zuckerman, S., & Plutchik, R. (1984). Suicidal behavior in normal school children: A comparison with child psychiatric inpatients. *Journal of the American Academy of Child Psychiatry, 23*, 416–423.

Polo, A.J., Bearman, S.K., Short, K.H., Ho, A. & Weisz, J.R. (2006). Strengthening school-research collaborations while developing effective youth depression programs. *Emotional & Behavioral Disorders in Youth, 6, 27–46.*

Poznanski, E.O., & Mokros, H.B. (1996). Children's Depression Rating Scale—Revised (CDRS-R) Manual. Los Angeles: Western Psychiatric Services.

Puig-Antich, J., Kaufman, J., Ryan, N.D., Williamson, D.E., Dahl, R.E., Lukens, E., et al. (1993). The psychosocial functioning and family environment of depressed adolescents. *Journal of the American Academy of Child and Adolescent Psychiatry, 32*, 244–253.

Rehm, L.P., Kaslow, N.J., & Rabin, A.S. (1987). Cognitive and behavioral targets in a self-control therapy program for depression. *Journal of Consulting and Clinical Psychology, 55*, 60–67.

Reinecke, M.A., Ryan N.E., & DuBois, D.L. (1998). Cognitive–behavioral therapy of depression and depressive symptoms during adolescence: A review and meta-analysis. *Journal of the American Academy of Child and Adolescent Psychiatry, 37*, 26–34.

Reynolds, W.M. & Coats, K.I. (1986). A comparison of cognitive–behavioral therapy and relaxation training for the treatment of depression adolescents. *Journal of Consulting and Clinical Psychology, 54*, 653–660.

Roberts, R.E., Roberts, C.R., & Chen, Y.R. (1997). Ethnocultural difference in prevalence of adolescent depression. *American Journal of Community Psychology, 25*, 95–109.

Rothbaum, F., Weisz, J.R., & Snyder, S. (1982). Changing the world and changing the self: A two-process model of perceived control. *Journal of Personality and Social Psychology, 42*, 5–37.

Schiffman, J., Becker, K.D., & Daleiden, E.L. (2006). Evidence-based services in a statewide mental health system: Do the services fit the problems? *Journal of Clinical Child and Adolescent Psychology, 35*, 13–19.

Stark, K.D., Reynolds, W.R., & Kaslow, N.J. (1987). A comparison of the relative efficacy of self-control therapy and a behavioral problem-solving therapy for depression in children. *Journal of Abnormal Child Psychology, 15*, 91–113.

Stolberg, R., Clark, D., & Bongar, B. (2002). Epidemiology, assessment, and management of suicide in depressed patients. In I. Gotlib, & C. Hammen (Eds.), *Handbook of Depression* (pp. 581–601). New York: Guilford Press.

Szigethy, E., Carpenter, J., Baum, E., Kenney, E., Baptista-Neto, L., Beardslee, W.R., et al. (2006). Longitudinal treatment of adolescents with depression and inflammatory bowel disease. *Journal of the American Academy of Child and Adolescent Psychiatry, 45*, 396–400.

Szigethy, E., Kenney, E., Carpenter, J., Hardy, D.M., Fairclough, D., Bousvaros, A., et al. (2007). Cognitive–behavioral therapy for adolescents with inflammatory bowel disease and subsyndromal depression. *Journal of the American Academy of Child and Adolescent Psychiatry, 46*, 1290–1298.

Szigethy, E., Whitton, S.W., Levy-Warren, A., DeMaso, D.R., Weisz, J.R., & Beardslee, W.R. (2004). Cognitive–behavioral therapy for depression in adolescents with inflammatory bowel disease: A pilot study. *Journal of the American Academy of Child and Adolescent Psychiatry, 43*, 1469–1477.

Weersing, V.R. & Weisz, J.R. (2002). Community clinic treatment of depressed youth: Benchmarking usual-care against CBT clinical trials. *Journal of Consulting and Clinical Psychology, 70*, 299–310.

Weinberg, W.A., Rutman, J., Sullivan, L., Penick, E.C., & Dietz, S.G. (1973). Depression in children referred to an educational diagnostic center: Diagnosis and treatment. Preliminary report. *The Journal of Pediatrics, 83*, 1065–1072.

Weisz, J.R. (2004). *Psychotherapy for children and adolescents: Evidence-based treatments and case examples.* New York, NY: Cambridge University Press.

Weisz, J.R., Jensen, A.L., & McLeod, B.D. (2005). Development and dissemination of child and adolescent psychotherapies: Milestones, methods, and a new deployment-focused model. In E.D. Hibbs & P.S. Jensen (Eds.), *Psychosocial treatments for child and adolescent disorders: Empirically based strategies for clinical practice* (2nd ed., pp. 9–39). Washington, DC: American Psychological Association.

Weisz, J.R., McCarty, C.A., & Valeri, S.M. (2006). Effects of psychotherapy for depression in children and adolescents: A meta-analysis. *Psychological Bulletin, 132*, 132–249.

Weisz, J.R., Rothbaum, F.M., & Blackburn, T.F. (1984). Standing out and standing in: The psychology of control in America and Japan. *American Psychologist, 39*, 955–969.

Weisz, J.R., Southam-Gerow, M.A., Gordis, E.B., & Connor-Smith, J. (2003). Primary and secondary control enhancement training for youth depression: Applying the deployment focused model of treatment development and testing. In A.E. Kazdin & J.R. Weisz (Eds.), *Evidence-based psychotherapies for children and adolescents* (pp. 165--183). New York: Guilford Press.

Weisz, J.R., Sweeney, L., Proffitt, V., & Carr, T. (1993). Control-related beliefs and self-reported depressive symptoms in late childhood. *Journal of Abnormal Psychology, 102*, 411–418.

Weisz, J.R., Thurber, C., Sweeney, L., Proffitt, V.D., & LeGagnoux, G.L. (1997). Brief treatment of mild-to-moderate child depression using primary and secondary control enhancement training. *Journal of Consulting and Clinical Psychology, 65*, 703–707.

Zalsman, G., Brent, D.A., & Weersing, V.R. (2006). Depressive disorders in childhood and adolescence: An overview of epidemiology, clinical manifestation, and risk factors. *Child and Adolescent Psychiatric Clinics of North America, 15*, 827–841.

Chapter 6

Resourceful adolescent program: A prevention and early intervention program for teenage depression

Ian M. Shochet & Rebecca Hoge

There is a need to find sustainable approaches to the prevention of adolescent depression. The Resourceful Adolescent Program (RAP) is a strengths-focused, resilience-building program designed to intervene when young people are aged 12–15 (just before the sharp increase in the incidence of depression). The aim of RAP is to facilitate development of positive coping and interpersonal skills to build resilience to help prevent the development of depressive symptoms in young people. RAP has been primarily designed as a universal school-based program to be run as an integral part of the school curriculum with students in grades 8–10 in groups of about 10–15 students. There is also evidence that RAP can be effectively applied as a selective or indicated prevention and early intervention program.

The program integrates elements of Cognitive–Behavioural Therapy (CBT) with interpersonal perspectives on depression, and has the overarching aim of assisting teenagers in self-regulation and managing the daily vicissitudes of self-esteem. It is an 11-session program that can be implemented by mental health professionals and teachers who have undergone training in the program. One of the essential features of the program is that *it is a very positively-focused program* that concentrates on 'building strengths' rather than 'repairing deficits'.

The efficacy and effectiveness of RAP have been systematically researched over the past ten years through randomized controlled trials. We have good evidence of program efficacy and some encouraging (although mixed) evidence of real world sustainability and effectiveness. In what follows, we describe our rationale for a universal approach to preventing teenage depression. We then describe the theoretical rationale for RAP, the intervention goals and approaches, a summary of the session-by-session content, the research findings in relation to RAP, special adaptations, and directions for the future.

Our rationale for a universal approach to prevention of teenage depression

As discussed in earlier chapters, depression is a pernicious disorder affecting approximately 20% of all teenagers, impacting on their development and future prospects. Even mild and subclinical symptoms of depression are associated with poorer outcomes and problems with lifetime trajectory (Garber, 2006). Thus, there is an urgent need world-wide to find sustainable prevention and early intervention approaches. While there has been some proliferation of research in the last five years, our knowledge in this regard is still very limited and there is some debate about the optimal approach.

The mental health intervention spectrum classifies preventive interventions into three categories: universal, selective, and indicated (Mrazek & Haggerty, 1994). Universal preventive interventions aim to reduce the incidence of new cases of a disorder in a whole population, while selective and indicated interventions target subgroups of a population who are identified as 'at-risk', and aim to prevent the disorder from developing in these individuals. Indicated interventions typically involve the use of screening measures (such as the Reynolds Adolescent Depression Scale—RADS; Reynolds, 1987) to identify students at elevated risk for depression, while selective interventions target students with a known population risk factor (e.g., parental psychopathology). When we began our research on RAP in 1997, we elected a universal approach to prevention (i.e., targeting a whole cohort of students irrespective of risk factors) for five reasons: (a) the population health benefits of universal approaches, (b) increased recruitment and reach in the universal approach, (c) benefit in preventing even mild symptoms of depression in previously healthy teenagers, (d) concerns about stigmatization in indicated (or selective approaches) where teenagers are singled out for intervention, and (e) the opportunity for symptomatic teenagers to obtain positive modelling experiences from some of their peers.

The population health argument: The proponents of the population-based approaches in the prevention science literature propose that there is great value in targeting not only the at-risk group, but also in keeping the healthy from becoming at-risk. This argument is based on the premise that a large group of people exposed to a low risk (e.g., minor depressive symptoms) will ultimately generate more clinical cases than a small group of individuals exposed to a higher risk (Rose, 1992). They provide a compelling argument that a population-based approach with even limited effect will ultimately reduce far more disorders than a highly effective targeted approach (Brown & Liao, 1999). Universal interventions aim to promote healthy behaviours and reduce risk factors for the entire population (Lopez et al., 2004). Rose states that a universal prevention strategy is necessary wherever risk is widely diffused, as is the case with depressive disorders. According to Andrews et al. (2002), if the distribution of depressive symptoms in the population is moved by a small amount, this will lead to a reduction in the number of overall cases of major depression.

Recruitment and Reach: Early indicated depression prevention trials reported low recruitment and retention rates. For example, Jaycox et al. (1994) and Clarke et al. (1995) achieved recruitment rates of less than 20% and 50%, respectively, and attrition rates of 30% and 27%, respectively. Offering universal interventions as an all-inclusive part of the normal school program increases participation rates. For example, Shochet et al. (2001) achieved an 88% recruitment rate and a low attrition rate of 5.8% and Merry et al. (2004b) reported a recruitment rate of 73% and attrition rates of 9% at six months and 28% at 18 months. According to Abrahms et al. (1996), the 'reach' of an intervention must be taken into account when evaluating its impact, rather than focusing solely on effect size. They argue that the 'impact' (I) of prevention is best judged on the product of the effect (E) and the recruitment rate or 'reach' (R) and not simply the effect size. To demonstrate, Abrahms et al. point out that a highly effective intervention with zero recruitment rate or an ineffective program with a 100% recruitment rate both produce an impact of zero.

Benefits of promoting and maintaining well-being in healthy and at-risk teenagers: The prevention of minor symptoms of depression in adolescents might not only be a means to an end in terms of altering the trajectory towards clinical depression, but is of value in and of itself if it results in amelioration of distress and dysfunction (Munoz et al., 1994). Minor depression can compromise functionality and quality of life and increase the utilization of medical services (Broadhead et al., 1987; Coulehan et al., 1990; Wells et al., 1989). In their meta-analysis, Horowitz and Garber (2006) concluded that the negative correlates of subclinical levels of depression and their tendency to persist over many years suggest that prevention of depression symptoms, regardless of whether a clinical diagnosis is warranted, is a goal worthy of study. This advantage of universal interventions has been supported by our own research on RAP. For example, Shochet et al. (2001) found that at 10-month follow-up, only 1.2% of initially healthy adolescents (those who recorded scores below the subclinical range on depression measures at pre-intervention) in the intervention conditions had moved into the subclinical or clinical range compared with 10.1% of initially healthy adolescents in the control group.

Screening and stigmatization: Targeted interventions rely on the availability and application of adequate screening procedures in order to accurately predict which individuals are at increased risk of developing a disorder. Screening is costly and difficult and must be conducted continually to detect new 'high-risk' individuals as they emerge (Lopez et al., 2004). Another disadvantage to targeted interventions that involve screening is that labelling individuals as 'at-risk' can lead to stigmatization. This is particularly important for adolescent populations for whom peer acceptance is critical. Until recently, the risk of stigmatization had not been empirically investigated. Rapee et al. (2006) compared the level of stigma perceived by participants in a universal and an indicated depression prevention program. Although effect sizes were small, results suggested that indicated delivery may be associated with greater levels of stigmatization. Specifically, level of embarrassment was consistently higher for the indicated intervention, and teasing by peers demonstrated a weaker and less consistent difference between conditions. As embarrassment and peer teasing are both important negative predictors of mental health, the risk of producing even small increases in stigma through indicated interventions is an important factor that must be considered in deciding how to implement prevention programs (Rapee et al.). One of the guiding principles in the development and evaluation of RAP was 'first, do no harm'.

Finally, we felt that the group process in universal approaches had the potential to provide the opportunity for symptomatic teenagers to obtain positive modelling experiences from some of their more functional peers. In addition, the inclusion of nonsymptomatic participants assists in ensuring that groups stay positively focused.

It is important to point out that since our first published trial (Shochet et al., 2001), there has been a proliferation of research and subsequent meta-analyses that suggest a targeted approach might be a better option than universal interventions (Merry et al., 2004a; Horowitz & Garber, 2006). While targeted trials have demonstrated greater effects than universal, it is premature to abandon universal programs for preventing depression (Horowitz & Garber). Merry et al. concluded that when accounting for the practical difficulties associated with targeted interventions, universal implementation is warranted.

Indeed, there have been some disappointing findings of program *effectiveness* with universal CBT approaches particularly when run by teachers in large classroom sizes (e.g., Spence et al., 2003). For the reasons outlined above, we believe that it is important to continue to research universal approaches (in addition to targeted approaches). Our view is that in the final analysis, universal approaches hold out the best prospects for a more sustainable real-world prevention approach. Our own results with universal trials of the RAP program (that integrates CBT with interpersonal perspective and is conducted in smaller group sizes than the Spence et al. studies) show good efficacy and mixed but some encouraging results with effectiveness. These issues are discussed more fully in the research section of this chapter.

Theoretical rationale of RAP

The RAP is a strengths-focused, resilience-building program based on the recognition and reinforcement of existing personal strengths and the development of additional skills and psychological resources. RAP was developed in 1997 by converting current knowledge at that stage about evidence-based practice for treatment of depression (drawn from Cognitive–Behavioural Therapy and Interpersonal Therapy) into a school-based preventive intervention. In addition, the program draws extensively on the parallel research on intrapsychic and interpersonal risk and protective factors. Finally, we integrated the interpersonal and individual components through a common focus on the management of the vicissitudes of the self. The latter was influenced by a self-psychological theoretical approach and supported by research that has consistently shown the mediation/proximal role of self-esteem in the onset of depressive symptoms.

Because RAP includes components of both CBT and interpersonal approaches (such as IPT), it addresses known psychosocial risk and protective factors for depression at both the individual and interpersonal level. Cognitive–behaviour therapy and interpersonal psychotherapy are the two best-validated psychosocial interventions for adolescent depression (Allen et al., 2006), with research trials showing both to be better than wait-list or treatment-as-usual approaches (Ryan, 2005). Further, there is some evidence that prevention programs that include an interpersonal component combined with strong cognitive–behavioural training (e.g., RAP and the Penn Prevention Program [Jaycox et al., 1994]) may be particularly effective (Garber, 2006).

The CBT components of the RAP program include cognitive restructuring (helping adolescents to identify and challenge negative or distorted thinking and develop positive self-talk), stress management using self-regulation and self-calming strategies, and problem-solving. Over the past couple of decades, Beck and other researchers at the Centre for Cognitive Therapy have provided extensive evidence of the link between what we think and how we feel (Burns, 1980). There is now converging evidence from correlational, predictive, and offspring studies that negative cognitions increase vulnerability to depression, and so it is not surprising that most depression prevention programs include cognitive restructuring as a central component. Stress management is an important component of depression prevention because stressful life events are a known risk factor for depression (Essau, 2004), and it has been demonstrated that relaxation training is as effective as CBT in reducing adolescent depressive symptoms (Reynolds & Coats, 1986). Finally, a problem-solving component was included because the ability to effectively solve problems has been proposed as a protective factor. In the short-term at least, improving adolescents' problem-solving skills has been shown to reduce depressive symptoms (Spence et al., 2003).

The broad interpersonal and IPT components (Klerman & Weissman, 1993; Mufson et al., 1993) include material that encourages participants to establish and draw on a network of social support, as well as develop skills necessary to deal with role transitions and roles disputes, and prevent and manage conflict ('Keep the Peace' and 'Make the Peace'). Interpersonal skills promoted in RAP include improved ability to understand the perspective of others, communication, and other interpersonal skills to prevent and manage conflict. The interpersonal components of RAP address known predictors of depression such as low social support (Galambos et al., 2004) and interpersonal conflict (Essau, 2004) that CBT-only programs may not directly address.

Family conflict, especially escalating parent–adolescent conflict, and parental over-control are major risk factors for depression during adolescence (Burbach et al., 1989; Lewinsohn et al., 1994b). There is good research to show that family conflict predates the onset of depression (Lewinsohn et al.). Further, severe parent–adolescent conflict is associated with elevated risk for chronicity and relapse in depressed adolescents (Birmaher et al., 1996). Parental psychopathology is another potent risk factor for adolescent depression, with children of a depressed parent being four times more likely to develop an affective disorder (Burns et al., 2002). Hammen et al. (2004) suggest an interaction between family conflict and maternal depression, based on their finding that when family discord is low, rates of depression do not significantly differ between offspring of depressed and nondepressed mothers. Thus, in the absence of family conflict, maternal depression alone does not appear to be a risk factor for depression.

In order for prevention strategies to successfully reduce the incidence of a disorder, it is important to not only identify a wide range of risk and protective factors, but also to understand how they interact with each other. Self-esteem appears to be a vital proximal variable that might funnel individual (e.g., cognitive styles, etc.) and interpersonal factors in teenage depression. For example, in their examination of nine possible predictors of depression in early adolescence, MacPhee & Andrews (2006) found that self-esteem accounted for the majority of variance in depression scores (31% for the total sample, 35% for females and 26% for males) and partially mediated the relationship of both parental nurturance and parental rejection to depression.

Similarly, studies conducted by Wilkinson (2004) involving both Norwegian and Australian samples showed that the effects of both parental and peer attachment were predominantly mediated by self-esteem. Several other studies have also reported that self-esteem or self-worth mediated the relationship between parental relationships and depression (Garber et al., 1997; Kenny & Sirin, 2006; Palosaari et al., 1996). Thus, it appears that self-esteem is not only an important single predictor of depression, but also mediates a number of important interpersonal predictors.

For this reason, a central hinge of the RAP program is to funnel skill-building through regulation of the self. Kohut's theory of self-psychology supports this. Kohut proposed that psychological well-being was contingent upon the development of a cohesive self structure able to act as a buffer against negative environmental stimuli. He identified three developmental needs, termed self-object needs, which must be fulfilled in the establishment of such a resilient self (Baker & Baker, 1987; Lynch, 1998; Romano, 2004). First is the sense of being among similar others, termed twinship or belonging. Second is the need to identify values, goals, and qualities to which one aspires, termed idealization. Third is the need for validation and acceptance, termed mirroring or grandiosity. Initially, these needs are fulfilled by others; however, in a healthy developmental trajectory, they are increasingly met by reference to the individuated intrapsychic self. This is congruent with the finding that peer rejection is only substantially related to depression in individuals who place high importance on peer appraisal (Prinstein & Wargo Aikins, 2004).

Thus, in summary, the RAP program draws on CBT and interpersonal perspectives to enhance the coping resources of adolescents to facilitate management of the vicissitudes of adolescent life and thus prevent or ameliorate depressive symptoms. Table 6.1 contains a summary of the skills taught in the RAP Program, the theory and research that guides each element, and the overarching integration of the program.

Intervention goals and methods

Thus far, we have described the approach and rationale of the RAP program, which is an experiential, resilience-building program designed to promote positive coping abilities and the maintenance of a sense of self in the face of stressful and difficult circumstances. We will now describe some of the key processes within the RAP program.

The RAP positive philosophy and metaphors

When adapting programs that are designed for use in treatment of clinical depression, it is important to avoid the risk of being too deficit or symptom-focused and quarantine against the effects of excessive or inappropriate self-disclosure. As a universal program, we were mindful that many of the students participating in the program were not necessarily symptomatic. In addition, RAP was not intended as group therapy, but as a resilience-building group. We also wanted to ensure that groups did not spiral into a contagion of deficits that became unmanageable for the facilitator. The authors of RAP placed a strong emphasis on the recognition and utilization of existing strengths and promotion of psychological skills and resources. Accordingly, the RAP program is embedded in positive language throughout, and all skills are framed in the

Table 6.1 Skills taught in the RAP program

Skill	Teaching strategies	Underlying theory		
		CBT	IP	Self
Personal strengths	Participants are helped to recognize and build on their existing strengths and personal resources. The aim of this part of the program is to help adolescents to focus on the importance of developing and maintaining good self-esteem.			✓
Cognitive restructuring	Participants are helped to recognize and challenge negative or distorted thinking and to develop positive self-talk.	✓		✓
Keeping calm	Strategies for keeping calm are taught including using self-management and self-regulation techniques. This involves learning to recognize physical symptoms, and how to manage these (e.g., through relaxation, humour and other stress reduction techniques).	✓		✓
Problem-solving	Participants are encouraged to define their problems, consider solutions, and use a step-by-step approach for carrying out and evaluating the solution.	✓		✓
Support networks	The importance of developing a support network is emphasized and participants are encouraged to seek help when necessary to maintain their emotional well-being.		✓	✓
Interpersonal component	This component covers a number of issues. Participants are encouraged to understand role transitions brought about by the adolescent developmental challenge of developing autonomy while maintaining connectedness. Participant's skills in perspective-taking are enhanced and they are taught ways of preventing and managing conflict.	✓	✓	✓

CBT, cognitive–behaviour therapy; IP, interpersonal perspectives; Self, self-management and preservation of self-esteem.

positive (e.g., 'Keep the peace', 'Positive self-talk', etc.). While the program was originally developed and funded as part of a national initiative to prevent depression and suicide, the program does not specifically mention depression or suicide at any point. Rather, the program is promoted to teenagers as an opportunity to learn skills that will increase their self-esteem, help them to manage and solve problems, and improve interpersonal relationships.

As part of this positive approach, RAP is written around a metaphor derived from the children's story, 'The Three Little Pigs'. The 'resourceful little pig' built a house out of bricks rather than straw or sticks, and being strong and resilient, was able to withstand the onslaught of the wolf. Throughout the RAP Program, participants develop their own personal 'RAP house' (see Figure 6.1) by laying down *personal resource* bricks (e.g., 'Personal Strength Bricks', 'Keeping Calm Bricks', and 'Problem-Solving Bricks').

In keeping with the strategy of funnelling coping skills through self-regulation and self-esteem, another device that we use throughout the program is to introduce students to the concept of the 'Selfenometer' (see Figure 6.2). This ten-point scale is introduced to students to help them regularly monitor their self-esteem level. At the beginning and end of each session, participants circle the number that relates to the way they feel on the Selfenometer printed in their Workbook. There are two main aims of the Selfenometer. First, the Selfenometer increases participants' awareness of fluctuations in their feelings of well-being from day to day and from situation to situation. Second, it normalizes this experience and encourages participants to be aware of their self-esteem, and to self-regulate in times of stress.

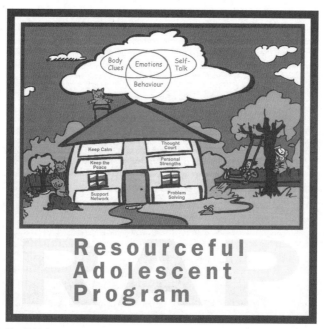

Figure 6.1 The RAP house.

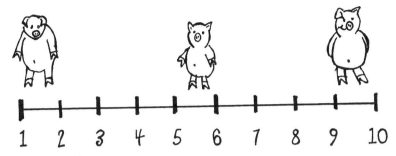

Figure 6.2 The Selfenometer.

Implementing RAP

Program structure, group size, and age of participants

RAP consists of eleven 50–60 minute sessions designed to be implemented in the classroom once a week for 11 weeks as part of the school curriculum. Ideally, RAP groups are limited to approximately 10–15 participants so that group leaders are able to provide individual attention and positive regard to all adolescents in the group. Groups are usually created by dividing a regular class in half. RAP was developed to be administered to 12–15-year-old (Year 8 and Year 9) adolescents as part of the school curriculum. Year 8 and Year 9 students are the primary target group as the incidence of depression increases sharply after age 15 years (Burke et al., 1990; Lewinsohn et al., 1994a), and the program is designed to forestall this acceleration in the development of depression. However, RAP has been implemented in a wide range of settings (e.g., detention centres, community mental health centres, employment services), and formats (e.g., three-day camps, five-day residential programs with adolescents from rural areas, indicated groups in mental health settings).

Group leaders and group processes

RAP is facilitated by mental health professionals or teachers who have completed an approved training course. Group leaders come from a range of professional backgrounds, including psychology, education, social work, and community mental health, and must be skilled in the areas of communication and group facilitation, and in managing potentially difficult situations. There is conflicting evidence regarding the effectiveness of teachers versus mental health professionals in delivering RAP. For example, Harnett & Dadds (2004) failed to find a positive effect for RAP when delivered by teachers, but the results of a subsequent placebo control trial by Merry et al. (2004b) indicated that when delivered by teachers, and compared to a placebo control, RAP-Kiwi (an adaptation for New Zealand teenagers) demonstrated a persisting effect on depressive symptomatology that was small but statistically significant. Further, in our initial effectiveness trial, the allied health support workers and teachers who had been appropriately trained were compared and no statistically significant differences were found. However, it is important when using teachers as groupfacilitators, to ensure that appropriate training and ongoing supervision are provided.

An important component of the RAP program is the group leader's unconditional positive regard, focus on strengths, and modelling of positive coping skills. The group process is experiential and positive throughout and creates many opportunities for the facilitator to validate and affirm participants. Group leaders work with participants in an empathic and encouraging way to demonstrate that they are not alone in the difficulties they may be experiencing and that they have access to support, encouragement, and understanding from their group leader. Skills such as active listening, step-by-step problem-solving, seeing the other person's point of view and focusing on strengths and resources are all processes that can be modelled by an effective group leader. Prompting and rewarding the use of skills being introduced in the RAP program is another important function of the group leader. The RAP process creates endless opportunities for group leaders to validate and affirm participants. We see this process component as a vital part of successfully implementing RAP.

Each session consists of group activities that enable participants to practice the skills being taught, experience how these skills can help, and relate each new skill to building their level of self-esteem as they respond to different situations. We do not make extensive use of homework exercises, but some sessions may have some brief homework components, centring around the identification of more positive coping resources.

Group composition

As mentioned, ideally RAP groups are limited to approximately 10–15 participants. Factors to consider in forming RAP groups include existing friendships, psychosocial functioning, and behaviour issues. For example, placing a number of students with conduct problems in a RAP group can be detrimental to the experience of other participants. However, diversity in RAP groups can be advantageous (e.g., if members of a RAP group vary in their level of coping skills, this can provide opportunities for less confident adolescents to learn from the responses and behaviours of their more resilient peers). Teachers are often an important resource for information about which adolescents will work well together in a RAP group.

Some researchers (e.g., Chaplin et al., 2006) have suggested that early adolescent girls achieve more positive outcomes from depression prevention interventions when they are in all-girl groups. In their study of 208 11–14 year olds, Chaplin et al. found that participants who completed the Penn Resiliency Program in either single-gender or co-ed groups reported significantly lower levels of depressive symptoms than the control group at post-intervention. Interestingly however, at post-intervention, girls in single-gender groups reported significantly lower levels of hopelessness than girls in co-ed groups and the control group. The single-gender group also exhibited higher attendance rates with girls in single-gender groups attending an average of two more sessions (of the 12-session program) than co-ed participants.

RAP resources

All the information required to run the RAP Program is detailed in a Group Leader's Manual (Shochet et al., 1997a). Each participant is given a Participant Workbook (Shochet et al., 1997b), which contains information and space to write responses to activities.

Participants are encouraged to keep their Workbook at the end of the program as a resource for them to refer to as required. A RAP DVD is provided with the Group Leader Manual, which presents scenarios that form the basis of some of the activities conducted in the program[1].

Recruitment

Successful implementation of RAP requires substantial groundwork in establishing a mutually trusting and supportive relationship with all stakeholders, in particular with school administration, teachers, and potential group leaders. If measures are used, it is essential that protocol is strictly followed in terms of obtaining appropriate permission from relevant authorities and consent from participants and their parents if required. If RAP is run as part of the school curriculum (without the use of any measures), such consent is not considered necessary by most school systems. Implementing RAP involves cost in terms of releasing staff from other duties, rearranging timetables, and organising rooms and other resources. To motivate schools to commit to this cost, it is important to stress the positive outcomes and potential benefits of implementing RAP. As stated earlier, RAP is promoted as a positively-focused resilience-building program.

Screening

Screening measures may be used for identifying changes in RAP participants' depressive symptomatology and coping skills after completing the program or to identify students at risk and limit participation to these individuals (indicated intervention). Screening measures used in the RAP research trials include The Child Depression Inventory (CDI; Kovacs, 1992), the Reynold's Adolescent Depression Scale (RADS; Reynolds, 1987), and the Beck Hopelessness Scale (BHS; Beck et al., 1974). It should be noted that while measurement is valuable from a clinical or research perspective, the ecological validity of routine screening in universal interventions must be considered in terms of the increased burden it places on schools.

Ethical issues in screening and conducting RAP

Participants' rights to privacy must be balanced with a duty of care to intervene when individuals are considered 'at-risk' (Shochet & O'Gorman, 1995). If screening procedures are implemented, participants are made aware of how the information they provide will be used and what will happen if their responses indicate the need for clinical intervention. Another process adopted is to obtain written consent from parents and students, agreeing that if an individual is identified as 'at-risk', a letter will be sent to their parents suggesting they seek further assessment.

Prior to screening or commencement of the RAP program, group leaders and their organization devise a procedure for responding if they become aware that a participant is in need of additional clinical intervention. In many cases, usual organizational procedures can be followed. For example, if a school psychologist running RAP identifies an at-risk student, they respond according to their standard procedures. Under some circumstances, group leaders make arrangements with other agencies (e.g., community mental health services) to provide individual intervention to adolescents if required.

[1] Further information about RAP Resources is available on the RAP website: www.rap.qut.edu.au

Session-by-session delivery of the RAP program

An overview of the RAP content is provided in Table 6.2. Each session is described in further detail below. Each RAP session begins with a review of the previous session, overview of the current session, and participants recording their Selfenometer rating. At the end of each session, the group leader briefly summarizes, and participants record their Selfenometer rating again.

Session One: Getting to know you

Key Messages: We're interested in you!

Let's work together in a team

Theoretical basis The aim of this session is to introduce the RAP program in an appealing, positive way and to establish an expectation that the RAP experience will be different to normal classes. In this session, the group leader begins to develop a working alliance with participants as this has been shown to correlate positively with therapeutic change (Castonguay et al., 2006). In the therapy literature, there is also good evidence to show that the alliance established early in an intervention is of primary importance (Klein et al., 2003). The establishment of the working alliance made possible in small groups is considered an indispensable part of the program and distinguishes RAP from universal programs that are conducted in large class-sized groups (e.g., Clarke et al., 1995; Spence et al., 2003).

Session content The RAP program is introduced to participants and rapport is built through 'getting-to-know-you' and team-building games. This is a very light-hearted session, which aims to create an atmosphere of trust and warmth that can be drawn on in later sessions. Examples of some exercises include brainteasers, word puzzles, and physical challenges (e.g., untying themselves from a knot formed by intertwining joined hands).

Session Two: Building self-esteem

Key Messages: I'm Ok. I'm building on my strengths

Theoretical basis Researchers and practitioners are increasingly focusing on strength-building strategies and it has been suggested that we must bring the building of strength to the forefront in the prevention of mental illness (Johnson, 2003). Further, the resiliency literature suggests that the promotion of self-esteem and self-efficacy in young people is probably the key ingredient in any effective intervention process (Werner & Johnson, 2004). This session has two major foci, namely to help students identify their existing strengths and coping resources, and to introduce the notions of self-esteem and managing self-esteem.

As research suggests that self-esteem may mediate many of the intrapsychic and interpersonal risk factors in depression, funnelling skills through improvement of self-esteem and self-regulation is a cornerstone of the RAP program. This second session therefore introduces the importance of self-esteem and self-regulation (but called self-esteem as adolescents are able to relate to this term). Through the

Table 6.2 Sessions, key messages and aims in the Resourceful Adolescent Program (RAP)

Session	Key message	Goals
1. Getting to know you	We're interested in you! Let's work together in a team.	Establish rapport and build trust between group members and group facilitator.
2. Building self-esteem	I'm OK. I'm building on my strengths.	Introduction to program elements, ground rules for group established, concepts of self-esteem, and personal strengths explored.
3. Introduction to the RAP model	Our body clues and our self-talk affect the way we feel and behave.	Links between behaviour, body clues, self-talk and emotions are explored, concepts of 'risky' and 'resourceful' responses are introduced.
4. Keeping calm	Be a detective. Find your body clues and keep calm.	Detailed exploration of body signals related to positive and negative feelings. Strategies to relax and manage stress and anger are explored.
5. Self-talk	I am what I think.	Exploration of how thoughts affect feelings and behaviour, and the skills of cognitive restructuring.
6. Thinking resourcefully	You can change your thinking.	Continues from Session 5 with a focus on challenging risky negative thoughts and promoting positive self-talk.
7. Finding solutions to problems	There are solutions to my problems.	Outlining of a problem-solving model and applying it to interpersonal situations.
8. Support networks	There is always help at hand.	Identification and development of a social support network for good times and bad times.
9. Considering the other person's perspective	There are two sides to every story. Take time out, stop and think.	Developing skills to identify the body clues, self-talk and emotions that the other person might be experiencing in interpersonal situations.
10. Keeping the peace and making the peace	Keep the peace and make the peace.	Strategies to prevent or manage conflict or to move on from conflict situations.
11. Putting it all together	Being a resourceful adolescent really works! Let's celebrate.	Review of program content, termination and celebration.

Selfenometer, participants are encouraged to develop self-reflection. This process also normalizes the notion of constant fluctuations in self-worth. Students develop skills of detecting changes to self-esteem and ways of regulating self-esteem. They become aware when their 'Selfenometer has taken a bit of a dive', and to take steps 'to improve the Selfenometer when experiencing a setback'.

Session content Session Two begins by providing an overview of the RAP Program content and explaining the RAP process. The idea of coping resources is introduced and RAP is presented as an opportunity for participants to increase their current resources. A group discussion explores what participants think RAP will teach them and how it will help them personally.

Ground rules are established by the group. This often includes establishing rules such as 'what is said in the group stays in the group', 'don't put each other down', 'don't interrupt', etc.

Participants then discuss questions about self-esteem. These questions aim to explain self-esteem and show how high self-esteem can help us to be resourceful and cope well in difficult situations. In this context, the 'Selfenometer' and the RAP metaphor of 'The Three Little Pigs' are introduced. The story is presented as a metaphor for the RAP house they will be building throughout the program. The RAP house consists of all the 'coping resource bricks' that they will build over the duration of the program. This activity is conducted in a light-hearted way with participants encouraged to help retell the popular children's story. It is important to note that the metaphor is not vital to the program's implementation and can be omitted or changed if it is considered inappropriate. For example, Indigenous Australians who adapted RAP replaced the house metaphor with a tree metaphor and participants developed resource leaves and branches to build a strong, resilient tree.

Session Two continues with participants filling in their 'Personal Strengths Bricks'. Students are helped to recognize that they already have many existing strengths and coping resources. Students then identify how their Selfenometer may have improved simply by recognising their various strengths. These Personal Strengths Bricks are illustrated in Participant Workbooks and cover several categories (creative, sporting, academic, achievements, family, personal, identity, recreational hobbies, humour, interpersonal, friendship, and other strengths). Examples of personal strengths are given in each category to prompt participants (e.g., Academic—I do my best at school, Personal—There are things I can do well, and Sporting—I am a good team member). Space is provided for individuals to write their own ideas. Prompts are particularly important for participants who are demoralized and for whom identification of strengths is compromised by their depressive lens. Listing personal strengths can be unfamiliar for adolescents, and so this activity is revisited in Session Three when participants have an opportunity to expand on their lists.

Session Three: Introduction to the RAP model

Key Message: Our body clues and our self-talk affect the way we feel and behave

Theoretical basis This session prepares participants for the cognitive-restructuring and other cognitive–behavioural components of the program. It is essentially an

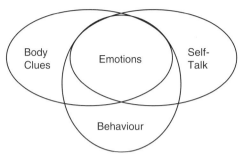

Figure 6.3 The RAP model.

introduction to CBT. Participants are introduced to the RAP Model (see Figure 6.3), a Venn diagram that was derived from the cognitive model of emotion and behaviour (Burns, 1980). Participants are given an overview of the RAP Model in this session and then have the opportunity to explore its components in greater detail in subsequent sessions.

Session content This session begins with a scenario (either from the supplementary DVD provided or a short video segment or role-play chosen by the group leader) that demonstrates a typical teenage situation (e.g., a friend breaks an agreement). The RAP Model is introduced in an interactive way, using language that adolescents understand and is used as a tool for exploring and understanding the way that body clues and self-talk interact with emotions and behaviours. Group leaders take this opportunity to normalize the problems many teenagers experience and use the RAP Model to demonstrate 'risky' and 'resourceful' ways of managing situations with reference to the three circles. This is further explored in a small group discussion.

The group leader asks participants to list some situations in which teenagers commonly feel stressed or worried or upset. As responses are given, the group leader relates them to the model and demonstrates how the circles of the model all fit together. Session Three ends on a positive note with participants expanding on their Personal Strengths bricks from Session Two.

Session Four: Keeping calm

Key Messages: Be a detective. Find your body clues and keep calm

Theoretical basis Stressful life events are a known risk factor for the development of depression and the way that individuals respond to stress can significantly impact on their future adjustment and psychopathology (Garber, 2006). The finding that the link between stress and depression increases in adolescence suggests that teaching stress management and emotional regulation skills in early adolescence is an important component of depression prevention. Relaxation training (in which participants learn the relationship between stress, muscle tension, and depression, and develop specific skills to facilitate self-calming) has been shown to be as effective as CBT in reducing adolescent depressive symptoms (Reynolds & Coats, 1986). Further, relaxation training reduces anxiety (Reynolds & Coats), which is a known risk factor for depression (Flannery-Schroeder, 2006).

Session content Session Four begins with another typical teenage scenario from the supplementary DVD or provided by the group leader. The scenario covers a situation that might provoke stress and anxiety, such as asking somebody out to the movies. The discussion then elicits an understanding of the 'Body clues' (i.e., physiological symptoms) invoked in this scenario. Participants generate a list of body clues that the adolescent might be experiencing in the situation being discussed. Students then identify their own personal stress indicators.

The next activity in Session Four involves asking participants to list the things they do to manage their body clues and help themselves to stay calm generally. Responses are written into the 'body clues' bubble of the RAP Model. The group leader self-discloses situations in which they have successfully used relaxation strategies to calm themselves down.

The session then gives participants an opportunity to try some common CBT relaxation techniques. The techniques provided include breathing exercises, deep muscle relaxations, visualizations, etc.

Session Four ends with participants filling in their 'Keep Calm Bricks' with ideas for strategies they can use to keep calm (some that they already use and some new ones from the list made earlier in the session). The Keep Calm Bricks cover a range of areas: relaxation, distraction, humour, support network, visualization, and other calming techniques.

Session Five: Self-talk

Key Message: I am what I think

Theoretical basis According to cognitive theories of depression, individuals who have negative beliefs about the self, world, and future, and make global, stable, internal attributions for negative events appraise stressors and their consequences negatively and are more likely to become depressed than those who do not have such a negative cognitive style (Garber, 2006). The aim of this session is to encourage participants to develop the habit of identifying negative thoughts, and learn appropriate ways to challenge these thoughts and replace them with more resourceful alternatives. Drawing extensively on the work of Beck (see Burns, 1980), this session provides a user-friendly way of encouraging participants to identify negative automatic thoughts.

Session content Session Five begins with the presentation of a potentially risky situation (using the DVD or role play). In this session, the focus is on the 'Self-talk' bubble of the RAP Model and participants are asked to generate a list of possible negative self-talk the teenager might be using in the situation.

Once a list of possible negative self-talk (negative automatic thoughts) has been compiled, the group leader sets up a 'Thought Court' activity (Wexler, 1991), where participants play the role of prosecutor and the group leader plays the role of the teenager. 'Thought Court Bricks' are distributed to participants, containing challenger questions including 'Are you exaggerating?', 'Are you jumping to conclusions?', 'Are you making things out to be worse than they really are?', and 'Is the way you're thinking helpful?'. The group leader works through the list of negative self-talk and responds to the questions as participants ask them. This activity provides a fun example of how we can challenge our negative self-talk.

A group discussion is held to explore ways in which teens can challenge their negative automatic thoughts. Participants record these, and are prompted to suggest alternative responses in terms of the CBT model. Participants discuss resourceful actions to take and complete the RAP Model by filling in the 'Behaviour' bubble.

Session Six: Thinking resourcefully

Key Message: You can change your thinking

Theoretical basis The focus of Session Six is on teaching cognitive restructuring skills. On the basis of Burns (1980), the technique employed involves completing a table consisting of seven columns: situation, risky thought, risky behaviour, risky feeling, resourceful thought, resourceful behaviour, and resourceful feeling.

Session content Each of the columns is explained to participants. Two completed examples (e.g., 'your friends have not invited you to the movies') are given in Participant Workbooks to demonstrate the kind of 'risky' and 'resourceful' responses that participants might write in each column. The group works through these examples together.

Next, participants are asked to work through the table, filling in each column for two common teenage situations: 'You get a bad mark for an assignment that you really worked hard on' and 'Your Mum shouts at you for something that you didn't do'. The group is given an opportunity to discuss their responses.

Finally, participants are asked to think of two situations of their own and fill in the table. Group leaders are encouraged to be particularly vigilant in this exercise, providing individual assistance and attention to each adolescent as they work independently on their chosen situation and identify their negative automatic thoughts and their challenges to these thoughts.

Session Seven: Finding solutions to problems

Key Message: There are solutions to my problems

Theoretical basis A positive problem-solving orientation provides protective factors that reduce the impact of negative life circumstances (d'Zurilla & Maydeu Olivares, 1995; Spence et al., 2003; Werner, 1995). Further, improving adolescents' problem-solving skills has been shown to reduce depressive symptoms, at least in the short-term (Spence et al.). The aim of this session is to introduce a model for effective problem-solving.

Session content After brainstorming a list of different ways of solving problems, participants are given a problem-solving task. They are given materials (such as a candle, a match box, and a thumb tack) and asked to attach the candle to the wall so that the candle is upright and able to be lit. In small teams, participants are given time to consider possible solutions and demonstrate their chosen strategy to the group. The group then discusses the techniques and processes that each team used to solve the problem and decide what the most effective ways of solving the problem were. Through this discussion, the group leader introduces the idea of a step-by-step problem-solving process and the need for divergent and creative thinking when solving problems. This idea is introduced to participants in the form of 'Problem-Solving Bricks' consisting of the following: the problem, possible solutions, possible consequences/outcomes, first choice, action plan, and did it work? The group leader explains that problem-solving fits into the Behaviour Bubble of the RAP Model.

The group then applies the problem-solving process to a typical teenage interpersonal problem (e.g., conflict with parents over appropriate volume for playing music). The problem is broken down using the Problem-Solving Bricks and participants write responses in their Workbooks.

Session Eight: Support networks

Key Message: There is always help at hand

Theoretical basis Social support is a significant predictor of depressive symptoms and these factors can reciprocally influence each other, creating feedback mechanisms that increase the risk of experiencing depression over time (Galambos et al., 2004). Late adolescence is particularly important for establishing support networks beyond the immediate family (Galambos et al.), and so prosocial coping is an important skill to impart to 12–15 year olds.

The inclusion of these components is supported by the resiliency literature. Children who thrive despite adversity are skilled in establishing a support network that provides positive role models and affectional ties that encourage trust, autonomy, and initiative (Werner, 1995). In addition to identifying social supports in difficult times, Session Eight also emphasizes the importance of sharing positive experiences. This is based on self-psychology's theory that we need people in our lives, who can provide a 'mirror' to reflect a sense of self-worth and value, creating internal self-respect (Baker & Baker, 1987).

Session content At the start of Session Eight, participants are asked to think about the people they like to have around when something really good happens and what they do to share in their excitement. Participants write these people's names into an appropriate 'Support Network Brick' in their Participant Workbook. Support Network Bricks include family, agencies, professional helpers, friends, and other people we know.

Next, participants are asked to brainstorm answers to the question: 'How can people in your support network help you when you are going through a bad time?' Group leaders introduce the idea of people in our support network being like emotional bandages that help us to heal when we are hurt. Participants are given time to think about who they would turn to in a number of different difficult situations listed in their Workbooks. For each situation, they list who they would turn to, why, and how this person would help. Participants are encouraged to be creative and generate a broad list of support people.

Each adolescent is asked to identify one person in their support network that they turn to when they are in a difficult situation and tell the group how they feel this person helps them. The group leader stresses the importance of continuing to find someone who can help if the first person approached isn't able to do so.

To end the session in a positive and light-hearted way, humour is introduced as a strategy for managing stress even though it is not technically related to the overall session content. Participants are shown a humorous excerpt from a video on the importance of humour in managing stress.

Session Nine: Considering the other person's perspective

Key Messages: *There are two sides to every story*

Take time out—Stop and think

Theoretical basis High levels of interpersonal conflict place adolescents at increased risk for depression. When conflict arises, adolescent behaviours that undermine autonomy (e.g., over personalising a disagreement, recanting a position, and appearing persuaded that their position is wrong) have been shown to predict increases in depressive symptoms (Allen et al., 2006). Behaviours that undermine relatedness (e.g., overt expressions of hostility, rudely interrupting, or ignoring) have also been shown to predict increases in depressive symptoms (Allen et al.).

Strategies for preventing and managing interpersonal conflict are important keys to the prevention of depression as social problems have been shown to have a reciprocal relationship with depression such that interpersonal difficulties precede depression and in turn, depression contributes to interpersonal difficulties (Garber, 2006). Late adolescence is a particularly important time for maintaining strong relationships with family members (Galambos et al., 2004), and a time when peer relationships become increasingly complex and intense (Allen et al., 2006), and so early adolescence is the optimal time to impart these skills.

Session content In Session Nine, the group leader encourages participants to apply the RAP Model to interpersonal situations. The message given to participants is that to manage situations resourcefully, it is important to understand the other person's perspective. Participants are introduced to the idea that being aware of the other person's body clues, self-talk, emotions and behaviour, facilitates the process of finding a solution that will satisfy all parties.

Participants are shown a series of optical illusions (e.g., the familiar picture that can be interpreted as a young lady or an old lady) to demonstrate that even though two people are looking at the same picture, they don't always see the same thing. This is used as a metaphor for interpersonal situations.

The group leader asks participants to brainstorm situations in which teenagers might have a problem with another person and they might go around in circles trying to solve it. They are also asked to think about what people's Selfenometer ratings might be when they are having interpersonal problems. The link between self-esteem and conflict is introduced by the group leader explaining that people fight when their Selfenometer is low and that their rating can go even lower as the conflict continues. The importance of solving interpersonal problems as soon as possible is stressed and the group leader explains that if we cannot solve a problem ourselves, then we turn to someone from our support network, who can help us to resolve the issue.

To apply these new ideas, the group selects a common dyadic interpersonal conflict situation and discusses what body clues and self-talk each person might be experiencing and how they might behave and feel. The group then brainstorms a list of things that make it difficult to see the two sides of a story when people are personally involved (e.g., becoming emotional, not listening properly). The group leader encourages discussion about the importance of the body clues, self-talk, emotions, and behaviours of each person in the situation, and the interaction between them. Participants are helped to draw the conclusion that neither person in the situation is necessarily right or wrong, they just see things differently because there are usually two sides to every story. Finally, participants fill in the diagram in their Workbooks with ideas for resourceful steps the people in the difficult situation explored earlier in the session could take to stop them from going around in circles.

Session Ten: Keeping the peace and making the peace

Key Messages: Keep the peace and make the peace

Theoretical basis While there is a commonly held myth that teenagers want nothing to do with their parents, the research literature indicates the exact opposite (Johnson, 2003). Teenagers need their parents, but the ways in which they need them evolves as they negotiate the major developmental task of adolescence: attaining autonomy while maintaining attachment. The strain associated with the task of establishing autonomy while maintaining positive relationships with their parents can lead to depressive symptoms in adolescents (Allen et al., 2006). Learning to manage negotiations around autonomy with parents and peers is a significant task with implications for the development of depressive symptoms (Allen et al.). The aim of this session is to increase participants' awareness and understanding of this developmental task, normalize the adolescent experience, and encourage resourceful ways of 'keeping the peace' and 'making peace' in relationships.

Session content Session Ten extends the material from Session Nine regarding finding ways to see the other person's perspective and to avoid going around in circles in conflict situations. The group leader asks participants to list some of the main things parents and teenagers disagree about, drawing out issues surrounding connectedness and independence, and the related anxieties parents might experience. The aim of this discussion is for participants to understand that there are two parts to the problem: the teenager wants to become more independent and the parents want to protect the adolescent by making decisions they think are best for them.

The group is then broken into two small groups to conduct a role-play of a conflict situation between an adolescent and their parent. One participant plays the teenager, one plays the parent and the remaining adolescents and group leader direct the play. Once it is obvious that the two actors are going around in circles, the teenager is to ask for 'Time Out'. The group leader stimulates a discussion about what happened in the role-play and normalizes conflict between teenagers and their parents.

Participants are directed to the 'Keep the Peace' and 'Make the Peace Bricks' in their Workbooks. These bricks give adolescents ideas for ways to deal with situations in more positive ways and help them to solve problems with other people resourcefully so that both parties are satisfied with the solution (e.g., strategies for overcoming conflict or signalling that a conflict is resolved). The participants act out the role-play again, this time using their Keep the Peace and Make the Peace Bricks. The group leader debriefs the role-play and stimulates discussion around the issues of keeping the peace and promoting harmony. Session Ten finishes with an individual activity in which participants are asked to think about a time when they had a disagreement with a parent where they were able to achieve a resourceful solution with which everyone was happy. Participants share and discuss their positive stories.

Session Eleven: Putting it all together

> Key Messages: Being a resourceful adolescent really works!
>
> Let's celebrate!

Theoretical basis The aim of this session is to give participants an opportunity to collate the skills learnt throughout the program, using their 'bricks' to build their resourceful RAP house. An important function of this session is to leave participants feeling that their contributions to the group were valuable and to feel confident about using their new skills. The group leader moves among the group and personally thanks every adolescent for participating in the program and provides positive feedback about their contributions.

Session content In Session Eleven, participants complete an evaluation of the program. The group leader then briefly goes through the Workbooks with participants, reviewing and discussing each session. Participants copy all of the Resource Bricks they can use to help them to be a more resourceful adolescent onto the integrated RAP house in their Workbooks. Once participants have completed their RAP house, the group celebrates their successes with a party. Optional games are provided in the Group Leader's Manual to be used if required.

Empirical support for the efficacy and effectiveness of the RAP program

Evaluation of the RAP Programs has been a priority. The efficacy and effectiveness of RAP have been investigated through several randomized controlled trials that statistically analysed intervention effects and clinical significance. The primary trials are summarized below. Taken together, the results suggest that RAP works well in the short- and medium-term when implemented by qualified mental health professionals or by trained teachers in small controlled studies. In larger rollouts using teachers, there are positive effects at post-testing but these are not as well-maintained at follow-up.

Initial efficacy trial

In 1997, an initial efficacy trial was conducted with 260 Year 9 students in a Brisbane high school (Shochet et al., 2001). This cohort-based randomized controlled trial compared two intervention conditions: RAP-A (in which adolescents received the RAP program), and RAP-F (in which RAP was provided to students and their parents were invited to take part in a three-session RAP Program for Parents [RAP-P]), with a no-intervention comparison group (Adolescent Watch [AW]). Successive Year 9 cohorts formed the comparison and intervention groups.

Three depression measures were administered at pre-intervention, post-intervention, and 10-month follow-up: The Children's Depression Inventory (CDI; Kovacs, 1992), the Reynolds Adolescent Depression Scale (RADS; Reynolds, 1987), and the Beck Hopelessness Scale (BHS; Beck et al., 1974) to provide convergent measures of depressive symptoms.

The RAP Program was delivered by specially trained mental health professionals or clinical psychology graduates. The recruitment rate for RAP in this trial (88%) was much higher than in previous indicated interventions (e.g., Clarke et al., 1995; Jaycox et al., 1994), and a low attrition rate of 5.8% was achieved. However, the recruitment rate for parents to the RAP-P Program was poor with only 10% of adolescent participants having one or more parents attending all three workshops. Because of the resulting small sample size, it was not possible to evaluate the impact of adding RAP-P, and so the two intervention conditions were merged.

The results of this trial indicate that RAP was effective in reducing depressive symptoms. At post-intervention and 10-month follow-up, adolescents in the intervention conditions reported significantly lower levels of depressive symptoms as measured by the CDI and BHS, but not the RADS.

The effects of RAP were also of clinical significance, indicated by movement between healthy, subclinical, and clinical ranges on the depression measures. Adolescents in the intervention groups who reported elevated, but subclinical symptoms at pre-intervention, were less likely than those in the control group to have moved into the clinical range and more likely to have moved into the healthy range of scores at post-intervention and 10-month follow-up. Examination of adolescents in the intervention group, who were in the subclinical range at pre-intervention, showed that none reported clinical levels of symptoms at post-intervention or follow-up, and 71.4% and 75% moved into the healthy range at post-intervention and follow-up, respectively. By comparison, a significant portion of initially subclinical control group members moved into the clinical range at post-intervention and follow-up (10.5% and 17.6%, respectively) and fewer reported scores in the healthy range at post-intervention and follow-up (31.6% and 41.2%, respectively).

Participating in RAP also benefited adolescents who initially scored in the healthy range and therefore would not have been included in selective or indicated interventions. This is one of the identified benefits of universal interventions. At follow-up, only 1.2% of initially healthy adolescents (those who recorded scores below the subclinical range on depression measures at pre-intervention) in the intervention conditions had moved into the subclinical or clinical range compared with 10.1% of initially healthy adolescents in the control group. Instability of risk status is a disadvantage of targeted interventions as the power to predict future disorder is generally weak (Offord et al., 1998). As depressive symptoms are a known risk factor for future depressive disorders (Clarke et al., 1995), preventing even minor depressive symptoms may alter the trajectory towards future depressive disorders.

This trial indicated that a school-based universal preventive intervention could achieve penetration and retention rates not achieved with indicated interventions and could have clinically significant effects on both 'at-risk' and 'healthy' adolescents. The above trial made use of psychologists as facilitators, which would not be sustainable. Such programs would only be sustainable if teachers could implement the interventions. A study conducted by Harnett & Dadds (2004) raised the possibility that teachers may not be able to effectively implement the RAP program. A number of subsequent controlled trials using teachers and school personnel as facilitators have been conducted with more encouraging (although mixed) results.

New Zealand randomized blind placebo-controlled trial

A version of RAP (RAP-Kiwi) was developed for dissemination in New Zealand (Merry et al., 2004b). The efficacy of RAP-Kiwi was evaluated in a randomized placebo-controlled trial. In this trial, 392 students aged 13–15 from two schools were randomized to intervention (RAP-Kiwi) or placebo-control condition. While the placebo was similar to RAP-Kiwi in time and structure, all active components of the intervention (e.g., CBT) were removed. The RAP-Kiwi intervention and the placebo program were delivered by specially trained teachers, and students who were blind to their condition. The results indicated that RAP-Kiwi was effective in reducing clinically significant adolescent depressive symptoms. This study achieved a high recruitment rate (73%) and retention was also high (91% at six months and 72% at 18 months). Depressive symptoms were measured before and after the program and at 6-, 12-, and 18-month follow-up using the Beck Depression Inventory II (BDI-II; Beck et al., 1996) and the Reynolds Adolescent Depression Scale (RADS; Reynolds, 1987).

Students who participated in RAP-Kiwi recorded significantly greater improvements in depressive symptoms at post-intervention on both measures of depression compared to those in the placebo condition. Follow-up testing indicated that RAP-Kiwi participants' scores on the RADS remained lower than the placebo-control condition at all time points. However, no such ongoing positive effect was measured by the BDI-II.

In clinical terms, movement of students between the BDI-II minimal/mild and moderate/severe categories at post-test indicated a net improvement of 11 students in the intervention group, compared with a net deterioration of three students in the placebo group. Merry et al. (2004b) concluded that when RAP-Kiwi was delivered by teachers, it was effective in reducing depressive symptoms and was a potentially effective public health intervention.

The results of this trial indicate that when delivered by teachers, and compared to a placebo control, RAP-Kiwi demonstrates a persisting effect on depressive symptomatology that is small but statistically significant.

Initial effectiveness trial

The two trials described above demonstrated the benefits of RAP in a controlled environment, with close supervision, and on a small scale. The next step was to establish whether RAP achieves its objectives in a cost-effective manner when conducted on a larger scale.

Montague and Shochet (2004) evaluated the effectiveness of RAP as a universal intervention with the use of school personnel (teachers and allied health support people, e.g., school psychologists, guidance officers, and nurses) as group leaders. The majority of group leaders were teachers, with mental health professionals used only in case of group leader absence or where schools were unable to provide sufficient teachers. Group leaders were trained as RAP facilitators in a one-day training course led by accredited RAP trainers. The effectiveness of teachers and allied health-support people was compared and no statistically significant differences were found.

Participants were drawn from five schools in the Catholic education system. Schools were allocated to the intervention group that received the RAP Program ($N = 525$) or a control group ($N = 481$). Recruitment rates were high (over 90%) and attrition was low. Depressive symptomatology was measured at pre-intervention, post-intervention, and six-month follow-up using the CDI (Kovacs, 1992), the RADS (Reynolds, 1987), and the BHS (Beck et al., 1974).

Preliminary analyses indicate that participants who received RAP recorded significantly lower levels of depressive symptoms at post-test than those in the control group. At follow-up, this effect was restricted to female participants only. Although the effect of RAP was much weaker in this trial than in the first efficacy trial, this study has provided some evidence that RAP can be effectively run using local resources under 'real world' conditions. There were no significant differences between school personnel and health professionals in their effect on depressive symptoms.

Three months after completion of the program, an independent interviewer asked 109 randomly selected RAP participants to provide behavioural examples of when they had used skills from the RAP Program. Qualitative results suggested that a large proportion of participants (60% of girls and 40% of boys) could identify important changes attributed to skills learnt in the RAP program. For example

> 'I had really low self-esteem about myself earlier this year. I'm not going to be big-headed or anything but we had this group thing and we had to write down about other people, what they're about and stuff and put in an envelope and I still look at it and stuff. I kind of think what do other people think about me. That's how my self-esteem boosts. When they write that about me—that I was nice—it really helped me out. I didn't realise people thought of me that way.'

> 'Like not thinking negatively, like if someone stands you up, don't think they don't like you, just think they missed the bus or something. Don't blame them. Someone stood me up twice. Before the program I would have been pissed and called her and just kept yelling at her. So it's a good program because it changed my life a bit.'
> 'I get into a lot of arguments with my brother and sister and sometimes my friends, but now I look to what will benefit me and say, 'okay, what are they going through?' so I don't get so upset as much. Before it always used to be my way.'

'With your parents and stuff, you should see their side of the story more.'

'Yes I was pretty stressed one night and I put on some really calm music and relaxed. Before I wouldn't have done anything.'

'That staying calm thing has helped me a lot. My dad, he's really angry and I've got his anger. I used to go around hitting people if I got angry or bashing in the wall in my room and I used to just yell and yell. Now I listen to music.'

'I wouldn't use it every day but I've used it before. At my best friend's party there was a bit of drug use … it got offered to me but I just passed it along and nothing was said. Before I would have probably used it if I didn't do RAP because I probably wasn't thinking then. Like afterwards it made me think about a lot of things like that'

It is interesting to note that the ability to increase self and other awareness was a common theme identified by the students. Thus, it appears that RAP also promotes mentalization, the ability to use knowledge about one's own and other's state of mind (Fonagy & Bateman, 2006).

Large multi-site effectiveness trial

To test the 'real world' effectiveness of RAP in a large rollout of the program using teachers as facilitators, a three-year multi-site effectiveness trial of RAP and our parallel parent program (RAP-P) was conducted. This randomized controlled trial was conducted with over 2,500 Year 8 students from two successive cohorts in 12 schools drawn from three Australian States. We are still in the early stages of examining the data using Multilevel modelling (which allows us to control for clustering effects of the data within schools) but we will briefly report some of our preliminary findings here.

Participants were randomly allocated on a matched schools basis to a control group or either RAP-A (in which adolescents received RAP) or RAP-F (in which students received RAP and their parents were invited to take part in three parent workshops and mailed a flexible delivery version of the parent program: RAP-P). Teachers of the Year 8 cohort who completed a one-day RAP group leaders' training workshop delivered the RAP program.

Depressive symptomatology and school connectedness were measured at pre-intervention, post-intervention (six months later), and 12-month follow-up. Results again suggested no additive effects of RAP-F over RAP-A, and so the two intervention groups were combined. Multilevel growth curve analysis, which uses hierarchical linear modelling (HLM; Bryk & Raudenbush, 1992), was conducted. HLM analyses showed an intervention effect (RAP vs. control) on a quadratic growth curve and not a linear growth curve at the three time points. This suggests that depression changed in a U-function across time. Individuals in the RAP condition had a decrease in depression at post-test. However, by follow-up, their depression had again increased. This contrasts the control group who did not experience a change in depression across time. Thus for the group as a whole, the intervention effect did not maintain at follow-up.

We examined the clinical significance of the findings for the at-risk group. Participants scoring in the clinical or subclinical range on the CDI (Kovacs, 1992) were classified as 'at-risk' (i.e., scores above 12). Scores of 12 and below were classified as 'healthy'. Approximately half (48%) of the at-risk students in the intervention group were healthy at post-intervention compared with 37% in the control group (a statistically significant difference). This pattern of results was similar at follow-up with 47% of initially at-risk RAP participants moving into the healthy range, compared with only 39% in the control group. However, chi-squared analysis revealed that the difference between intervention and control groups was no longer significant (probably because of the smaller sample size due to attrition at follow-up). We also examined the comparative number of at-risk participants that remained healthy at *both* post-intervention and follow-up. Over double the percentage of at-risk RAP participants remained healthy at both time points compared to the control (36% vs. 17%). This was statistically significant.

Thus, this study shows that a large roll-out using teachers has some significant impact for participants in the short-term that is clinically meaningful for the at-risk group. In the main, the effects generally wash out for the group as a whole but a significantly greater proportion of at-risk students become and stay healthy because of the RAP program.

Effectiveness of RAP in the Mauritian school environment

A small study using teachers that was conducted in Mauritius replicated the strong findings obtained in the first efficacy trial (Rivet, 2005). In this study, 80 Year 7 and 80 Year 9 students were randomly assigned to intervention and control (stratified by year level). Recruitment and retention rates of participants and completion of measures were exceptional (100%).

As hypothesized, RAP participants reported significant reductions in depression symptoms when compared to the control group. This study also demonstrated the clinical significance of RAP in terms of movement between clinical, subclinical, and healthy ranges of depressive symptomatology (as measured by the RADS-II; Reynolds, 2002; BHS; Beck et al., 1974; Hopelessness Scale for Children; Kazdin et al., 1983). None of the RAP participants who were in the healthy category at pre-intervention moved into the combined category (subclinical and clinical) at post-intervention compared to 11.3% of control group adolescents. By follow-up, these rates had increased to 16.1% for the control group compared to only 6.1% in the RAP Group. Further, 65.6% of RAP participants who scored in the subclinical or clinical range at pre-intervention moved into the healthy category at post-intervention compared to only 22.2% of the control group. Similarly, at six-month follow-up, 56.2% of initially subclinical or clinical RAP participants scored in the healthy range compared to 27.8% of control group participants.

Importantly, all teachers reported that they considered examples given in the manual to be culturally appropriate to the Mauritian context, and as a result felt able to deliver the program effectively without having to adapt material. However, a small proportion of students (26.3%) and teachers (12.5%) strongly agreed that a French version of the program would be beneficial as it is one of the most commonly spoken languages in Mauritius. A French translation of RAP has subsequently been developed. Qualitative findings in the Mauritian study were also positive with most components of the program being ranked positively by students. Participants graded cognitive skills as the most useful aspect of the program, specifically commenting on the RAP Model and challenging self-talk components. The majority of students (82.5%) enjoyed having their teacher as the group leader, and commented positively on the teacher's ability to listen, understand, and support them throughout the program.

Dutch indicated trial of RAP

A pilot study was conducted using a Dutch translation of RAP in an indicated trial with adolescents who met diagnostic criteria for an anxiety disorder and/or a major depressive episode (Muris et al., 2001). Analysis of pre- and post-intervention data showed that RAP participants reported decreases in anxiety and depression scores and an increase in self-efficacy. This trial indicates that the concepts of RAP translate well to the Dutch culture and is also suggestive of RAP's possible potential as an indicated intervention.

Summary of findings

In summary, the findings suggest we can be confident about RAP's efficacy in the short- and medium-term. (Like all presently available strategies these effects will probably diminish in the long-term in the absence of follow-up interventions.) There is good evidence of efficacy when conducted by mental health professionals. There is also evidence of effectiveness of the program when conducted by teachers, particularly in smaller trials. The program effects with teachers were better than placebo (Merry et al., 2004b) and a small trial in Mauritius using teachers (where there was a remarkable level of student and teacher compliance) showed results similar to the initial efficacy trial. In large trials using teachers, the results are more mixed with intervention effects at post-testing, but sustained effects only for subgroups of students. Thus, RAP is effective when conducted in a controlled environment by trained or carefully selected teachers, but large, unsupervised implementation has demonstrated small, but not necessarily sustained effects. These findings suggest the need for increased focus on teacher selection and training to ensure they are comfortable in presenting the RAP Program and the management of organizational issues that impact on schools in large scale implementation. It is important to note that quantitative results probably underestimate the perceived value to participants as indicated by their qualitative responses.

RAP has a number of characteristics that may explain why it has demonstrated relatively more promising intervention effects. To date, most universal depression prevention programs have focused on the use of cognitive–behavioural strategies (Spence & Shortt, 2007). However, because depression is a complex disorder with many causes, prevention programs need to target multiple components (Horowitz & Garber, 2006). RAP includes components of both cognitive–behavioural therapy and interpersonal components. We have also developed an over-arching integration of these frameworks by funnelling skills through self-regulation and management of self-esteem. This may offer a partial explanation for more promising efficacy and effectiveness of RAP.

In addition, while universal interventions for prevention of depression are typically conducted in schools as large-group presentations (Horowitz & Garber, 2006; Spence & Shortt, 2007), RAP is an experiential program and trials have been conducted with small groups (10–15 adolescents). This ensures that group leaders are able to connect with participants and offer sufficient time and attention to each individual. It is our view that running interventions in large class sizes that is typical of the usual composition for subject curricula would relegate interventions to surface level only. The smaller groups allow non-specific 'common factors' (e.g., increased connectedness to group leaders) to be harnessed with the skills-building components.

Dissemination and adaptations of RAP

RAP has been endorsed at the Australian Commonwealth level as an evidence-based program for preventing adolescent depression and has become widely used throughout Australia and internationally. The program has been translated into Chinese, Dutch, French, and Braille and we have specific adaptations for a New Zealand-based program to make it suitable for Maori students. Programs appear to have translated well culturally into other countries, with the notable exception of two well-conducted trials in China. In the Chinese trials (Wang & Shu, 2004), very good qualitative evaluations did not translate into measurable effects on depressive symptoms and raises the question of whether pathways to teenage depression are different in Chinese culture.

Within Australia, we have been mindful of the need to adapt the program for indigenous students. In response to regular requests since the RAP Programs were developed in 1997, a project was undertaken to develop an indigenous supplement for RAP. The demand for an indigenous adaptation had inspired a number of indigenous organizations and community groups from around Australia to develop their own resources and adapt the RAP program to suit their young people. For example, a community in Kempsey, New South Wales, felt the concepts in the RAP program could be readily translated and adapted into Aboriginal culture and folklore and generously gave us documented examples of their adaptation. Similarly, community workers in Woorabinda and elders in Kununurra in the Kimberleys, Western Australia, felt the RAP concepts translated well into existing concepts of coping. We contacted group leaders throughout the country who had conducted RAP with indigenous adolescents, surveyed the aspects of the program that worked well or needed adaptation, and collated the various adaptations from across the country.

Given the diversity of indigenous communities throughout Australia, it was not appropriate to develop a manual to be used universally with indigenous teenagers. Rather, the *RAP-A Indigenous Supplement: Guidelines for the Adaptation and Implementation of the RAP Program for Indigenous Adolescents* (Shochet et al., 2004) is a collection of ideas and adaptations derived from people's experiences in running RAP with indigenous teenagers throughout Australia. On the basis of knowledge of their participants and input from elders and other respected community members, RAP group leaders choose the most appropriate activities and adaptations from the Indigenous Supplement for each session.

Another highly successful adaptation and implementation of the RAP program is the *school camp structure*. The RAP Program has been adapted and facilitated in a school camp format in Queensland and Tasmania. For example, Lehman & Cowles (2001) conducted five three-day camps with 170 Year 9 students from schools in Tasmania. A participation rate of 98% was achieved and qualitative evaluations were extremely positive with participants' average overall evaluation of the program at 4.52 on a five-point scale. Student feedback indicates that RAP camps are beneficial to participants. For example

> 'In the camp you get to know all the people, teachers, guidance officers and social workers a lot better than you would just by going to single sessions and you get to meet new people'.
> 'RAP was great. It built my confidence and made me feel better about myself and accept the way I am. The time between sessions at camp gave us time to relax and calm down'.
> 'RAP made us realise that we have control over our thoughts and can make changes'.

Lehman & Cowles (2001) describe many advantages to conducting RAP in a camp format, including the provision of additional time, building relationships, increased self-referrals for support, personal enjoyment, and the opportunity to generalize skills to other camp activities outside of the RAP sessions. While RAP camps overcome some of the more commonly cited implementation difficulties (e.g., timetabling and room availability), they also present unique difficulties in terms of increased costs, and heavy workload for group leaders.

Future directions

Developing a computerized RAP to increase teacher-implemented effectiveness

Researchers have identified teacher variability with regard to program fidelity (accuracy and skill of program delivery) as a potential impediment to effective RAP dissemination. Our own surveys also suggest that teachers vary considerably in terms of their comfort level with the material and the process elements of managing groups. Based upon recent evidence regarding successful outcomes for interactive computer-based augmentation of cognitive–behaviour therapy for childhood anxiety (e.g., Spence et al., 2006), we hypothesize that a computerized version of RAP may offer a novel solution to the above mentioned constraining variables. The RAP team is currently developing an interactive CD ROM that involves a teacher-facilitated program of RAP but with students working in small groups around computers in the classroom. The model that we are developing involves a mix of interactive work on the computer, interspersed with teacher led discussions, and summaries in small and larger groups. Our plan is to use the computer to engagingly and creatively deliver the more technical aspects of RAP in a standardized format. This will free up the teachers to focus upon developing a positive teacher–student relationship—a 'common factor' that plays a significant role in the success of many interventions (Lambert and Ogles, 2004). Thus, we see that computerized implementation of RAP by teachers has the potential to optimally harness both specific skills and common factors of the 'therapeutic relationship' in the intervention.

Promoting school connectedness (RAP-T)

Related to the above emphasis of the teacher–student relationship, our research into the effectiveness of RAP has highlighted the importance of school connectedness (i.e., the extent to which students feel accepted, valued, respected, and included in the school), as a major variable not specifically addressed by the RAP program. We have published data from our multi-site effectiveness trial that shows that school connectedness is particularly important for depression (Shochet et al., 2006). School connectedness correlated extensively with depression (between 38% and 55% covariation) and predicted depressive symptoms one year later even after controlling for prior symptoms of depression. It is our view that school connectedness is arguably one of the most important variables in adolescent depression. In a subsequent study (Shochet et al., 2008), we found that school connectedness had an even stronger correlation to depression than parental attachment.

Consequently, a Resourceful Adolescent Program for Teachers (RAP-T) was developed, which aims to provide teachers with skills to foster school connectedness in their students. RAP-T was developed to increase teachers' recognition of the importance and value of school connectedness and their skills in promoting school connectedness. A trial of the RAP-T only (i.e., without the adolescent RAP program) has been funded by the Australian Research Council. While teachers describe a change in their teaching practices, this does not appear from the initial results to be impacting on teenage reports of school connectedness or on their depressive symptoms. (This trial did not involve all school personnel and thus limited the potential sources of impact on the students.)

Given the vital importance of school connectedness, our future research is aimed at 'unpacking' further the predictors of school connectedness at both the individual and school level. We believe that a subsequent comprehensive package of interventions might include some additions to the adolescent RAP program that focus on developing skills to enhance school connectedness, plus the RAP-T interventions for teachers delivered in a whole-of-school approach.

Summary and conclusion

We have developed the RAP as a positively-focused group program for prevention and early intervention of depressive symptoms in the early teenage years. We believe that one of the program strengths is that it integrates CBT and interpersonal perspectives. We have also been very mindful of the importance of positive relationships in the group process and therefore insist on manageable group sizes.

The evidence suggests that when delivered appropriately either by mental health professionals or by adequately trained and supervised teachers, the RAP program is effective in preventing clinically meaningful depressive symptoms in the short- and medium-term. While our research has mostly focused on universal interventions, we have some evidence that the program also works effectively as a targeted early intervention program for at-risk students.

The evidence of this integrative perspective in prevention of teenage depression seems to be more promising than CBT interventions on their own. Increasingly, we are becoming aware of the extent to which interpersonal factors are particularly salient for teenage depression (more so than for other disorders). Vicissitudes of interpersonal relationships seem to go hand in hand with vicissitudes of self-esteem and depressive symptoms. CBT skills play an important role when harnessed in the service of self-regulation and maintaining positive interpersonal relationships. The development of social supports, perspective-taking, and other interpersonal skills are important additional components to a comprehensive intervention.

The interpersonal processes needed in the optimal delivery of prevention and early intervention programs for teenage depression requires much more comprehensive research. In a disorder in which interpersonal issues are so germane, a more detailed understanding of the 'therapeutic' relationship needed in different delivery contexts will prove to be very important. Good program content will be substantially more effective when delivered with warmth, vitality, autonomy, support, and opportunities for individual connection (in the case of group programs).

Finally, no single psychosocial prevention intervention is likely to maintain effects over an extended period of time and a series of timely 'booster' interventions should be an integral part of any comprehensive early intervention approach.

References

Abrahms, D.B., Orleans, C.T., Niaura, R.S., Goldstein, M.G., Prochaska, J.O., & Velicer, W.F. (1996). Integrating individual and public health perspectives for treatment of tobacco dependence under managed healthcare. *Annals of Behavioral Medicine, 18*, 290–304.

Allen, J.P., Insabella, G., Porter, M.R., Smith, F.D., Land, D., & Phillips, N. (2006). A social-interactional model of the development of depressive symptoms in adolescence. *Journal of Consulting and Clinical Psychology, 74,* 55–65.

Andrews, G., Szabo, M., & Burns, J. (2002). Preventing major depression in young people. *British Journal of Psychiatry, 181,* 460–462.

Baker, H.S. & Baker, M.N. (1987). Heinz Kohut's self psychology: An overview. *The American Journal of Psychiatry, 144,* 1–9.

Beck, A.T., Steer, R.A., & Brown, G.K. (1996). *BDI-II Beck depression inventory* (2nd ed). San Antonio: The Psychological Corporation.

Beck, A.T., Weissman, A., Lester, D., & Trexler, L. (1974). The measurement of pessimism: The hopelessness scale. *Journal of Consulting and Clinical Psychology,* 42, 861–865.

Birmaher, B., Ryan, N.D., Williamson, D.E., Brent, D.A., Kaufman, J., Dahl, R.E., et al. (1996). Childhood and adolescent depression: A review of the past 10 years. Part 1. *Journal of the American Academy of Child and Adolescent Psychiatry, 35,* 1427–1439.

Broadhead, W.E., Blazer, D.G., George, L.K., & Tse, C.K. (1987). Depression, disability days, and days lost from work in a prospective epidemiologic survey. *Journal of the American Medical Association, 264,* 2524–2528.

Brown, C.H. & Liao, J. (1999). Principles for designing randomized preventive trials in mental health: An emerging developmental epidemiology paradigm. *American Journal of Community Psychology, 27*, 673–710.

Bryk, A.S. & Raudenbush, S.W. (1992). *Heirarchical linear models: Applications and data analysis methods.* Thousand Oaks, CA: Sage Publications.

Burbach, D.J., Kashani, J.H., & Rosenberg, T.K. (1989). Parental bonding and depressive disorders in adolescents. *Journal of Child Psychology and Psychiatry and Allied Disciplines, 30*, 183–204.

Burke, K.C., Burke, J.D., Regier, D.A., & Rae, D.S. (1990). Age at onset of selected mental disorders in five community populations. *Archives of General Psychiatry, 47*, 511–518.

Burns, D.D. (1980). *Feeling good: The new mood therapy.* New York, N.Y.: New American Library.

Burns, J.M., Andrews, G., & Szabo, M. (2002). Depression in young people: What causes it and can we prevent it? *Medical Journal of Australia, 177*, S93–S96.

Castonguay, L.G., Constantino, M.J., & Grosse Holtforth, M. (2006). The working alliance: Where are we and where should we go? *Psychotherapy: Theory, Research, Practice, Training, 43*, 271–279.

Chaplin, T.M., Gillham, J.E., Reivich, K., Elkon, A.G.L., Samuels, B., Freres, D.R., et al. (2006). Depression prevention for early adolescent girls: A pilot study of all girls versus co-ed groups. *Journal of Early Adolescence, 26*, 110–126.

Clarke, G.N., Hawkins, W., Murphy, M., Sheeber, L.B., Lewinson, P.M., & Seeley, J.R. (1995). Targeted prevention of unipolar depressive disorder in an at-risk sample of high school adolescents: A randomised trial of a group cognitive intervention. *Journal of the American Academy of Child and Adolescent Psychiatry, 34*, 312–321.

Coulehan, J.L., Schulberg, H.C., Block, M.R., Janosky, J.E., & Arena, V.C. (1990). Depressive symptomatology and medical comorbidity in a primary care clinic. *International Journal of Psychiatry in Medicine, 20*, 335–347.

D'Zurilla, T.J. & Maydeu Olivares, A. (1995). Conceptual and methodological issues in social problem-solving assessment. *Behavior Therapy, 26*, 409–432.

Essau, C.A. (2004). Primary prevention of depression. In D.J.A. Dozois & K.S. Dobson (Eds.). *The prevention of anxiety and depression: Theory, research, and practice* (pp. 185–204). Washington, DC: American Psychological Association.

Fonagy, P. & Bateman, A.W. (2006). Mechanisms of change in mentalization-based treatment of BPD. *Journal of Clinical Psychology, 62*, 411–430.

Flannery-Schroeder, E.C. (2006). Reducing anxiety to prevent depression. *American Journal of Preventive Medicine, 31*, S136–S142.

Galambos, N.L., Leadbeater, B.J., & Barker, E.T. (2004). Gender differences in and risk factors for depression in adolescence: A 4-year longitudinal study. *International Journal of Behavioral Development, 28*, 16–25.

Garber, J. (2006). Depression in children and adolescents: Linking research and prevention. *American Journal of Preventive Medicine, 31*, S104–S125.

Garber, J., Robinson, N.S., & Valentiner, D. (1997). The relation between parenting and adolescent depression: Self-worth as a mediator. *Journal of Adolescent Research, 12*, 12–33.

Hammen, C., Brennan, P.A., & Shih, J. (2004). Family discord and stress predictors of depression and other disorders in adolescent children of depressed and nondepressed women. *Journal of the American Academy of Child and Adolescent Psychiatry, 43*, 994–1002.

Harnett, P.H. & Dadds, M.R. (2004). Training school personnel to implement a universal school-based prevention of depression program under real-world conditions. *Journal of School Psychology, 42*, 343–357.

Horowitz, J.L. & Garber, J. (2006). The prevention of depressive symptoms in children and adolescents: A meta-analytic review. *Journal of Consulting and Clinical Psychology, 74*, 401–415.

Jaycox, L.H., Reivich, K.J., Gillham, J., & Seligman, M.E.P. (1994). Prevention of depressive symptoms in school children. *Behavior Research and Therapy, 32*, 801–816.

Johnson, N.G. (2003). On treating adolescent girls: Focus on strengths and resiliency in psychotherapy. *Journal of Clinical Psychology/In Session, 59*, 1193–1203.

Kazdin, A., French, N., Unis, A., Esvelt-Dawson, K., & Sherick, R. (1983). Hopelessness, depression, and suicidal intent among psychiatrically disturbed inpatient children. *Journal of Consulting and Clinical Psychology, 51*, 504–510.

Kenny, M.E. & Sirin, S.R. (2006). Parental attachment, self-worth, and depressive symptoms among emerging adults. *Journal of Counseling & Development, 84*, 61–71.

Klein, D.N., Schwartz, J.E., Santiago, N.J., Vivian, D., Vocisano, C., Castonguay, L.G., et al. (2003). Therapeutic alliance in depression treatment: Controlling for prior change and patient characteristics. *Journal of Consulting and Clinical Psychology, 71*, 997–1006.

Klerman, G.L. & Weissman, M.M. (1993). The place of psychotherapy in the treatment of depression. In G.L. Klerman & M.M. Weissman (Eds.). *New applications of interpersonal psychotherapy* (pp. 51–71). Washington, DC: American Psychiatric Press.

Kovacs, M. (1992). *The children's depression inventory*. New York: Multi-Health Systems.

Lambert, M.J. & Ogles, B.M. (2004). The efficacy and effectiveness of psychotherapy. In M.J. Lambert (Ed.). *Bergin and Garfield's handbook of psychotherapy and behavior change* (5th ed., pp. 139–193). New York: John Wiley & Sons.

Lehman, P. & Cowles, S. (2001, March). *Resilience-building camps using the Resourceful Adolescent Program*. Australian Infant, Child, Adolescent and Family Mental Health Association Fourth National Conference, Brisbane, Australia.

Lewinsohn, P.M., Clarke, G.N., Seeley, J.R., & Rohde, P. (1994a). Major depression in community adolescents: Age at onset, episode duration, and time to recurrence. *Journal of the American Academy of Child and Adolescent Psychiatry, 33*, 714–722.

Lewinsohn, P.M., Roberts, R.E., Seeley, J.R., Rhode, P., Gotlib, I.H., & Hops, H. (1994b). Adolescent psychopathology II: Psychosocial risk factors for depression. *Journal of Abnormal Psychology, 103*, 302–315.

Lopez, A.D., Ezzati, M., Rodgers, A., Vander Hoorn, S., & Murray, C.J.L. (2004). Conclusions and directions for future research. In M. Ezzati, A.D. Lopez, A. Rodgers, & C.J.L. Murray (Eds.). *Comparative quantification of health risks: Global and regional burden of disease attributable to selected major risk factors* (pp. 2231–2234). Geneva: World Health Organisation.

Lynch, G. (1998). The application of self-psychology to short-term counselling. *Psychodynamic counselling, 4*, 473–485.

MacPhee, A.R. & Andrews, J.J.W. (2006). Risk factors for depression in early adolescence. *Adolescence, 41*, 435–466.

Merry, S., McDowell, H., Hetrick, S., Bir, J., & Muller, N. (2004a). Psychological and/or educational interventions for the prevention of depression in children and adolescents. Cochrane Database of Systematic Reviews, Issue 2. Art. No.: CD003380. DOI: 10.1002/14651858.CD003380.pub2.

Merry, S., McDowell, H., Wild, C.J., Bir, J., & Cunliffe, R. (2004b). A randomized placebo-controlled trial of a school-based depression prevention program. *Journal of the American Academy of Child and Adolescent Psychiatry, 43*, 538–547.

Montague, R. & Shochet, I.M. (2004, September). *Preventing adolescent depression with sustainable resources: What have we learnt?* Fourth International Conference on Child and Adolescent Mental Health, Berlin.

Mrazek, P.J. & Haggerty, R.J. (1994). *Reducing risks for mental disorders: Frontiers for preventive intervention research.* Washington, DC: National Academy Press.

Mufson, L., Moreau, D., Weissman, M.M., & Klerman, G.L. (1993). Interpersonal psychotherapy for adolescent depression. In G.L. Klerman & M.M. Weissman (Eds.), *New applications of interpersonal psychotherapy* (pp. 130–166). Washington, DC: American Psychiatric Association Press.

Munoz, R.F., Hollon, S.D., McGrath, E., Rehm, L.P., & VandenBos, G.R. (1994). On the AHCPR depression in primary care guidelines: Further considerations for practitioners. *American Psychologist, 49*, 42–61.

Muris, P., Bogie, N., & Hoogsteder, A. (2001). Effects of an early intervention group program for anxious and depressed adolescents: a pilot study. *Psychological Reports, 88*, 481–482.

Offord, D.R., Kraemer, H.C., Kazdin, A.E., Jensen, P.S., & Harrington, R. (1998). Lowering the burden of suffering from child psychiatric disorder: Trade-offs among clinical, targeted and universal interventions. *Journal of the American Academy of Child and Adolescent Psychiatry, 37*, 686–694.

Palosaari, U., Aro, H., & Laippala, P. (1996). Parental divorce and depression in young adulthood: Adolescents' closeness to parents and self-esteem as mediating factors. *Psychiatrica Scandinavica, 93*, 20–26.

Prinstein, M.J. & Wargo Aikins, J. (2004). Cognitive moderators of the longitudinal association between peer rejection and adolescent depressive symptoms. *Journal of Abnormal Child Psychology, 32*, 147–158.

Rapee, R.M., Wignall, A., Sheffield, J., Kowalenko, N., Davis, A., McLoone, J., et al. (2006). Adolescents' reactions to universal and indicated prevention programs for depression: Perceived stigma and consumer satisfaction. *Prevention Science, 7*, 167–177.

Reynolds, W.M. (1987). *Reynolds adolescent depression scale: Professional manual.* Odessa, FL: Psychological Assessment Resources Inc.

Reynolds, W. (2002). *Reynolds adolescent depression scale* (2nd edition). Lutz, FL: Psychological Assessment Resources Inc.

Reynolds, W.M. & Coats, K.I. (1986). A comparison of cognitive-behavioral therapy and relaxation training for the treatment of depression in adolescents. *Journal of Consulting and Clinical Psychology, 54*, 653–660.

Rivet, E. (2005). *Preventing adolescent depression in Mauritius: The efficacy of a universal school-based program.* Unpublished master's thesis, University of Sydney.

Romano, D.M.C. (2004). A self-psychology approach to narcissistic personality disorder: A nursing reflection. *Perspectives in Psychiatric Care, 40*, 20–28.

Rose, G. (1992). *The strategy of preventive medicine.* Oxford: Oxford University Press.

Ryan, N.D. (2005). Treatment of depression in children and adolescents. *The Lancet, 366*, 933–940.

Shochet, I.M., Dadds, M.R., Ham, D., & Montague, R. (2006). School connectedness is an underemphasized parameter in adolescent mental health: Results of a community prediction study. *Journal of Clinical Child and Adolescent Psychology, 35*, 170–179.

Shochet, I.M., Dadds, M.R., Holland, D., Whitefield, K., Harnett, P., & Osgarby, S. (2001). The efficacy of a universal school-based program to prevent adolescent depression. *Journal of Clinical Child Psychology, 30,* 303–315.

Shochet, I., Hoge, R., & Wurfl, A. (2004). *RAP-A indigenous supplement: Guidelines for the adaptation and implementation of the RAP program for indigenous adolescents.* Brisbane: Queensland University of Technology.

Shochet, I.M., Homel, R., Cockshaw, W.D. & Montgomery, D.T. (2008). How do school connectedness and attachment to parents interrelate in predicting adolescent depressive symptoms? *Journal of Clinical Child and Adolescent Psychology, 37,* 676–681.

Shochet, I., Holland, D., & Whitefield, K. (1997a). *The Griffith early intervention depression project: Group leader's manual.* Brisbane: Griffith Early Intervention Project.

Shochet, I.M. & O'Gorman, J. (1995). Ethical issues in research on adolescent depression and suicidal behaviour. *Australian Psychologist, 30,* 183–187.

Shochet, I., Whitefield, K., & Holland, D., (1997b). *The Griffith early intervention depression project: Participant's workbook.* Brisbane: Griffith Early Intervention Project.

Spence, S.H., Holmes, J.M., March, S., & Lipp, O.V. (2006). The feasibility and outcome of clinic plus internet delivery of cognitive–behavior therapy for childhood anxiety. *Journal of Consulting and Clinical Psychology, 74,* 614–621.

Spence, S.H., Sheffield, J.K., & Donovan, C.L. (2003). Preventing adolescent depression: An evaluation of the Problem Solving for Life Program. *Journal of Consulting and Clinical Psychology, 71,* 3–13.

Spence, S.H. & Shortt, A.L. (2007). Research review: Can we justify the widespread dissemination of universal, school-based interventions for the prevention of depression among children and adolescents? *Journal of Child Psychology and Psychiatry, 48,* 526–542.

Wang, W. & Shu, M. (2004). *A controlled trial of an early intervention program for depression in Chinese schools.* 28th International Congress of Psychology, Beijing, China.

Wells, K.B., Stewart, A., Hays, R.D., Burnam, M.A., Rogers, W., Daniels, M., et al. (1989). The functioning and well-being of depressed patients. *Journal of the American Medical Association, 262,* 914–919.

Werner, E.E. (1995). Resilience in development. *Current Directions in Psychological Science, 4,* 81–85.

Werner, E.E. & Johnson, J.L. (2004). The role of caring adults in the lives of children of alcoholics. *Substance Use and Misuse, 39,* 699–720.

Wexler, D.B. (1991). *The PRISM workbook: A program for innovative self-management.* New York: W.W. Norton & Company Inc.

Wilkinson, R.B. (2004). The role of parental and peer attachment in the psychological health and self-esteem of adolescents. *Journal of Youth & Adolescence, 33,* 479–493.

Chapter 7

Improving care for depression: Integrating evidence-based depression treatment within primary care services

Joan Rosenbaum Asarnow, James McKowen, & Lisa H. Jaycox

Major depression is predicted to become the second leading cause of disability in the world by 2020 (Murray and Lopex, 1996). Depression increasingly afflicts young people. Between 15 and 20% of youth are estimated to suffer from depressive disorders by the age of 18 (Lewinsohn, 2002); 30-day prevalence rates are estimated at 6.1% (Kessler et al., 2001); and 28.3% of high school students in the United States report periods of depression during the past year that interfered with usual activities and lasted at least 2 weeks (Centers for Disease Control, 2002). Suicide, the third leading cause of death in the United States for youth aged 15–24 years, is frequently associated with depression (American Academy of Child and Adolescent Psychiatry et al., 2000), and depression during adolescence is associated with a high rate of completed and attempted suicide in adulthood (Weissman et al., 1999) as well as a cluster of negative outcomes including recurrent depression, psychosocial and role impairments, drug and alcohol abuse, early parenthood, school failure and drop out, and adult depression (Fergusson & Woodward, 2002; Paradis et al., 2006). These data, in conjunction with observations that adult depression frequently begins during adolescence (Lewinsohn, 1999; Weissman et al., 1999) underscores the importance of recognizing and treating depression in youth.

Recognition of the difficulties in reaching and treating the large number of depressed youth through mental health specialty services has led to increased focus on other service sectors as part of national efforts to improve depression care and outcomes. This chapter focuses on primary care and efforts to integrate evidence-based depression treatment within primary care clinics. We emphasize cognitive–behaviour therapy and antidepressant medications as the two most established forms of evidence-based treatments for youth depression and draw heavily on our recently completed study evaluating a quality improvement intervention for improving access to these evidence-based treatments through primary care clinics (Asarnow et al., 2005a). Other chapters in this volume emphasize schools and other service sectors, as well as other approaches to depression treatment.

Why primary care?

Primary care visits provide a critical gateway for detecting, preventing, and treating depression in youth. While access to specialty care is limited, particularly among poor and uninsured youth, most youths have some contact with a primary care provider each year for well-child visits, school physicals, or acute care (Gans et al., 1991; Kramer et al., 1997; Monheit & Cunningham, 1992; Ziv et al., 1999). Further, frequent users of primary care are likely to have elevated levels of mental health problems, suggesting that primary care settings offer an enriched setting for detecting youth with mental health problems (Mehl-Madrona, 1998). Despite the promise of primary care settings for improving care for youth depression, rates of detection and treatment are generally low, with current studies indicating that paediatricians identify mental health needs in only a small subgroup of youth who need services (Asarnow et al., 2000; Briggs-Gowan et al., 2000; Costello, 1988; Horwitz et al., 1992; Kramer et al., 1999; Kramer & Garralda, 1998; Lavigne et al., 1998). Moreover, even with adult depression, which is frequently treated in primary care settings, quality of care is frequently moderate to poor with resultant poor outcomes (Mehl-Madrona, 1998; Sturm and Wells, 1995; Wells et al., 1996, 1999), underscoring the need for quality improvement efforts to be included in programs designed to increase access to treatment through primary care services.

Although detection and treatment of mental health problems within primary care settings is feasible, there are also significant challenges to service delivery in these settings. First, primary care visits occur within the context of a patient provider relationship that emphasizes physical health care and patients generally view these visits as emphasizing physical vs. mental health. Second, primary care visits tend to be brief (averaging 10–15 minutes) in comparison to the lengthier visits typically scheduled in specialty mental health care. Within this relatively brief time period, providers must balance competing needs and the relative importance of screening for mental health needs, psychosocial risk factors, and addressing a wide range of health issues including medical problems, inoculations, and the diverse array of health risk behaviours (e.g., substance use, risky sexual behaviour, safe practices, seat belt use, and obesity risk). It is not possible for all primary care providers to do everything and some primary care clinicians are reluctant to add mental health problems to the already wide range of health conditions that they are treating. However, since a substantial proportion of youth fail to follow up on specialty mental health referrals or lack access to specialty mental health care, other primary care providers feel a need to address mental health problems within the primary care setting.

Figure 7.1 illustrates the pathways to care through primary care. As shown in Figure 7.1, the first step in this pathway is detection of depressive symptoms or disorder at the time of a primary care visit. Once these problems are identified, the primary care provider must evaluate the severity of the identified condition and develop a management/treatment plan. Some providers may elect to refer most of these patients to specialty care. However, others may opt to treat the condition initially with or without consultation with mental health specialists. Typical primary care options include watchful waiting where the youth is followed and monitored to assess the need for further treatment, primary care counselling, medication, or some combination of these options.

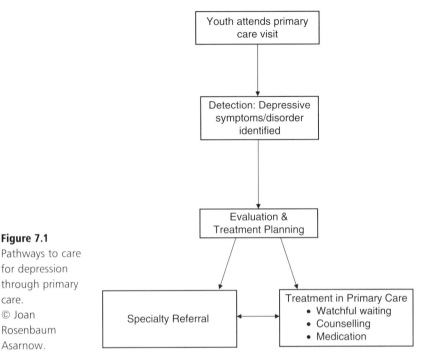

Figure 7.1
Pathways to care
for depression
through primary
care.
© Joan
Rosenbaum
Asarnow.

The youth partners in care model

Youth Partners in Care (YPIC) is a multi-site randomized effectiveness trial that compared a quality improvement (QI) intervention with usual care (UC). The study screening results, baseline sample, and 6-month outcomes have been described elsewhere (Asarnow et al., 2005a,b; Fordwood et al., 2007; Goldstein et al., 2007). In brief, the project was implemented in 6 different sites from 5 major health care organizations. Sites were selected to include two managed care sites, two public sector sites, and two academic medical centre sites. The YPIC QI model aimed to improve detection of depression; access to evidence-based depression treatment, specifically cognitive–behaviour therapy and pharmacotherapy; and quality of care. Our approach was modelled after the approach used in the Partners in Care Study, which was successful in improving outcomes for adult patients suffering from depression (Wells et al., 2000), and was also successful in improving outcomes for youth patients at the end of the 6-month intervention period.

Detection

First, to address problems with low detection in primary care, we developed a system for in-clinic screening while patients were waiting to see their providers. We demonstrated the feasibility of using a brief 15–20 minute written screening questionnaire that youth could complete in the waiting room or in the exam room while waiting to see their providers (Asarnow et al., 2005b). Consecutive adolescent and young adult patients, aged 13–21 years, were invited to complete the screener. The older 18–21 year-old group was included to parallel typical adolescent medicine practices where these late adolescent/young adult patients are typically included.

Across sites, a total of 4,783 youth were eligible for screening. Most youth took the screener (4182/4783, 87%), and most who took the screener completed the depression and health items (3471/4,182, 83%). Thus, screening appeared feasible, with 73% of patients approached for screening completing most of the screening questionnaire. When youth did not complete the screener, the major reasons given were not interested, not enough time, too ill, and parent did not want youth to complete the screener. An additional subgroup also passively refused by handing in incomplete questionnaires.

Questionnaire items were designed to screen *for probable depressive disorder* and *depressive symptoms.* We used stem items (E1,2,34) for DSM-IV major depressive and dysthymic disorder derived from the 12-month Composite International Diagnostic Interview Version 2.1 (CIDI-12,2.1) (World Health Organization, 1997). These items ask about the presence of a period of 2-weeks or more of daily depressed mood or lack of interest during the past year (Major Depression screener), or a period of 1 year or more when the patient experienced nearly daily depression or lack of interest extending into the past year (Dysthmia screener). Consistent with diagnostic criteria for adolescents (American Psychiatric Association, 2000) items were adapted to require a duration of one year of depressed mood for dysthymic disorder and include irritability as an indicator of depressed mood. Youth were classified as having *probable current depressive disorder* if they endorsed (1) the major depression or dysthmia screener, and (2) endorsed current depression on either of two items asking about the presence of 1 week or more of daily depressed mood or lack of interest in the past month. Positive predictive validity against the CIDI 2.1 12-month diagnosis was 43% in a sub-study with our adolescent sample (Asarnow et al., 2005b). This is a high predictive value for a depression screener (Burnam et al., 1988) and is generally comparable with results on adult samples; specifically, positive predictive validity of a similar screener in the adult Partners in Care Study was 55% against the CIDI 2.1 12-month diagnosis (Wells et al., 2000). The Centre for Epidemiological Studies—Depression Scale (CES-D) (Radloff, 1977) was also included in the screener to provide a dimensional measure of *depressive symptoms* during the past week. This widely used 20-item self-report scale, ranges from 0 to 60, and has been shown to be reliable and valid in adolescents (Clarke et al., 1995; Roberts et al., 1990). The internal reliability was high in this study (Cronbach alpha = 0.91).

Table 7.1 presents the screening results for the overall sample and the sample at each site. As expected, given the diversity of our sites, patients varied in age, ethnicity, and gender; and these demographic variables varied across sites. Age ranged from 13 to 21 years, with a mean of 16.89 years (SD, 2.00). Over half of patients identified themselves as Latino or Hispanic. The overall rate of probable depressive disorder was 31%, but rates across sites varied from 27–40%, with the highest rates occurring in sites where patients tended to be older and female. Given a positive predictive value of 43% on our screener, this suggests rates of true depressive disorder in the range of 11–18%. This is consistent with other research, which found that 12–20% of adolescents seen in primary care met criteria for depressive disorders (Kramer & Garralda, 1998). In this

Table 7.1 Results of screening across sites

	Sites						
	A (N = 542)	B (N = 617)	C (N = 1046)	D (N = 440)	E (N = 484)	F (N = 342)	Total (N = 3471)
Age							
Mean (SD) years	16.22 (1.96)	17.25 (1.97)	16.34 (1.51)	17.22 (2.31)	17.54 (1.81)	17.61 (2.44)	16.89 (2.00)
Range	13.0–21.77	13.0–21.99	13.0–20.73	13.04–21.89	13.30–21.97	13.0–22.0	13.0–22.0
Female No., (%)	300, 55%	465, 75%	640, 61%	267, 61%	335, 69%	253, 74%	2260, 65%
Ethnicities							
Latino/Hispanic No., (%)	116, 21%	7, 1%	685, 65%	354, 80%	379, 78%	256, 75%	1797, 51.77%
African-American No., (%)	52, 10%	368, 60%	68, 7%	3, 1%	20, 4%	12, 4%	523, 15.07%
Asian No., (%)	31, 6%	3, 0.5%	54, 5%	22, 5%	12, 2%	5, 1%	127, 3.66%
Mixed No., (%)	111, 20%	77, 12%	163, 16%	39, 9%	29, 6%	37, 11%	456, 13.14%
White No., (%)	215, 40%	146, 24%	29, 3%	12, 3%	28, 6%	24, 7%	454, 13.08%
Other No., (%)	17, 3%	16, 3%	47, 4%	10, 2%	16, 3%	8, 2%	114, 3.28%
CES-D							
Mean (SD)	14.24 (11.10)	16.13 (11.91)	14.82 (10.72)	13.71 (10.55)	16.05 (10.81)	18.83 (11.78)	15.39 (11.18)
Range	0–57.0	0–55.0	0–55.0	0–54.0	0–49.0	0–55.0	0–57.0
Probable Depression No. (%)	166, 31%	198, 32%	290, 28%	118, 27%	157, 32%	136, 40%	1065, 31%

Note: Due to rounding of decimals, totals may not exactly equal sum of cells. © Joan Rosenbaum Asarnow. Table adapted from Asarnow, J.R., Jaycox, L.H., Duan, N., LaBorde, A.P., Rea, M.M., Tang, L., et al. (2005) Depression and role mpairment among adolescents in primary care clinics. *Journal of Adolescent Health*, 37(6), 477–483.

context, it is important to note that research has demonstrated that subsyndromal depression is associated with increased risk for depressive disorder as well as social and role impairments comparable to those seen in syndromal depression (Clarke et al., 1995; Gotlib et al., 1995; Lewinsohn et al., 2000). Brief screening protocols are also more feasible within the context of primary care practices, where the average visit length is 15 minutes, as compared to longer diagnostic interviews. Thus, broad screening for syndromal and subsyndromal depression, such as we did in YPIC, is likely to be the most useful and feasible approach for identifying adolescents who may respond to treatment or preventive interventions.

Eligibility for the YPIC intervention was based on either (1) youth responses indicative of probable current depressive disorder, defined as a positive response to the CIDI depression screener items described above and a CES-D score of 16 or greater, or (2) severe current depressive symptoms, defined as a CES-D score of 24 or greater. Once youth screening positive were identified and appropriate informed consent and assent obtained for participation in the randomized trial, youth were randomized to either (1) the quality improvement (QI) intervention, or (2) usual care (UC). Youth in the UC condition received treatment as usual at the site. However, all depression care at project sites was enhanced in that all primary care providers were offered training and educational materials (manuals, pocket-cards) on depression evaluation and treatment (Asarnow et al., 1999c). Patients in the UC condition had access to treatment as usual at the site, but did not have access to the specific mental health providers who were trained in the study CBT and care management strategies.

Quality improvement intervention

In addition to the primary care provider training in depression evaluation and management, the QI intervention included four major components: (1) expert leader teams at each site that collaborated with the study team to develop and implement the intervention at the site, (2) care managers who supported the primary care provider with on-site patient evaluation, education, treatment, monitoring, and linkage with specialty mental health services, (3) training for care managers in rigorous manualized cognitive–behaviour therapy for depression with care managers available to deliver therapy at the primary care clinics, and 4) patient and provider choice of treatment modalities (CBT, medication, combined CBT and medication, Care Manager monitoring, no contact).

Our strategy for disseminating/exporting the QI intervention to the sites proceeded in phases with some overlap in time across phases. Phase 1 emphasized building the culture to support the intervention implementation. Although the intervention was designed centrally by the study, it could not be adopted within the practices until the intervention was adapted to the needs of each participating clinic and operationalized for each clinic structure. This phase began with a series of meetings at each site aimed at (1) explaining the study rationale, objectives, and procedures, (2) building enthusiasm and support, and 3) developing an 'expert leader team' to collaborate with the central study team in adapting the intervention to the needs of the practice and clinic patients. Although collaboration and leadership by the site 'expert leader team' was crucial, minimizing the burden on leaders at the sites was critical to the success of the study.

Unlike researchers whose primary focus is on the 'research project', site leaders were confronted with multiple demands on their time, had roles that did not allow for significant reduction in responsibilities, and consequently accepted responsibilities for the project with minimal relief from other clinical and administrative duties. The role of the expert leaders was generally to teach the central study team about the needs of the practice setting, develop a plan for implementing the intervention at the clinics, support the project through enthusiasm and staff education, develop and implement strategies for integrating the study intervention model with usual care procedures, trouble shoot, and problem-solve around implementation and quality assurance issues.

Second, with input from participating sites and 'expert leader teams', we developed manuals and other materials to guide and support intervention implementation (Albright & Asarnow, 1999; Asarnow et al., 1999a,b,c, 2003a,b). A detailed manual was developed for primary care providers that presented patient evaluation strategies, algorithms for determining when patients required immediate hospitalization or urgent referral to specialty mental health referral and/or protective services (e.g., suicidal risk, abuse), algorithms for adapting the management plan to address frequent mental health and medical comorbidities, algorithms for choosing treatment modality (CBT, medication, CM follow-up, combined medication and CBT), algorithms for medication management (acute, continuation, and maintenance treatment), and guidelines for evaluating patient response and modifying treatment based on the quality of the patient's response. Pocket cards were developed to highlight major points and distributed to the PCPs, CMs, and made available at the clinics for easy reference.

A similar manual guided the CM interactions, which emphasized supporting the PCP with patient evaluation, education, choosing the preferred treatment modality, and monitoring patient progress and needs (Albright & Asarnow, 1999). Brochures entitled 'Stress & Your Mood' were developed for the initial patient evaluation session. These brochures provided information on links between stress, depression, and other mood problems; depressive symptoms; and available treatment options. Additionally, the process of reviewing the brochure provided a semi-structured format for eliciting information on stresses and supports in the youth's life, depressive and other mental health symptoms, and treatment preferences. The 'Stress & Your Mood' brochure provided a brief assessment and psychoeducation tool that facilitated integration of the YPIC sessions within the relatively brief appointments that were typical in the primary care clinics.

The study CBT was based on the Adolescent Coping with Depression Course (Clarke et al., 1990). A CBT manual and workbook were developed that could be used in either group or individual format (Asarnow et al., 1999a,b, 2003a,b). To address potential access problems, the manual was developed in three 4-session modules, with modules focusing on behavioural activation and building social support, cognitions, and communication and problem-solving. This format enabled new group members to join every 4 weeks (vs. 12 week waiting periods), thus increasing the feasibility of the group format. Finally, standard clinical note forms were developed to increase the focus on intervention components and allow quality assurance monitoring.

Third, provider trainings were conducted to guide providers through the manuals, provide demonstrations and role-play opportunities, and train each provider on their component of the intervention. Separate trainings were held for the expert leader teams, primary care providers, and CMs/CBT therapists. Trainings were generally held at the sites.

Fourth, to maximize adherence to the intervention model and enhance quality of care, ongoing training/intervention support and quality assurance procedures were developed for each site. Because the CM was the central link in the intervention, and in all sites the same individuals served as CMs and CBT therapists, the continuing training and quality assurance emphasized the CMs. CMs were providers with either a masters or Ph.D. in a mental health field (social work, psychology, marriage, and family counselling) or nursing. Regular contacts were scheduled during which all cases were reviewed and additional training and support provided by the central study team. The mode of contact depended on the site and the needs of the CM/CBT therapist; but varied from monthly lunch meetings with supplemental calls when needed, to weekly telephone contacts. Additional quality assurance procedures included chart reviews and review of audiotapes of sessions to monitor adherence to the model. Despite the initial agreement to audiotape, relatively few audiotapes were submitted in this naturalistic effectiveness trial, underscoring the challenges involved in transporting research-based quality assurance protocols to routine practice settings.

Patient components

As shown in Figure 7.2, for patients and families, the QI condition began with an invitation to come into the clinic for an initial visit with the Care Manager, at no charge. The purpose of this initial visit was to evaluate patient and family needs, educate the patient/family about treatment options, and develop a treatment plan (CBT, medication management, combined CBT and medication, referral and linkage with services, or Care Manager follow-up). This treatment plan was reviewed and finalized with the Primary Care Provider and, as appropriate, efforts were made to schedule a primary care visit to review and finalize the treatment plan with youths and family members. The Care Manager followed the patient during the 6-month intervention period and coordinated care with the Primary Care Provider, with adjustments made to the treatment plan as needed during the 6-months of the intervention.

Table 7.2 summarizes the intervention components received by participants in the QI condition. These data are abstracted from patient charts for the full QI sample, and therefore, differ somewhat from previous reports based on self-report data and the 6-month outcome sample (Asarnow et al., 2005a). As shown in Table 7.2, most (71%) intervention patients completed an initial evaluation. However, almost half of these evaluations were completed by telephone (67/149, 45%) rather than in person at the clinic. The most common form of study treatment was Care Manager Follow-Up, which occurred in 70% of patients. Consistent with results indicating that youth tended to express a preference for psychosocial vs. pharmacologic treatment (Jaycox et al., 2006), CBT was more common (45% of patients) than was medication (15.1%). However, 24% of patients received CBT contacts by telephone only, 56% in person only, and 20% received a mixture of both. Fewer than half of patients (40%) received more than 3 CBT contacts, which could be considered a minimal 'dose' of treatment,

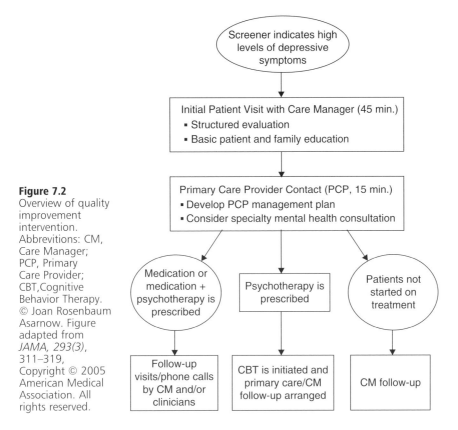

Screener indicates high levels of depressive symptoms

Initial Patient Visit with Care Manager (45 min.)
- Structured evaluation
- Basic patient and family education

Primary Care Provider Contact (PCP, 15 min.)
- Develop PCP management plan
- Consider specialty mental health consultation

Medication or medication + psychotherapy is prescribed

Psychotherapy is prescribed

Patients not started on treatment

Follow-up visits/phone calls by CM and/or clinicians

CBT is initiated and primary care/CM follow-up arranged

CM follow-up

Figure 7.2
Overview of quality improvement intervention. Abbrevitions: CM, Care Manager; PCP, Primary Care Provider; CBT,Cognitive Behavior Therapy. © Joan Rosenbaum Asarnow. Figure adapted from *JAMA, 293(3)*, 311–319, Copyright © 2005 American Medical Association. All rights reserved.

and only 5.1% had 12 or more contacts, which could be considered a full course of treatment. The mean number of sessions for patients receiving any CBT contact was 3.85 (SD = 3.69; range 1–16), when in-person only 3.69 (SD = 3.8, range 1–16), when by telephone only 1.86 (SD = 1.28; range 1–5), and when in combination 6.57 (SD = 3.7, range 3–16). Thus, a combination of individual and phone sessions yielded the greatest dosage of therapy.

Although we and expert leaders at the sites had anticipated that group CBT would be more cost-effective and practical for the sites, group treatment was relatively rare and occurred at only 3 sites. In total, twelve patients received group CBT, with the mean number of sessions being 3.66 (SD = 2.7, range 1–9).

We also found that relatively few providers had contacts with parents and youth together, occurring in only 27 patients. Further, only 28 cases included provider contact with parents alone. Overall, however, involvement with parents was associated with increased frequency of contact.

Examination of barriers to treatment revealed that CMs described 'scheduling problems' as the most common barrier to treatment, occurring in 81% of patients. The patient not being interested in treatment was described by 23% of patients, and a parent being unsupportive of treatment was described in 5% of patients.

Table 7.2 Treatment given during QI intervention-based on chart review

	Total *N* = 211 Frequency (%)
Initial evaluation	149 (71%)
In-person	82 (55%)
Telephone	67 (45%)
Total receiving any treatment	151 (72%)
Total CBT treatment	94 (45%)
Received CBT in-person only	53 (56%)
Received CBT by telephone only	22 (24%)
Received mixture of both	19 (20%)
Total CM treatment	147 (70%)
Received CM in-person only	21 (14%)
Received CM telephone only	96 (65%)
Received mixture of both	21 (14%)
Total psychiatric medication	32 (15.1%)
Psychiatric medication through study	10 (31%)
Psychiatric medication through external provider	18 (56%)
Psychiatric medication through both	4 (12.5%)
Combination treatment	100 (47%)
Psychiatric medication + CBT + CM	22 (22%)
Psychiatric medication + CM only	9 (9%)
Psychiatric medication + CBT only	0 (0%)
CBT + CM (no medication)	69 (69%)
CBT only	3 (1.4%)
CM only	47 (22%)
Medication only	1 (0.5%)
Total external provider therapy	33 (16%)
Post-study F/U care	123 (59%)
Continue with PCP f/u only	95 (77%)
Continue with study PCP plus:	
Study MH provider	1 (1%)
Non-study MH provider	6 (5%)
Specialty MH care	4 (3%)
Continue with study MH provider only	1 (1%)
Continue with non-study provider only	9 (7%)
Referred to specialty MH provider only	7 (6%)

Note: These numbers differ from those in other reports due to differences in available sample and data. No data were available on 3 intervention cases. Data were missing on type of contact for 9 CM cases. © Joan Rosenbaum Asarnow.

After the 6-month intervention period, the chart review data indicate that 59% of cases received continuing care for mental health issues. The majority of these cases continued with their primary care provider (86%), and 22% of cases received ongoing mental health care either alone or in combination with PCP treatment. Only two cases continued treatment with a study mental health provider.

CES-D at 6 Months

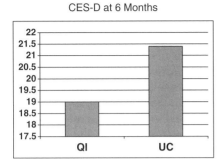

Severe depression at 6 Months

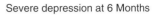
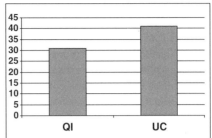

MCS-12 at 6 Months

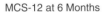
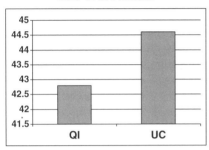

Satisfaction with mental health care

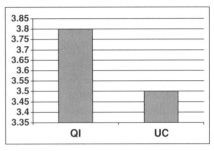

Figure 7.3 Youth partners in care 6-month outcomes. © Joan Rosenbaum Asarnow. See Asarnow et al. 2005a for more information.

Patient outcomes

Consistent with our hypothesis that increasing rates of evidence-based treatment would lead to improved patient outcomes, at the 6 month outcome assessment patients in the QI condition reported significant improvements in depressive symptoms and quality of life, compared to UC patients. Additionally, QI patients reported greater satisfaction with available mental health care (Figure 7.3) (Asarnow et al., 2005a).

Conclusions

The YPIC results underscore both the potential benefits and feasibility of interventions designed to improve quality of care for adolescent depression in primary care settings. We demonstrated that brief screening protocols like those used in YPIC are feasible in primary care clinics with the vast majority of patients completing screening questionnaires during their visits. Further, the value of screening was underscored by the relatively high prevalence of depression among primary care patients: roughly 31% of patients were found to have symptoms of sufficient severity to require further evaluation, with 11–18% of patients estimated to meeting criteria for current major depressive disorder and/or dysthymic disorder (Asarnow et al., 2005b). Given the morbidity and mortality associated with depression, these data highlight the potential public health value of screening if treatment is available.

The YPIC outcome results lend support to the report of the US Preventive Services Task Force, which recommends screening for depression in primary care when combined with access to effective treatments (US Preventive Services Task Force, 2002). The YPIC QI intervention was associated with improved depression and quality of life outcomes as well as higher levels of patient satisfaction with mental health care. Although not all patients chose to begin treatment, 71% had some study treatment contact and an additional 2 patients had treatment through non-study providers, resulting in 72% of patients receiving some mental health contact based on our chart review. Thus, while patients in the QI condition generally had some mental health follow-up, either in-person or by telephone, these data underscore that even when evidence-based mental health treatments are available and relatively easy to access, many patients will choose not to pursue treatment.

When offered depression treatment through the YPIC study, roughly 23% of patients expressed no interest in treatment. However, most (81%) of the YPIC patients declining treatment noted difficulties in scheduling. This highlights the point that patients and their families struggle with competing demands on their time and resources and this may result in limited treatment uptake even when it is available. On the one hand this means that a proportion of patients who would benefit from treatment do not receive it. However, from the perspective of health care organizations, this suggests that costs will be limited by the relatively small number of patients electing to receive treatment if offered.

Telephone services are less burdensome for patients to access, and therefore, provide one strategy for engaging patients in treatment and delivering treatment for youth and families where transportation, time, or other barriers impede treatment in a clinic setting. For these reasons, in YPIC outreach and service delivery by telephone was frequently used to engage patients in treatment and increase treatment rates. Although future research is needed to evaluate the efficacy of treatment contacts delivered by telephone, telephone services provide one strategy for supplementing more traditional clinic-based services.

When given a choice of treatment modality in YPIC, CBT was selected more frequently than was medication, with 45% of patients choosing CBT and only a small minority of patients choosing medication treatments (15%). These data are consistent with analyses of our baseline data on treatment preferences. When asked what treatment they would prefer if they should suffer from depression, youth tended to express a preference for psychosocial treatment rather than medication (Jaycox et al., 2006). These data are also consistent with data suggesting a tendency for youth to discontinue medication treatment when given a psychosocial treatment option (Clarke et al., 2005). It is important to note that the YPIC study was conducted prior to the FDA advisories regarding the risk of possible suicidality with antidepressant medications (www.fda.gov). Recent findings of a decrease in youth antidepressant prescriptions after the FDA advisories and black box warnings (Libby et al., 2007; Nemeroff et al., 2007; Olfson et al., 2003) suggest that this tendency to prefer psychosocial treatment is likely to be even stronger at the present time.

Although the YPIC results are encouraging and support the promise of efforts to integrate evidence-based depression care within primary care services, these results should be viewed in the context of the study limitations. First, although YPIC is to our knowledge the largest trial to evaluate an intervention for adolescent depression in primary care settings and included a broad and diverse sample from multiple sites, future research is needed to test the YPIC approach across a broader and more diverse group of clinics and patients. Second, the sample included youth with a wide range of depressive symptoms, and while some youth met criteria for depressive disorders, others fell below these criteria and had depressive symptoms but no depressive disorder. The use of broad inclusion criteria, as well as minimal exclusion criteria, enhanced feasibility within primary care clinics where time for screening was limited. Third, while depression outcomes were improved in the QI condition compared to UC, almost a third of QI patients continued to show severe depressive symptoms at the 6-month outcome assessments and longer term follow-up is needed to further clarify intervention impact. On the basis of results of the Treatment of Adolescent Depression Study, it would appear that combined medication and psychosocial treatment is optimal for moderate to severe depression (March et al., 2004). Despite the relatively low use of medications among YPIC patients, we did find a higher rate of medication treatment among youth meeting criteria for depressive disorders (vs. subsyndromal depressive symptoms), suggesting that medication treatments were more common among those with greatest need (Asarnow et al., 2005a). However, additional research is needed to develop and evaluate strategies for enhancing rates of combined treatment among youth with more severe depressive disorders.

In conclusion, the YPIC results provide clear support for the value of current depression treatments. Although results from the Treatment of Adolescent Depression Study (March et al., 2004) have raised questions regarding the value of CBT alone (without medication) for severe to moderate depression in adolescents, the YPIC results indicate that when offered within the context of a QI intervention (1) patients and providers are more likely to chose CBT over medication, and (2) the combination of care management and supported CBT and medication treatments within primary care settings can lead to improved youth outcomes. These data underscore the potential benefits of future efforts to improve quality of care through primary care. Given the current shortage of specialty mental health providers for youth, limited access to specialty mental health services, and reluctance of many youth and families to seek mental health services due to perceptions of stigma and other factors, the YPIC QI intervention offers a model for future efforts to improve youth mental health outcomes through primary care systems.

References

Albright, A. & Asarnow, J. (1999). *Youth partners in care: Guidelines and resources for the care manager (cm). (adapted from rubenstein, unutzer, miranda, et al. Partners in care: Guideline and resources for the depression nurs specialist, 1996.).* Los Angeles: UCLA School of Medicine.

American Academy of Child and Adolescent Psychiatry, Shaffer, D., Pfeffer, C.R., & Issues, W.G.o.Q. (2000). *Practice parameters for the assessment and treatment of children and adolescents with suicidal behavior.* Washington, DC: AACAP Communications Department.

American Psychiatric Association. (2000). *Diagnostic and statistical manual of mental disorders (4th edition)*. Washington DC: American Psychiatric Association.

Asarnow, J., Jaycox, L.H., Clarke, G., Lewinsohn, P., Hops, H., & Rohde, P. (1999a). *Stress and your mood: A workbook*. Los Angeles, California: UCLA School of Medicine.

Asarnow, J., Jaycox, L.H., Rea, M., Clarke, G., Lewinsohn, P., Hops, H., et al. (1999b). *Stress and your mood: A manual for groups*. Los Angeles: University of California.

Asarnow, J., Jaycox, L.H., Rea, M., Clarke, G., Lewinsohn, P., Hops, H., et al. (2003a). *Stress and your mood: A manual for individuals*. Los Angeles, California: UCLA School of Medicine.

Asarnow, J., Jaycox, L.H., Rea, M., Clarke, G., Lewinsohn, P., Hops, H., et al. (2003b). *Stress and your mood: A workbook for individuals*. Los Angeles, California: UCLA School of Medicine.

Asarnow, J.R., Carlson, G., Schuster, M., Miranda, J., Jackson-Triche, M., & Wells, K.B. (1999c). *Youth partners in care: Clinician guide to depression assessment and management among youth in primary care settings (adapted from rubenstein, unutzer, miranda, et al. Partners in care: Clinician guide to depression assessment and management in primary care settings; 1996.)*. Los Angeles: UCLA School of Medicine.

Asarnow, J.R., Jaycox, L., Duan, N., LaBorde, A., Rea, M., Anderson, M., et al. (2005a). Effectiveness of a quality improvement intervention for adolescent depression in primary care clinics: A randomized controlled trial. *Journal of the American Medical Association, 293(3)*, 311–319.

Asarnow, J.R., Jaycox, L., Duan, N., LaBorde, A., Rea, M., Tang, L., et al. (2005b). Depression and role impairment among adolescents in primary care clinics. *Journal of Adolescent Health, 37(6)*, 477–483.

Asarnow, J.R., Jaycox, L., Rea, M., LaBorde, A., Carlson, G., Albright, A., et al. (2000). Quality improvement for depression among adolescents in primary care. Paper presented at the annual meeting of the american academy of child and adolescent psychiatry. New York, New York.

Briggs-Gowan, M.J., Horwitz, S.M., Schwab-Stone, M.E., Leventhal, J.M., & Leaf, P.J. (2000). Mental health in pediatric settings: Distribution of disorders and factors related to service use. *Journal of American Academy of Child and Adolescent Psychiatry, 39(7)*, 841–849.

Burnam, M.A., Wells, K.B., Leake, B., & Landsverk, J. (1988). Development of a brief screening instrument for detecting depressive disorders. *Med Care, 26(8)*, 775–789.

Centers for Disease Control. (2002). Youth risk behavior surveillance-united states, 2001.

Clarke, G., Debar, L., Lynch, F., Powell, J., Gale, J., O'Connor, E., et al. (2005). A randomized effectiveness trial of brief cognitive-behavioral therapy for depressed adolescents receiving antidepressant medication. *Journal of American Academy of Child and Adolescent Psychiatry, 44(9)*, 888–898.

Clarke, G.N., Hawkins, W., Murphy, M., Sheeber, L.B., Lewinsohn, P.M., & Seeley, J.R. (1995). Targeted prevention of unipolar depressive disorder in an at-risk sample of high school adolescents: A randomized trial of group cognitive intervention. *Journal of the American Academy of Child and Adolescent Psychiatry, 34(3)*, 312–321.

Clarke, G.N., Lewinsohn, P.M., Hops, H., & Seeley, J.R. (1990). Adolescent Coping with Depression Course. Eugene, OR: Castalia Press.

Costello, E.J., Edelbrock, C., Costello, A.J., Dulcan, M.K., Burns, B.J., & Brent, D. (1988). Psychopathology in pediatric primary care: A new hidden morbidity. *Pediatrics, 82*, 415–424.

Fergusson, D.M. & Woodward, L.J. (2002). Mental health, educational, and social role outcomes of adolescents with depression. *Archives of General Psychiatry, 59(3)*, 225–231.

Fordwood, S.R., Asarnow, J.R., Huizar, D.P., & Reise, S.P. (2007). Suicide attempts among depressed adolescents in primary care. *Journal of Clinical Child and Adolescent Psychology, 36(3),* 392–404.

Gans, J.E., McManus, M.A., & Newacheck, P.W. (1991). *Adolescent health care: Use, costs, and problems of access* (Vol. 2). Chicago, IL: American Medical Association.

Goldstein, R.B., Asarnow, J.R., Jaycox, L., Shoptaw, S., & Murray, P. (2007). Correlates of "non-problematic" and "problematic" substance use among depressed adolescents in primary care. *Journal of Addictive Diseases, 26(3),* 39–52.

Gotlib, C., Lewinsohn, P.M., & Seeley, J.R. (1995). Symptoms versus a diagnosis of depression: Differences in psychosocial functioning. *Journal of Consulting & Clinical Psychology, 63(1),* 90–100.

Horwitz, S.M., Leaf, P.J., Leventhal, J.M., Forsyth, B., & Speechley, K.N. (1992). Identification and management of psychosocial and developmental problems in community-based, primary care pediatric practices. *Pediatrics, 89(3),* 480–485.

Jaycox, L.H., Asarnow, J.R, Sherbourne, C.D., Rea, M.M., LaBorde, A.P., & Wells, K. (2006). Adolescent primary care patients' preferences for depression treatment. *Administration and Policy in Mental Health, 33,* 198–207.

Kessler, R.C., Avenelovi, S., & Merikangas, S.K. (2001). Mood disorders in children and adolescents: An epidemiological perspective. *Biological Psychiatry, 49,* 1002–1014.

Kramer, T. & Garralda, M. (1998). Psychiatric disorders in adolescents in primary care. *British Journal of Psychiatry, 173,* 508–513.

Kramer, T., Gledhill, J., Garralda, M.E., & Iliffe, S. (1999). *Identification and management of adolescent depression in primary care: Feasibility and efficacy.* Paper presented at the Paper presented at the International Society for Research on Child and Adolescent Psychopathology, Barcelona, Spain.

Kramer, T., Iliffe, S., Murray, E., & Waterman, S. (1997). Which adolescents attend the gp? *British Journal of General Practice, 47(418),* 327.

Lavigne, J.V., Arend, R., Rosenbaum, D., Binns, H.J., Christoffel, K.K., Burns, A., et al. (1998). Mental health service use among young children receiving pediatric primary care. *Journal of American Academy of Child Adolescent and Psychiatry, 37(11),* 1175–1183.

Lewinsohn, P. (2002). Depression in adolescents. In C. Hammen & Gotlib, I. (Ed.), *Handbook of depression* (pp. 541–553). New York: Guilford Press.

Lewinsohn, P.M., Rohde, P., & Seeley, J.R. (1999). Natural course of adolescent major depressive disorder: I. Continuity into young adulthood. *Journal of American Academy of Child and Adolescent Psychiatry, 38,* 56–63.

Lewinsohn, P.M., Solomon, A., Seeley, J.R., & Zeiss, A. (2000). Clinical implications of "subthreshold" depressive symptoms. *Journal of Abnormal Psychology, 109(2),* 345–351.

Libby, A.M., Brent, D.A., Morrato, E.H., Orton, H.D., Allen, R., & Valuck, R.J. (2007). Decline in treatment of pediatric depression after FDA advisory on risk of suicidality with ssris. *American Journal of Psychiatry, 164(6),* 884–891.

March, J., Silva, S., Petrycki. S. et al. (2004). Fluoxetine, cognitive-behavioral therapy, and their combination for adolescents with depression: Treatment for Adolescents With Depression Study (TADS) randomized controlled trial. *Journal of the American Medical Association, 292(7),* 807–820.

Mehl-Madrona, L.E. (1998). Frequent users of rural primary care: Comparisons with randomly selected users. *J Am Board Fam Pract, 11(2),* 105–115.

Monheit, A.C. & Cunningham, P.J. (1992). Children without health insurance. *Future Child, 2*, 154–170.

Murray, C.J. & Lopex, A.D. (1996). *The global burden of disease: A comprehensive assessment of mortality and disability from disease, injuries, and risk factors in 1990 and projected to 2020.* Boston, Mass: The Harvard School of Public Health on behalf of the World Health Organization and the World Bank.

Nemeroff, C.B., Kalali, A., Keller, M.B., Charney, D.S., Lenderts, S.E., Cascade, E.F., et al. (2007). Impact of publicity concerning pediatric suicidality data on physician practice patterns in the united states. *Archives of General Psychiatry, 64(4),* 466–472.

Olfson, M., Shaffer, D., Marcus, S.C., & Greenberg, T. (2003). Relationship between antidepressant medication treatment and suicide in adolescents. *Archives of General Psychiatry, 60(10),* 978–982.

Paradis, A.D., Reinherz, H.Z., Giaconia, R.M., & Fitzmaurice, G. (2006). Major depression in the transition to adulthood: The impact of active and past depression on young adult functioning. *Journal of Nervous and Mental Disorder, 194(5),* 318–323.

Radloff, L.S. (1977). The ces-d scale: A self report depression scale for research in the general population. *Applied Psychological Measurement, 1,* 385–401.

Roberts, R.E., Rhoades, H.M., & Vernon, S.W. (1990). Using the ces-d scale to screen for depression and anxiety: Effects of language and ethnic status. *Psychiatry Research, 31(1),* 69–83.

Sturm, R. & Wells, K.B. (1995). How can care for depression become more cost-effective? *Journal of the American Medical Association, 273(1),* 51–58.

US Preventive Services Task Force. (2002). Screening for depression: Recommendations and rationale. *Annals of Internal Medicine, 136(10),* 760–764.

Weissman, M.M., Wolk, S., Goldstein, R.B., Moreau, D., Adams, P., Greenwald, S., et al. (1999). Depressed adolescents grown up. *JAMA: Journal of the American Medical Association, 281(18),* 1707–1713.

Wells, K.B., Sherbourne, C.D., Schoenbaum, M., Duan, N., Meredith, L., Unutzer, J., et al. (2000). Impact of disseminating quality improvement programs for depression in managed primary care: A randomized controlled trial. *Journal of the American Medical Association, 283(2),* 212–220.

Wells, K.B., Schoenbaum, R., Sherbourne, C.D., & Meredith, L. (1996). Caring for depression. *Harvard University Press.*

Wells, K.B., Schoenbaum, M., Unützer, J., Lagomasino, I.T., Rubenstein, L.V. (1999). Quality of care for primary care patients with depression in managed care. *Archives of Family Medicine, 8(6),* 529–536.

World Health Organization. (1997). *Composite international diagnostic interview (cidi) core version 2.1 interviewer's manual.* Geneva.

Ziv, A., Boulet, J.R., & Slap, G.B. (1999). Utilization of physician offices by adolescents in the United States. *Pediatrics, 104(1 Pt 1),* 35–42.

Part 3

Family interventions

Chapter 8

Family-based approaches to the prevention of depression in at-risk children and youth

Catherine M. Lee & Veronica Asgary Eden

Major Depressive Disorder is the most common of the DSM IV disorders, with a lifetime prevalence rate of 16% (Kessler et al., 2005a), and a 12-month prevalence rate of 6.7% in the United States (Kessler et al., 2005b). Although depression is diagnosed in children and adolescents, the median age of onset is 30 (Kessler et al., 2005a). Nevertheless, epidemiological studies indicate that Major Depressive Disorder is almost as common in adolescence as it is in adulthood (Lewinsohn & Clarke, 1999). US data indicate that, by the age of 18, one in five young people will have experienced an episode of Major Depressive Disorder (Clarke et al., 2003).

The majority of those with diagnoses of Major Depressive Disorder experience other mental disorders, including over half with at least one lifetime anxiety disorder, almost a third with a lifetime externalizing disorder, and approximately a quarter with a lifetime substance abuse disorder (Kessler et al., 2007). Of great concern, less than a third of those suffering from mood disorders receive services from a mental health professional (Wang et al., 2005b). The median delay between onset of the disorder and seeking services is eight years (Wang et al., 2005a). This recurrent disorder is highly disruptive both to the affected individual, and to his or her family (Goodman, 2007; Seligman et al., 2004). It is also associated with an increased rate of suicide (Clarke et al., 2003). World-wide, depression is associated with a substantial economic burden including direct costs, morbidity costs, and mortality costs (Luppa et al., 2007).

Experts agree that the only sustainable way to reduce the burden of mental disorders is through prevention (World Health Organization, 2001). Prevention programs have been defined as *universal*, *selective*, and *indicated* (Mrazek & Haggerty, 1994). As the name implies, universal preventive interventions are applied to an entire population. For example, during the 2003 Severe Acute Respiratory Syndrome (SARS) crisis, universal prevention programs included television advertising campaigns reminding the public to reduce contagion by frequent and thorough hand-washing. Selective preventive interventions, on the other hand, target people who are at elevated risk of developing a particular disorder or problem. So, to continue the SARS example, selective prevention programs required people entering hospitals to wear masks. Indicated preventive interventions target people who do not meet criteria for a disorder, but who have elevated risk and may show detectable, but subclinical signs of the disorder.

Those who had come into contact with a confirmed case of SARS were targets for indicated preventive interventions requiring a period of quarantine. Despite the common belief that universal programs reduce the stigma that may be associated with indicated programs, recent research suggests that stigma effects are small (Rapee et al., 2006).

The risk reduction model of prevention relies heavily on research to guide interventions (Mrazek & Haggerty, 1994). Risk factors are characteristics of the individual or the environment that render a person more vulnerable to the development of a problem or disorder, or that are associated with more severe symptoms. Once at-risk individuals are identified, they are the target of prevention programs designed to protect them from developing the problem or disorder. The other side of the coin is the identification of factors associated with resilience—those characteristics that protect high-risk individuals from developing the problem or disorder. If we understand the variables that are protective, then we can use such knowledge in developing effective prevention programs. Family-centred prevention efforts are based on research that has underlined the key role played by the family in the development of children and youth (Spoth et al., 2002). Risk factors for the development of depression include individual variables such as interpersonal skills deficits and cognitive errors, family variables such as parental depression, marital conflict and parent–adolescent conflict, as well as contextual factors such as negative life events (Barrett & Turner, 2004; Dozois et al., this volume).

Most successful prevention programs for young people have several common features (Biglan et al., 2003). Often a slightly diluted version of an effective treatment intervention is offered to those with sub-clinical problems. Efficacious family-based treatment programs targeting externalizing behaviour problems (Hunsley & Lee, 2007) and internalizing problems (Diamond & Josephson, 2005) may form the basis for prevention programs. As prevention programs are designed to prevent the development of problems, the demonstration of program efficacy requires programmatic research carried out over many years (Nation et al., 2003). Successful programs are offered in a milieu that minimizes obstacles to participation, by using schools, community centres, and home visits, as well as by offering childcare services so that parents can participate (Carr, 2002). Finally, the developers of effective prevention programs all stress the importance of program fidelity in adopting their interventions (e.g., Webster-Stratton, 2006). A key issue in the development of efficacious and effective programs is ensuring that they meet the needs of an ethnically diverse population (Miranda et al., 2005).

Despite the strong evidence of family factors in the development and maintenance of depression in children and adolescents, there is a paucity of evidence that family-based approaches are effective in preventing depression. In an incisive analysis of this apparent paradox, Shochet and Dadds (1997) proposed that in addition to developmental issues around adolescents' willingness to include their parents, some interventions may inadvertently increase family conflict and erode adolescent self-esteem by engaging parents in the role of co-therapists or cognitive–behavioural coaches. Shochet and Dadds proposed that the evidence base could be enhanced by greater attention to clinically informed interventions that are sensitive to the complexities of the parent–adolescent relationship.

In this chapter, we review risk factor research on family variables that have been associated with elevated risk of depression (psychopathology in family members, child abuse and neglect, and family disruption) as well as mechanisms by which risk is transmitted (biological processes; parent–child interaction patterns, including conflict, parental control, and lack of support; and parental cognitive styles). We also examine family factors that have been identified as protective or that are associated with resilience in youth (such as availability, support, and monitoring). Next, we highlight recent findings on aspects of treatment that focus on family factors. Subsequently, we review prevention programs that have been developed to modify family factors that are associated with depression. We include in our review universal prevention programs that have included a parental component, as well as programs that were designed to prevent the development of depression in young people who are at-risk by virtue of being the offspring of depressed parents. Next, we describe programs that have been developed to prevent depression in young people who are at-risk by having experienced family disruption such as parental separation, divorce, or death. In the final section, we draw conclusions and make recommendations for both program development and research.

Family risk factors

One of the major challenges in prevention research is developing a sophisticated understanding of the nature of risk factors as well as a framework for how such knowledge can be translated to particular types of prevention strategies (Zvolensky et al., 2006). It is important to identify causal risk factors, which produce systematic change in the dependent variable when modified by an intervention (Kraemer et al., 1997) and to differentiate between risk factors that cannot be changed or fixed markers and risk factors that can be changed or variable risk factors (Kraemer et al., 2005).

Psychopathology in family members

Parents

One of the key risk factors for youth depression is parental psychopathology (e.g., Lee & Gotlib, 1991, 1994; McCauley Ohannessian et al., 2004; Rohde et al., 2005; Sarigiani et al., 2003; Weissman & Jensen, 2002). Not surprisingly, one of the strongest predictors of depressive disorders in children and adolescents is parental depression (Beardslee et al., 1998), particularly maternal depression (Coyne & Downey, 1991; Gotlib & Lee, 1996; Goodman, 2007).

Maternal depression. Two methodological approaches have been used in examinations of adolescents with depression and their family members. 'top-down' studies investigate the children of depressed parents or grandparents and 'bottom-up' studies are family studies of depressed adolescents (Birmaher et al., 1996).

Consistent links have been found between depression in mothers and in their children. Top-down studies reveal that maternal history of depression is linked to greater symptoms of depression and poorer adaptive interpersonal functioning in adolescence (Hammen et al., 2003). Bottom-up studies indicate that adolescent depression is associated with an elevated rate of having a depressed mother (Essau, 2004). Moreover, maternal Major Depressive Disorder (MDD) is associated with MDD recurrence, chronicity, and severity in offspring (Rohde et al., 2005). Adolescents with depressive symptoms and nondepressed mothers do not display the same chronic interpersonal difficulties as do those with depressed mothers (Hammen et al., 2003). Maternal depression appears to have stronger links to depressive symptoms in daughters than in sons (Burt et al., 2005; Fergusson et al., 1995). Although the effects of maternal depression are well documented, the role of paternal psychopathology has received less attention (Phares & Compas, 1992). Maternal depression interacts with both paternal depression and paternal substance abuse in predicting youth depression (Brennan et al., 2002).

Paternal depression. In the last 20 years, researchers have increasingly examined the role of fathers in children's development (Bouchard et al., 2007; Marsiglio et al., 2000). The quality of the father–child relationship is a significant determinant of child functioning (Lamb & Tamis-Lemonda, 2004). Although the majority of North American youth live in households with two parents, substantial numbers of fathers do not reside with their children. The fact that a father does not live with his child does not preclude him from having a meaningful role in his child's life. The majority of nonresident fathers maintain at least some contact with their children (Phares & Lum, 1997; Walter, 2000) and there is consistent evidence that authoritative parenting by nonresident fathers is associated with having fewer externalizing and internalizing problems (Amato & Gilbreth, 1999).

With increasing recognition that fathers contribute significantly to the development and outcome of their children, there has been growing attention paid to links between adolescent depression and paternal psychopathology. Connell and Goodman (2002) conducted a meta-analysis of the literature on the association between psychopathology in mothers and father and internalizing and externalizing behaviour problems in offspring. The review yielded 134 independent samples, including over 60,000 parent–child dyads. Children's internalizing problems were more closely related to the presence of psychopathology in mothers than to paternal psychopathology, although the magnitude of this difference was small. Interestingly, there was an interaction between parental gender and child age. Paternal psychopathology was more closely related to emotional problems in samples examining older children, whereas maternal psychopathology was more closely related to emotional problems in samples investigating younger children.

In another important meta-analysis that exclusively examined the effects of fathers' depression on child functioning, Kane and Garber (2004) found that paternal depression was significantly related to offspring depression and father–child conflict. Paternal depressive symptoms may also make unique contributions to negative child outcomes above and beyond maternal contributions (Kane et al., 2002). Echoing the findings for maternal depression, there are stronger links between paternal depression and depression (Compton et al., 2003) and recurrence of depression in daughters than in sons (Rohde et al., 2005). Studies examining adolescent depression rarely assess psychopathology in both parents. Although maternal and paternal depression each contributes to youth adjustment, few studies have assessed functioning in both parents.

Assortative mating. The tendency for individuals who have similar phenotypes to pair off together more frequently than would be expected by chance is referred to as assortative mating. Meta-analysis has revealed that assortative mating occurs in both bipolar and major depression (Mathews & Reus, 2001). The combined effects of paternal and maternal depression, rather than depression in either parent alone, may be linked with worse child outcomes (Foley et al., 2001; Kane & Garber, 2004). Fathers' depression has been reported to exacerbate risk for child internalizing problems in families with a depressed mother (Mezulis et al., 2004). Additionally, maternal depression has been found to interact with paternal depression and substance abuse in predicting youth depression (Brennan et al., 2002). Given assortative mating patterns, it is possible that many samples examining the effects of maternal depression on youth depression are also inadvertently examining the effects of paternal depression. Future research should consider the group differences between youth with one or more depressed parents. Overall, parental depression can be conceptualized as a variable risk factor for youth depression. Interventions that target parental psychopathology while children are still young may have a preventative effect for youth depression.

Comorbidity. As depression is comorbid with other disorders, a growing body of research has examined the impact of other types of parental psychopathology on adolescent depression. For example, longitudinal studies have found that having a high familial loading for bipolar disorder or depression and a mother with an anxiety disorder contributes to the risk of developing adolescent depression (Williamson et al., 2004). In a top-down study, McCauley Ohannessian et al. (2004) examined a large sample of 665 13–17 year-olds and their biological parents recruited over a five-year period. Parents with diagnosed substance abuse problems were recruited from inpatient and outpatient alcoholism programs, whereas comparison parents without psychopathology were recruited from the community (McCauley Ohannessian et al., 2004). Adolescents with parents diagnosed with alcohol dependence and either comorbid drug dependence or depression were more likely to exhibit higher levels of psychological symptomatology, including depression, than were adolescents with parents diagnosed with alcohol dependence only or nondisordered parents. These findings highlight the importance of examining comorbid parental psychopathology when examining the effects on offspring.

In a cross-sectional bottom-up study examining the clinical features of depression among depressed adolescents, Essau (2004) asked adolescents with any lifetime depressive disorders to report on their parents' psychopathological symptoms. Fifty-four percent of these adolescents reported that their parents had depressive symptoms, 22% had alcohol problems, 11% had illicit drug problems, and 32.4% had anxiety problems. Overall, depressed adolescents with depressed parents experienced more recurrent depressive episodes than did depressed adolescents with nondepressed parents.

Grandparents

Although there has been very limited investigation of multiple generations, two recent studies yielded compelling results. An ambitious longitudinal study of three generations has drawn attention to the long lasting generational effects of depression on offspring (Warner et al., 1999; Weissman et al., 2005). Weissman et al. (2005) reported on a 20-year follow up of families at high risk for depression during which the first two generations were interviewed four times. Grandchildren ($n = 161$) with a mean age of 12 were included along with their parents and grandparents. Forty percent of grandchildren with at least one grandparent and one parent diagnosed with Major Depressive Disorder (MDD) were diagnosed with a mood disorder (Weissman et al., 2005). The association between parental MDD and child diagnosis was moderated by grandparental MDD status (Weissman et al., 2005). These findings suggest that a history of depression spanning several generations is a fixed marker for youth depression.

The second study that investigated the effects of grandparental depressive symptoms used women's reports of their parents' psychiatric status. Hammen et al. (2004) examined the transmission of depression in a community sample of nearly 800 depressed and never-depressed women and their 15-year-old children. Maternal grandmothers' depression affected the mothers' depression and the mothers' chronic stress (in the areas of marital relationship, close friends, and relationships with parents and siblings). Both maternal and grandmaternal depression affected youth depression; this link was mediated by interpersonal stress processes (in the areas of social life, close friendships, romantic relationships, relations with family members, academic performance, and school behaviour). These preliminary data highlight the importance of investigating the intergenerational effects of depression.

Siblings

Within the burgeoning literature on psychopathology in first degree relatives of depressed adolescents, there has been relatively little examination of sibling psychopathology. There is preliminary evidence, however, that depressed youth affect and are affected by their siblings. Klein et al. (2002) examined 268 adolescents with MDD, 401 adolescents without MDD, and their 2,202 first degree relatives, including parents and siblings. The authors found that rates of MDD were highest among relatives of adolescents with recurrent episodes and greater impairment (Klein et al., 2002). Coercive family interactions with an antisocial older brother are associated with increases in depressive behaviour in girls (Compton et al., 2003).

Preliminary studies have found that the effects of parental psychopathology on siblings are complex. For example, although maternal MDD is associated with concordance for MDD in siblings, this was not observed for paternal psychopathology (Olino et al., 2006). The differential impact may indicate that mothers' influence on their offspring may be more pervasive and uniform than fathers' influence (Olino et al., 2006).

Child abuse and neglect

Although the family should provide a safe context for a child to develop, many children are exposed to a harsh or rejecting family environment. A history of childhood abuse or neglect significantly increases the risk of depression in adolescence (Kaplan et al., 1999; Nicholas & Rasmussen, 2006). A large longitudinal study, which examined 776 children over a 17-year period found that adolescents and young adults with a history of childhood maltreatment were three times more likely to become depressed or suicidal compared to individuals without such a history (Brown et al., 1999). Moreover, risk of repeated suicide attempts was eight times higher for youth with a history of sexual abuse (Brown et al., 1999).

The links between harsh or abusive parenting and adolescent depression are well documented (Bender et al., 2007; Cicchetti et al., 1994; Sheeber et al., 2001). Longitudinal research (Stuewig & McCloskey, 2005) has shown that parents who are physically harsh towards their young children develop into rejecting parents of adolescents. Parental criticism, rejection, and shaming behaviour towards the adolescents were inversely correlated with warm receptive behaviour. High rejection and low warmth were in turn linked to youths' propensity to experience shame, which was linked to ensuing depression. These findings suggest that the reduction of abusive parenting would be effective in reducing adolescent depression. In addition to the effects of being the direct target of abusive parenting, it is clear that violence in the family has indirect effects. Exposure to marital violence is related to higher levels of depression and depressive symptoms in school-aged children and young adults (Hughes & Luke, 1998; McCloskey et al., 1995; Nicholas & Rasmussen, 2006).

Researchers have consistently found that early adversity predicts depression because of a heightened sensitivity to the environment (Hammen et al., 2000; Harkness et al., 2006; Rudolph & Flynn, 2007). In adolescents with a history of childhood abuse and/or neglect, a first depressive episode may be triggered by a lower level stressful event than is necessary to provoke depression in adolescents without such a history (Harkness et al., 2006; Phillips et al., 2005).

Family disruption

The links between early parental death and risk for depression were highlighted in the seminal research conducted by Brown and Harris (1978) who found that the loss of a mother during childhood potentiated a woman's sensitivity to stressful life events. A large body of research has confirmed that episodes of depression are frequently preceded by interpersonal loss. Furthermore, among adolescent women with a history of childhood adversity, depressive episodes are triggered by a lower level of stress than is required to trigger depression in those who did not experience childhood adversity (Hammen et al., 2000). Although bereavement may be a potent trigger for a depressive episode, the loss of a parent does not inevitably lead to child or adolescent depression (Hammen, 2005). Although many mental health professionals assume that the death of a parent would be an appalling blow that would provoke serious mental health problems for any child who experienced such loss, a substantial minority of bereaved children are resilient in the face of such deaths and do not show any signs of adjustment problems (Lin et al., 2004). Furthermore, there is no evidence to support the assumption that a person who does not show an overt grief reaction is an emotional time bomb who will inevitably one day experience a delayed grief reaction (Bonanno, 2004). Genetic factors may also moderate the effects of exposure to early family adversity on later depression (Caspi et al., 2003). Early loss may therefore play a role in later reactivity to stress, but the mechanisms of risk transmission are multifaceted. It is clear that in our efforts to identify those who are suffering psychological pain, we must be careful to identify those who are at-risk, but we must not overlook the many people who are resilient in the face of adversity. By searching to better understand the qualities, behaviours, and resources of these individuals—who despite enduring suffering maintain their equilibrium and lead satisfying lives—we may be in a better position to mount effective prevention programs to reduce the likelihood that those who experience the risk will develop the disorder.

The adjustment of children of divorced and separated parents has been the subject of hundreds of studies (Lee & Bax, 2000). Adults who are in the process of separation and divorce may experience the gamut of emotions, increased anxiety, depression, and substance use, increased accident-proneness, as well as changes in immune functioning (Kelly & Emery, 2003). It is inevitable that children of all ages are affected by the disruption in their lives as parents shift from living in one home to living in two separate homes. Meta-analyses of this literature by Amato and Keith (1991) and Amato (2001) revealed significant differences between children whose parents were divorced and children whose parents were continuously married. However, the magnitude of these differences was modest, reflecting considerable variability among children of divorced parents. The most robust differences between children from divorced and continuously married families are in terms of externalizing problems, with smaller differences in terms of depression and anxiety (Kelly & Emery, 2003). Although parental separation and divorce are painful stressors for most children and adolescents, the intensity of the reaction is of clinical significance in only a minority of young people (Kelly & Emery, 2003).

Research has consistently underlined the deleterious consequences on child adjustment of parental conflict (Amato & Keith, 1991; Amato & Sobolewski, 2004). There is compelling evidence that a conflictual coparental relationship can undermine good parenting. High conflict parental relationships are associated with less maternal warmth, greater maternal criticism and rejection, and greater paternal withdrawal than in low conflict relationships (Krishnakumar & Buehler, 2000). Given the strong links between marital conflict and parental depression, children may also be exposed to greater parental psychopathology. Furthermore, once the parents separate, the opportunity for a healthy non-resident parent to act as buffer, protecting the child from the effects of the other parent's psychopathology, is reduced (Kelly & Emery, 2003). Maternal depressive symptoms are associated with lower maternal warmth and greater child problems (Whiteside & Becker, 2000). Similar to the pattern found in continuously married families (Lee et al., 2005), the effects of parental conflict are particularly pernicious when parents involve the child in their exchanges, with these young people experiencing greater depressive and anxious symptoms than do their counterparts whose parents shield them from their angry exchanges (Buchanan et al., 1991).

Variables that predict healthy adjustment in children in continuously married families play a similar role in protecting children in divorced families. Children benefit from competent parenting by both their primary caregivers (Kelly & Emery, 2003; Leon, 2003). Authoritative parenting by non-resident fathers is negatively associated with externalizing and internalizing problems (Amato & Gilbreth, 1999). Children take their cues from the adults who are significant in their lives, so that parental adjustment to the transition facilitates the child's adjustment (Leon, 2003).

A respectful coparental relationship is beneficial to both parents and children (Cummings et al., 2004).

Risk factors for childhood problems are not randomly distributed, so that the same child may be exposed to a pile up of stressors. A recent study using the comparison sample for the Fast Track program that was designed to prevent conduct disorder tracked adjustment trajectories in 369 children and their parents, investigating the role of family instability, including residential moves, death of a family member, separation, divorce or marital reconciliation, entry into home of new partner or new child, and parental job loss (Milan et al., 2006). Teacher and parent ratings revealed that children who experienced the greatest accumulated family instability over a six-year period showed more externalizing problems at home and school, and more internalizing problems at home. Analyses of structured diagnostic interviews revealed that cumulative family instability was associated with increased risk of diagnosis of externalizing disorders, and comorbid internalizing and externalizing disorders, but not with internalizing disorders only. These findings highlight the importance of considering the comorbidity of conduct problems and depression in childhood and adolescence (Wolff & Ollendick, 2006).

Transmission mechanisms

Family factors affect youth depression by several pathways. These include biological factors, environmental factors, family interactions and conflict, and parental support and control. Resilience is also related to various aspects of family functioning, including parental support, low parental control, parental warmth, high family cohesion, and parental monitoring.

Transmission of maternal depression

In a seminal review, Goodman and Gotlib (1999) proposed four mechanisms that may explain the transmission of maternal depression to youth, including (a) genetics, (b) neuroregulation difficulties that impact affect regulation, (c) exposure to negative maternal affect and behaviours, and (d) stress and the environmental context within which the youth lives. Offspring of mothers with early-onset depression may carry a higher heritability for depression than do children whose mothers' depression occurs later in life. Additionally, depressed youth of depressed mothers have an earlier mean onset (12.7 years) than do depressed youth of nondepressed mothers (mean onset 16.8 years; Weissman et al., 1987).

Second, Goodman and Gotlib (1999) examined the hypothesis that children with depressed mothers are born with dysfunctional neuroregulatory mechanisms that disturb emotional regulation processes and increase vulnerability to depression. Abnormal neuroendocrine functioning during pregnancy in depressed women exposes foetuses to an increase in cortisol levels and a decrease in blood flow (Field, 2002; Glover, 1997; Glover et al., 1998). Nevertheless, no studies have examined prospectively the role of these abnormalities in explaining links between maternal depression and youth depression (Goodman, 2007; Goodman & Gotlib, 1999). Recent preliminary findings suggest an association between foetal exposure to maternal depression and neuroregulatory dysfunctions across the first year of life (Goodman, 2007), but these findings have not been extended to older children and adolescents.

The third mechanism proposed by Goodman and Gotlib (1999) that maternal depression can be transmitted to offspring through the exposure to negative cognitions, affect, behaviours, and parenting practices has received the greatest investigation. A meta-analysis of 46 observational studies (Lovejoy et al., 2000) revealed that maternal depression is strongly associated with hostile and coercive parenting behaviour and moderately associated with disengaged parenting. Social learning processes such as modelling, observational learning, and reinforcement may facilitate the acquisition of these maladaptive mechanisms by youth of depressed mothers (Goodman, 2007). Depressed parents are also more hostile, less involved with, and less affectionate towards their children (Garber, 2006). Lower maternal social support mediates the relationship between maternal depression and internalizing problems in 11 and 12 year olds (McCarthy & McMahon, 2003). Dysfunctional communication between 8–16 year olds and their depressed mothers mediates the relationship between maternal depression and negative youth self-concept (Hammen et al., 1990). In addition, parental criticism mediates the relationship between maternal depression and depressive disorder in 12–14 year olds (Hilsman, 2001).

In contrast to the large literature on transmission of risk in families with a depressed parent, relatively less work has examined protective factors. A notable exception is the study by Brennan et al. (2003), which examined the relationship between maternal depression, parent–child relationships, and resilient outcomes in a cross-sectional study of 816 fifteen year olds. These investigators reported that low levels of parental psychological control, high levels of maternal warmth, and low levels of maternal over-involvement all interacted with maternal depression to predict resilience outcomes in adolescents.

Finally, the fourth mechanism in the Goodman and Gotlib (1999) model refers to stressors and the environmental context within which the youth lives. Consistent findings have shown that children of depressed mothers are exposed to a more stressful environment than that experienced by children of nondepressed mothers. This stressful environment may include inadequate parenting, the symptoms and episodic course of maternal depression (Compas et al., 2002), the chronic and episodic stressors that are often the context for depression (Monroe & Hadjiyannakis, 2002), and the creation of stress such as marital conflict that is linked with depression (Hammen et al., 1991). The occurrence of one or more of these four risk mechanisms is associated with vulnerabilities in youth in numerous categories of functioning, including psychobiological, cognitive, affective, and behavioural or interpersonal. These vulnerabilities interact and affect one another (Goodman & Gotlib, 1999).

Finally, Goodman and Gotlib's model (1999) included three potential moderators that interact with the aforementioned vulnerabilities. These include the father's health and involvement with the child, the course and timing of the maternal depression, and characteristics of the child, such as gender and temperament.

Family climate

Even in the absence of parental psychopathology, ongoing exposure to adverse family environments including the absence of supportive and facilitative behaviour and the presence of high levels of conflictual, critical, and angry interactions is a significant risk factor for adolescent depression (Sheeber et al., 2001). These negative family relationships are chronic and mostly inescapable stressors.

Youth perception of low parental support, impaired quality of parent–child relationships, and parental rejection have been consistently linked to depression (Garber, 2006; Pavlidis & McCauley, 2001; Stice et al., 2004). Observational data have also linked low parental support to youth depression. Pineda, Cole, and Bruce (2007) observed 72 mother–adolescent dyads discussing controversial topics and found that mothers of adolescents with symptoms of depression provided lower rates of positive parenting and were less likely to respond to adolescents' distress with supportive parenting than were mothers of adolescents without depressive symptoms. In examining mechanisms by which family processes may increase adolescents' vulnerability to depression, the most commonly reported finding is that depression is negatively linked to level of support, attachment, and approval provided by the family environment (Sheeber et al., 2001). This finding has been replicated in studies of community, clinical, and at-risk samples.

A recent investigation examined family relationships in adolescents with unipolar depressive disorder and subdiagnostic depressive symptoms (Sheeber et al., 2007). Results based on multiple sources indicated that both depressed youth and adolescents with subdiagnostic symptoms experienced less supportive and more conflictual relationships with both their mothers and their fathers than did healthy adolescents (Sheeber et al., 2007). Interestingly, the association between parent–adolescent conflict and depression was not moderated by a supportive parent–adolescent relationship with either the same parent or the second parent.

Reviews of the literature have found consistent evidence that family conflict predicts risk for depression among youth (Kane & Garber, 2004; Sheeber et al., 2001). Parent–offspring conflict is associated with self-reported depressive symptoms in adolescents and children (Forehand et al., 1988; Garber, 2006; George, Herman, & Ostrander, 2006). Brendgen et al. (2005) found that a problematic relationship with parents increased the odds of an elevated trajectory of depressed mood in young adolescents regardless of individual temperament. Parent–child conflict has been found to be a mediator of the link between parental substance abuse and offspring internalizing problems (El-Sheikh & Flanagan, 2001).

As previously mentioned links have also been found between interparental conflict and adolescent internalizing problems (Bosco et al., 2003). On the other hand, high levels of parental support serve as a buffer between marital discord and youth depressive symptoms (Davies & Windle, 2001).

High levels of parental control have been implicated in youth depression. Several studies have found that low family cohesion and high affectionless control are associated with youth and young adult symptoms and diagnoses of depression (e.g., George et al., 2006; Nomura et al., 2002).

Moreover, recent findings have suggested that high family cohesion and connection are also resilience factors for youth depression (Hjemdal et al., 2007; Locke, Newcomb, Duclos, & Goodyear, 2007). Other parenting behaviour has also been associated with lower depression scores in young adolescents, including high levels of parental care and monitoring and low levels of parental indifference (Formoso et al., 2000; Kim & Ge, 2000; Liu, 2003). On the basis of these findings, targeting maternal and paternal parenting qualities may increase resilience in at-risk youth.

Research has suggested that parents may inadvertently teach their children to behave in a depressed manner. In a community sample of 86 families with depressed adolescents and 408 families of nondepressed adolescents, parents of adolescents with elevated levels of depressive symptoms were more likely to reinforce depressive behaviour than were parents of adolescents without depressive symptoms (Sheeber et al., 1998). More specifically, mothers of depressed adolescents were more likely to increase facilitative behaviour and fathers of depressed adolescents were more likely to decrease aggressive behaviour in response to adolescent depressive behaviour (Sheeber et al., 1998).

Children and adolescents develop cognitive styles as a function of their parents' behaviour towards them (Sheeber et al., 2001). For example, mothers' criticism of their children has been associated with children's negative attributional style and negative self-view (Jaenicke et al., 1987). Depressed mood and maladaptive behaviour associated with depressive symptoms are reinforced by causal attributional styles (Garber & Flynn, 2001). Moreover, children's self-denigrating comments during family problem-solving interactions have been associated with fathers' critical statements toward them (Hamilton et al., 1999). There is a need to examine the role of parents' inferential messages and attributions for causality that they communicate to their children in order to understand the impact on youth depression and how prevention programs can target these parenting factors (Sanders & McCarty, 2005). Many of these risk factors are variable and may be modified by changes in parent coping, parental behaviour, and parental cognitions (Eley et al., 2004). Prevention strategies targeting these mechanisms could reduce the risk for adolescent depression.

Taken together, these studies underline the salience of the family context in child and youth development. Early exposure to loss and conflict may provoke sensitization so that the child is increasingly vulnerable to the effects of subsequent stressors. Parents have both direct and indirect effects on their children, through their interactions and through the modelling of ways of interacting with others, dealing with emotions, and reacting to challenges. Early risk may set in motion an escalating cycle in which the child's reactions may in turn trigger depressogenic responses.

Interventions for the treatment of depression

Despite depression prevalence rates of 2–8%, only 1% of children and adolescents in the United States receive outpatient treatment for depression (Olfson et al., 2003). Although adolescent depression is a serious problem, in contrast to the wealth of research on the treatment of adult depression, the literature with respect to depression in young people is less extensive. Reviews of this literature have concluded that there is support for both Cognitive–Behaviour Therapy (CBT) and Interpersonal Therapy (IPT) in the treatment of adolescent depression (Chorpita et al., 2002; Kazdin, 2003, 2004).

Guidelines for the treatment of depression in children (National Institute for Health and Clinical Excellence, NICE, 2005) recommend that the initial assessment should address risk and protective factors in the child's social networks. Recognizing the multiple risk pathways (Dozois et al., this volume), mental health professionals are encouraged to consider whether it is necessary that parental psychopathology be treated in parallel with the services offered to the young person. The young person should be advised of the benefits of lifestyle factors including regular exercise, adequate sleep, and good nutrition. The NICE guidelines recommend that antidepressant medication should not be prescribed in the treatment of mild depression. Instead monitoring, non-directive supportive therapy or group CBT are recommended. The first line of treatment for youth with moderate or severe depression is individual CBT, IPT, or short-term family therapy.

CBT interventions are based on the assumption that there are genetic risk factors for depression, which, when combined with maladaptive learned thoughts and behaviours, heighten the chances of experiencing clinically significant depressive symptoms (Asarnow, this volume; Clarke et al., 2003). Parents may be involved in the role of coaches to reinforce therapeutic interventions, or may be involved in learning skills in parenting, conflict resolution, and communication. Compelling evidence regarding the interpersonal difficulties experienced by those suffering from depression fuelled interest in developing a therapy that addressed those interpersonal factors associated with this disorder (Klerman et al., 1984). Interpersonal psychotherapy (IPT) for depression focuses on changing interpersonal problems that are related to the onset, maintenance, and relapse of depressive symptoms. Mufson and her colleagues (Mufson et al., 1999; Mufson & Dorta, 2003) developed IPT-A for adolescents by including attention to developmental issues such as separation from parents, exploration of parental authority, the development of dyadic relationships, and peer pressure.

Echoing the observations made 10 years ago by Shochet and Dadds, only a minority of interventions for depressed children and youth are explicitly labelled as having a family focus. For example, less than a quarter of the studies in a meta-analysis of studies that included random assignment of depressed children and youth to a psychotherapy condition or comparison condition were identified as having a family component (Weisz et al., 2006). Studies listed as including a family, interpersonal, or parent component yielded a broad range of effect sizes, from −0.12 to 0.72, making it difficult to make summary statements about the efficacy of family-based interventions for youth depression. The majority of these family-based interventions were based on cognitive–behavioural (Asarnow et al., 2002; Brent et al., 1997; Clarke et al., 1999; Lewinsohn et al., 1990), or interpersonal approaches (Mufson et al., 1999, 2004; Rosello & Bernal, 1999), with one research group examining attachment-based family therapy (Diamond et al., 2002). A comparison of the efficacy of CBT and systemic behavioural family therapy (SBFT) revealed that although CBT showed greatest post-treatment effects in changing dysfunctional cognitions, at two-year follow up, advantages of SBFT were evident in terms of reducing family conflict and parent–child relationship problems (Kolko et al., 2000).

Given the strong evidence for family factors in the aetiology and maintenance of adolescent depression, many cognitive–behavioural interventions now routinely include parent education sessions in their programs (Wells & Albano, 2005). However, in general, findings are contradictory with respect to the added benefits of including a parent component to CBT. It is clear that despite its intuitive appeal, the inclusion of parents in treatment of youth depression poses many challenges. As a central developmental task in adolescence is the negotiation of increasing autonomy, therapists must find that delicate balance that engages the distant parent and that allows the adolescent sufficient space from a parent who may be over-involved (Wells & Albano, 2005). Although it would be desirable to engage parents in reinforcing the skills that are being taught in CBT, parents of depressed youth have a greater likelihood to experience their own psychopathology that may interfere with their capacity to take on a constructive role. Furthermore, family disruption brings complex family constellations, with residential and nonresidential parents, and blended families.

Cultural issues in parenting have received relatively little attention in the treatment of adolescent depression. Given concerns that some ethnic groups are less likely to access services than are others, efforts are being made to address barriers to service experienced by depressed African American adolescents (Breland-Noble et al., 2006). Breland-Noble and colleagues have developed an intervention that includes a collaboration with parents that includes not only psychoeducation and skill-building, but also attempts to address the impact of previous negative experiences with mental health professionals.

There is evidence that treatments that focus on family functioning hold promise in the treatment of adolescent depression. However, there is stronger evidence for the value of targeting family functioning, rather than for engaging parents as coaches for their offspring. Given the high personal and economic costs of depression, it is important to consider strategies that can prevent its development.

Prevention

In reviewing the literature on cognitive–behavioural and family interventions to prevent depression Gillham et al. (2000) highlighted the work of Beardslee and his colleagues (Beardslee et al., 1992, 1993) in developing and evaluating two family-based programs for the prevention of adolescent depression. Gillham et al. also reported that targeted cognitive–behavioural interventions showed promise in preventing depression. In a recent meta-analytic review, Horowitz and Garber (2006) examined a wide range of programs designed to prevent depressive symptoms in children and adolescents. Studies were included in the review if they had an explicit focus on preventing depression in participants under age 21 who were randomly assigned to an active intervention or to a control group, and if they included a generally accepted measure of depression. Thirty studies reported in published articles, doctoral dissertations, and conferences presentations were identified. Five of these studies involved parent participation.

Horowitz and Garber's analyses of effect sizes revealed that across the range of programs, indicated and selective interventions yielded larger effect sizes than did universal programs. Studies with a greater percentage of female participants had larger effect sizes. The authors defined a prevention effect as occurring when there was an increase in depressive symptoms in the control group and either no change or a decrease in the intervention group. Decreases in symptoms in the intervention group in the absence of increases in the comparison group were labelled as treatment effects. Using this definition, Horowitz and Garber concluded that there was little evidence that these programs are effective in preventing depression. Their recommendations include a focus on at-risk groups, such as being a female adolescent, offspring of depressed parents, with elevated levels of depressive or anxious symptoms, and being exposed to family-related stress such as divorce or bereavement.

An important issue in engaging youth in services is the challenge of recruiting them to services and retaining them throughout the course of the program. A study by Hawley and Weisz (2005) investigated the therapeutic alliance in young people receiving outpatient mental health services and their parents. The *parent*–therapist alliance was related to participation in therapy, with those parents who reported a stronger alliance participating more in services and cancelling fewer sessions. The *youth*–therapist alliance was related to reports of improvements in symptoms. The results of this study nicely illustrate that unless parents are convinced that the therapy is useful, it will be difficult for the youth to participate; but, unless the young person is collaboratively engaged with the therapist, there will be limited change in his or her symptoms. It is likely that these effects will be even more pronounced with respect to preventive programs. One strategy to access young people more directly is to offer services through the schools. Table 8.1 presents prevention studies that have included a parent component.

Including parents in universal prevention programs

Given the strong evidence of family factors in development and maintenance of adolescent depression, there have been attempts to enhance school-based programs by including a family component. Ialongo et al. (1999, 2001), for example, compared a classroom-centred program to a program designed to promote partnerships between school and home. The *Family–School Partnership* (*FSP*; Ialongo et al., 1999) was conducted as part of a universal program with first and second grade children. Families assigned to *FSP* were invited to attend a series of four workshops designed to foster a collaborative partnership, as well as five workshops based on Webster-Stratton's *Parents and Children* series, to promote effective parenting. Analyses of participation rates revealed that parents of children with the highest ratings for behaviour problems and the lowest achievement ratings attended the fewest sessions. Although there was no identifiable effect of FSP on teacher ratings of children's total problems rated in first grade, a positive program effect was evident in grade two. No effects were evident with respect to parent ratings of behaviour problems. Benefits in terms of lower teacher ratings for behaviour problem were maintained at follow-up when the children were in sixth grade (Ialongo et al., 2001). Although it was hypothesized that this intervention would have a long-term effect on depression, no data addressing this issue were reported. No data were presented addressing the efficacy of the program in enhancing parent–teacher communication or in parenting skills.

Shochet et al. (2001) examined the utility of adding to the *Resourceful Adolescent Program* (RAP) a three session family component (RAP-F) designed to reduce family conflict and promote a responsive, warm relationship between adolescent and parent. The RAP is a universal prevention program delivered as part of the curriculum to students in grade 9. To facilitate parental attendance in RAP-F, each three-hour session was conducted in the evening. Students were assessed on three occasions, two weeks before the start of the program, within three weeks after the end of the intervention, and ten months post-intervention. Their scores were compared with those of the

Table 8.1 Family approaches to prevention of depression

Study	Sample & recruitment	Sample, groups, and assignment	Age of child	Goals	Change in risk & protection	Depression outcomes	Comments
Universal programs							
Ialongo et al., 1999	First grade children and their parents	678 families. Randomized block design comparing Classroom-centred and Family–school partnership interventions	5.3 years– 7.7 years	Improving parent–teacher communication, parental teaching, and behaviour management in order to enhance achievement and reduce poor achievement, shy, and aggressive behaviour	Little relation between parent-participation and child achievement; effect on child behaviour problems evident in second grade	N/A	No direct evaluation of whether program was effective in changing risk and protection.
Shochet et al., 2001	Year 9 students	Random assignment to Resource-Adolescent Program (n = 68), RAP + family component (n = 56) and comparison untreated cohort from the previous year (n = 118)	12–15	Family component designed to address family conflict and promote warm parent–adolescent relationship	Very low attendance by parents	Lower levels of depression and hopelessness in both treated groups	No direct evaluation of whether program was effective in changing risk and protection.

Children of depressed parents

Beardslee et al., 1997	Parents with affective disorder and their nondepressed child	Random assignment to 6–10 session clinician-facilitated family intervention (n = 18) ; or 2 lecture discussion for parents only (n = 18)	8–15	To enhance understanding of depression, youth's interpersonal relationships and independence	Parent reported: Increased parent–child communication; increased understanding of depression	K-SADS-E-R, CDI, CBCL. Children in clinician group reported to be functioning better	Severe risk; small sample size
Clarke et al., 2001	Moderate risk adolescents of depressed parents	Random assignment to group CBT (n = 49) or TAU (n = 49)	13–18	Cognitive restructuring with focus on having a depressed parent	N/A	CES-D, HAM-D, K-SADS-E Improvements. CBCL—no change	Unknown effect of parental involvement, fading of effects
Sanford et al., 2003	Outpatient	44 depressed parents randomly assigned to parenting program (n = 21) or wait list (n = 23)	6–13	8 weekly 2-hour sessions with 8–12 parents (alone or with partner) psychoeducation & parenting	Decrease in family conflict; decrease in parent disagreements	CDI—no significant differences	High attrition, small sample size, lower drop-out rates among less depressed parents

grade 9 cohort from the previous year who had been assessed, but had not received any intervention. Both RAP and RAP-F were very successful in engaging and retaining youth, with all participants attending at least 9 of the 11 sessions, and only 2% attrition. In contrast, only 36% of parents in the RAP-F group attended at least one session, and only 10% attended all three sessions. Analyses of youth depressive symptoms revealed that youth in both active intervention conditions improved their scores on both the Child Depression Inventory and the Beck Hopelessness Scale; no intervention effects were evident on the Reynolds Adolescent Depression scale. No differences were found between those participating in RA and RAP-F. Given the low parental participation rates, the authors interpreted the program effects as due to adolescent participation in the program.

Although it makes sound theoretical sense to engage parents in services to ensure that they understand and can reinforce the themes addressed in preventions programs, there has been only limited study of the benefits of inclusion of parents in universal prevention programs for their children and currently there is no empirical support. Consistent with findings for parenting interventions, it appears to be most difficult to recruit and retain those parents who may be in greatest need of the program. Parents who are themselves depressed often live in conflictual, stressful environments that provide little support; in addition to family stressors, they may experience financial hardship and socio-economic disadvantage (Hammen, 2005). For such parents, attendance at workshops, lectures, or group sessions may be unappealing due to shame or hopelessness, and may also present obstacles in terms of transportation, child-care, and time management.

Selective prevention programs

Beardslee and his colleagues have developed and evaluated interventions for youth who are at-risk for depression due to affective disorder in one or both of their parents (Beardslee & Gladstone, 2001; Beardslee et al., 1997; Focht-Birkerts & Beardslee, 2000). Two interventions were designed to reduce risk of depression in youth by reducing family risk factors and promoting resilience. A clinician-based program included 6–10 sessions conducted with parents that culminated in a family session. The mean number of sessions was 7.1. The family session was a forum for discussion of information of depression, designed to shift understanding of depressive behaviours. Ideally, the family session was also a spring-board for ongoing dialogue between family members. A refresher session was offered six months later. A two-session lecture and discussion program was offered to groups of parents. Both interventions produced positive results, with the more intense, clinician intervention yielding stronger findings. Children in the clinician group reported higher levels of functioning than did children in the lecture group, although there were no differences in child self-reported symptoms. Families in the clinician group evidenced improvement in protective factors, such as communication, supportiveness, and understanding of affective disorder.

This approach is based on the premise that parental affective disorder is associated with parental behaviours that arouse negative affect in their children. The tendency to constrict affect is a risk factor for adolescent depression, whereas the tendency to express affect serves a protective function. Parents with affective disorders can therefore play an important role in promoting their children's resilience by facilitating communication about affect the child or youth experiences as a result of the parent's illness-related behaviour. In the second phase of the project, families are offered consultation about their offspring on an annual basis. Focht-Birkerts and Beardslee (2000) provided case examples of families with parents suffering recurrent serious psychopathology who have successfully engaged in a process that enables them to talk about the role of depressive disorder in the lives of all family members.

Sanford et al. (2003) reported on a preliminary trial of a group treatment for depressed parents. Groups were delivered in eight weekly 2-hours sessions. The intervention included two components: family psychoeducation modelled after the approaches used for families dealing with schizophrenia and behavioural parent training. Sanford et al. reported high levels of attrition, so that the participant pool dwindled from 65 patients referred to the study, to 44 who were randomly assigned to groups, 32 who completed post-treatment measures, and 25 who completed follow-up data. Despite the small sample size, positive group effects were found in terms of decreasing conflict and disagreement, and enhancing sense of parenting competence. There were no positive effects in terms of child outcome.

Indicated prevention programs

Clarke et al. (2001) reviewed records of a health maintenance organization to identify depressed adults with adolescent offspring. Youth were categorized as low ($n = 233$), medium ($n = 123$), or high ($n = 116$) depression severity. Medium severity youth (those reported symptoms of depression that were at below the threshold for diagnosis of a mood disorder) were randomly assigned to a cognitive–behavioural treatment condition or to a usual care condition. Prior to randomization, 29 declined to participate. Randomized sub-syndromal youth were more likely to be female than youth from the initial pool. The active intervention consisted of 15 one-hour sessions offered to groups of 6–10 youth. Youth attended an average of 9.5 sessions. Cognitive restructuring was used to identify and challenge dysfunctional thoughts, with a particular focus on having a depressed parent. In addition, three parent information meetings were offered towards the beginning, middle, and end of the course of groups for adolescents. No data are presented on parental attendance at parent meetings. Positive program effects were found in terms of youth ratings of depression (CES-D), clinician ratings of depression (Hamilton Depression Rating Scale), but not in terms of parent ratings (CBCL). Survival analyses of incidence of major depressive episodes indicate a significant advantage to participating in the intervention. The preventive effects were evident, but less dramatic at 18- and 24-month follow-up. The authors cautioned that although this trial provides strong evidence of efficacy, the durability of effects is less clear, and the effectiveness in standard clinical settings is unknown. Furthermore, it is unknown whether the three parent sessions contributed to program efficacy.

To address the dilemma of how to reach and recruit depressed mothers into a program designed to prevent depression in their children, Boyd et al. (2006) conducted focus groups with mothers receiving services for a mood disorder at a community mental health agency, as well as with mental health providers. Themes identified in this process are used to inform the development of a new program, the *Protecting Families Program* that will offer concurrent services to mothers, including psychoeducation about depression and its impact on children, as well as parenting skills for emotion regulation and behavioural control, and a modified version of the Penn Optimism Program for their children.

It is clear that the design of prevention programs must take into account obstacles to parent participation. Strategies to engage stressed adults in parenting programs include the timing and location of sessions, the provision of transport, childcare, and meals. Although these appear to be costly services to offer, they should be considered within the context of the significant savings that will accrue if depressive symptoms are reduced, or an episode of major depression averted.

Table 8.2 describes prevention programs that were designed to prevent depression in young people exposed to parental separation, divorce, and death. Programs can be divided according to the focus on the program, into those that involved children only, parents only, and those that provided services separately for adults and their children.

A number of school-based programs offered services for children whose parents had experienced separation or divorce (Lee et al., 1994). These programs were designed to help child understand their parents' divorce, to express their feelings about it, to problem solve, and to seek support. Diverse measures of child adjustment included depression (Gwynn & Brantley, 1987; Roseby & Deutsch, 1985), internalizing problems (Alpert Gillis et al., 1989), and affective symptoms (Stolberg & Mahler, 1994). Although these programs reported success in terms of enhancing divorce-related knowledge, with the exception of Stolberg and Mahler, these changes were not accompanied by reductions in children's symptomatology. The fact that program participants were relatively healthy children who had not been identified as having problems limits the extent to which any positive program effects would be found (Lee et al., 1994). In addition, the programs may have been weakened by their failure to draw on the substantial body of knowledge of mediators of children's adjustment to parental separation and divorce (Grych & Fincham, 1992).

Two programs (Forgatch & DeGarmo, 1999; Wolchik et al., 1993) contacted recently divorced mothers through court records. Wolchik et al. excluded from their program mothers who were in treatment for psychological problems, as well as families who scored highly on the putative mediating variables of the quality of the mother–child relationship and the divorce-related events. Mothers and children who reported clinical range depressive symptoms were also excluded. In both study group, parenting sessions focused on putative mediators of the risk for children of divorced parents—ineffective parenting, parental distress, and poor parent–child relationships. Parenting skills were taught in an effort to reduce coercive parenting (Patterson, 1982). To reduced barriers to participation, childcare and meals were provided and transportation was available if required (Forgatch & DeGarmo, 1999). Mothers who missed a number of group sessions were offered individual sessions to cover material that had been missed. Both programs reported relatively low attrition rates, with less than a third of program participants dropping out before the end of a one-year follow up. Both programs reported efficacy in reducing risk factors and enhancing protective factors by improving parenting, and decreasing coercive interactions. Within a year of the program, there were no evident

Table 8.2 Programs to prevent depression in children exposed to parental separation, divorce, or death

Study	Sample & recruitment	Sample, groups, and assignment	Age of child	Intervention	Change in risk and protective factors	Change in depression outcomes
Adult-focused						
Forgatch & DeGarmo, 1999	Recently separated mothers of sons; recruited through media and divorce records	Random assignment to rx ($n = 153$) or no rx ($n = 85$). Attrition rate of 18% in each group	1st to 3rd graders	Parenting groups	Decrease in coercive parenting in rx group	No change in CDI or in mother rating
Wolchik et al., 1993	Divorced mothers	Random assignment to rx ($n = 48$) or wait list ($n = 48$). Attrition 29% from rx, 22% from wait-list	8–15	10 group session and 2 individual sessions for mothers	Rx group showed improved parent–child relationships; effective discipline; better maternal mental health; improved attitude towards father.	No change in maternal or child ratings of depression within a year.
Child-focused interventions						
Alpert-Gillis et al., 1989	Children whose parents had separated	Assignment procedure not mentioned. 52 rx 52 no rx. 81 no rx intact comparison	2nd & 3rd graders	16 week- promotes support. Encourages expression of feelings	Improvement on Children's divorce adjustment scale	Parent rated problems decreased. 0.77 No change in teacher ratings

(continued)

Table 8.2 (continued) Programs to prevent depression in children exposed to parental separation, divorce, or death

Study	Sample & recruitment	Sample, groups, and assignment	Age of child	Intervention	Change in risk and protective factors	Change in depression outcomes
Gwynn & Brantley, 1987	Children whose parents had been separated at least a year. Unspecified matching to no-treatment children	Assignment procedure not mentioned. Paired groups 30 boys 30 girls 30 received rx; 30 no rx.	9–11 4th and 5th graders	8 weeks of Educational support group	All children decreased negative feelings about divorce	Rx group significantly reduced symptoms of depression
Roseby & Deutsch, 1985	Children who had experienced parental separation or divorce Schools randomly assigned as rx or no rx.	Schools randomly assigned to rx or no rx. Rx: n = 27 No rx: n = 19.	9–11	10-week group treatment social role taking	Improved knowledge of divorce	No change in depression
Stolberg & Mahler, 1994	Children whose parents had separated or divorced	Schools randomly assigned to 1 of 3 rx conditions or no rx. Transfer, skills + support: n = 29; skills + support: n = 28; support: n = 23; no rx. n = 23	8–12	14 week inter-vention: support, skill-building, skills transfer	N/A	NS. Significant decrease in internalizing behaviours p. 151

Adult and child-focused

Sandler et al., 1992	Bereaved parents recruited through death certificates and referrals from community agencies	Random assignment of families to rx (n = 35) or wait list (n = 37). 24 completed the program	7–17	9 family and 6 parent only sessions demoralization; warmth; cohesion; routines; coping; support	Increased warmth in parent–child relationships; increased satisfaction with social support; discussion of grief-related issues	No change in self-report or clinician rating of depression Reduced parent reported depression for older children
Wolchik et al., 2000	Divorced mothers recruited through court records	Random assignment to mother only program: n = 81; dual: n = 83;self-study for mothers: n =76 Attrition: mother: 20%; dual 12%	9–12	11 sessions	Rx had enhanced mother–child relationship quality, effective discipline, attitudes towards noncustodial parent	Lower internalizing problems in 2 rx conditions 0.34

effects in terms of reducing depressive symptoms in the child, according to either mother or child report. However, follow-up analyses 30 months later revealed that parenting changes were first evident, followed by changes in boys' behaviour, followed by changes in maternal depression. Intervention effects in terms of boys' externalizing behaviours were mediated by changes in boys' internalizing behaviours (DeGarmo et al., 2004).

Two programs included conditions in which both parents and children were offered services to help them deal with the family disruption of parental divorce (Wolchik et al., 2000) or bereavement (Sandler et al., 1992). These programs reported that the interventions were effective in changing putative mediators of child and youth outcome. In turn, the programs reported a reduction in depressive symptoms among child and youth participants.

In conclusion, the evidence-base for family-based prevention efforts has not changed dramatically since Shochet and Dadds (1997) first identified the paradox that despite the strong predictive power of family variables, there is limited evidence that family-based interventions are effective in reducing adolescent depression. Programs that hold the greatest promise are those that build on knowledge of risk and protection factors. Assessment of the capacity to change hypothesized mediators is a necessary pre-condition to demonstrate a prevention effect. It is clear that the pathways to resilience are complex and that some family changes are not evident until months or years after the program. This requires the provision of lengthy follow-up evaluations, and the possibility of providing booster sessions to reinforce positive patterns at times of transition.

In considering any intervention, mental health professionals must be sensitive to iatrogenic effects. Generally, psychological services have a low risk of causing harm. It is difficult to imagine, for example, contexts in which a person would be disadvantaged by learning to label emotions, to deal constructively with conflict, or to express interpersonal needs. However, given the volatile and fragile family interaction patterns within which depression can develop, it is possible that family-based interventions may run the risk of inadvertently increasing problems. As eager coaches, parents may inadvertently undermine the young person's esteem or self-confidence.

Some of the obstacles to family-based preventions have been identified throughout this chapter. First, it is likely that the families with the greatest need to change may be the least likely to attend. So parents experiencing depression, marital conflict, poverty, and isolation may be the hardest to reach. Furthermore, parental psychopathology may interfere with the parent's capacity to play a supportive role. It may be necessary to address the parent's difficulties before the parent can be engaged to help the young person. It may also be necessary to address conflict between the parents, before they can work together to help the young person. In the final section of the chapter, we explore programs that have not been explicitly developed to prevent child and adolescent depression, but which target risk factors, and therefore hold the possibility of reducing child and adolescent depression.

Untested, but promising strategies to prevent child and youth depression: promoting evidence-based parenting

Throughout the chapter we have highlighted research that emphasizes the key role parents play in their children's socialization. Harsh or inconsistent discipline, poor supervision and monitoring of a child, parental abuse, and neglect are risk factors that are associated with the development of a wide range of child and adolescent psychopathology. On the other hand, the availability of supportive, caring parents can protect children and youth from the development of psychopathology. Although the responsibilities of child-rearing can be daunting at times to all parents, some parents are particularly vulnerable due to their age, isolation, distress, conflict, or limited socio-economic resources. Children's functioning is challenged by poor parenting, conflict in the family, and parental psychopathology (Biglan, 2003). We describe below three evidence-based programs that have been developed to promote good parenting and therefore to decrease risk factors for diverse child problems. The effects of these programs on child and adolescent depression have not been evaluated.

The *Triple-P Positive Parenting Program* is an evidence-based parenting program designed to (a) enhance knowledge, skills, and confidence of parents; (b) promote safe environments for young people; and (c) promote children's competence through positive parenting practices (Sanders, 1999; Sanders et al., 2003; Sanders et al., 2004). Consistent with the idea of adapting programs to offer different dosages of intervention according to participants' needs, the *Triple-P program* is a multi-level system that provides interventions of gradually increasing intensity, according to the level of need (Collins et al., 2004). We focus here on preventive interventions.

The universal Triple-P program is offered to all interested parents using a variety of media to provide evidence-based information about general parenting strategies to deal with everyday issues and challenges. The next step in the program hierarchy is to offer brief (one or two session) individualized services by phone or face to face to address parents' specific concerns. Moving one step further, parents of children with mild to moderate problems may benefit from a program delivered over four sessions by a primary health care provider. Program materials are adapted for five different developmental stages (infants, toddlers, preschoolers, children in elementary school, and teenagers). The program is designed to enhance protective factors and to decrease risk factors for the child problems. Consequently, parents are trained to develop positive relationships with their children, encourage desirable behaviour, teach new skills, and manage misbehaviour. Parents are encouraged to adopt developmentally appropriate expectations about their child's behaviour. The importance of taking care of oneself as a parent is also stressed. The *Triple-P* approach involves intense training of practitioners as well as continuing education for those who deliver the program. The developers of *Triple P* approach have conducted a series of randomized controlled trials comparing *Triple P* interventions with wait-list control groups, as well as comparing different formats of *Triple P* (Sanders et al., 2004). Results of this research indicate that *Triple P* is effective in helping parents to adopt positive parenting practices, which in turn is associated with fewer child problems, greater parental confidence, and enhanced parental well-being (Sanders et al., 2004). Currently, the *Triple P* program is being adapted for use in diverse populations in several countries and evaluations of those programs are underway. The efficacy in preventing depression has not been examined.

A number of programs have demonstrated impressive results in targeting at-risk parents. In a 25-year long program of research, Olds and his colleagues have developed, implemented, tested, and replicated a program offering services to low income teenage single mothers expecting their first child (Olds, 2002). Home visits were conducted by trained nurses beginning during the pregnancy and continuing after the child's birth. During these visits nurses addressed women's concerns about the pregnancy, delivery, and care of the child. They taught skills in both self care and child care and promoted women's use of the healthcare system. In randomized controlled trials, Olds and his colleagues have found that the home visit program is effective in achieving the immediate goal of improving parental care. In the middle term, this has benefits for children in terms of reducing child abuse and neglect, and in the long-term, reducing the number of arrests, convictions, substance abuse problems, and sexual promiscuity in the children when they reached the age of 15. Furthermore, the program has positive effects in terms of improving a young mother's life course by increasing labour force participation and her economic self-sufficiency. These positive effects are all the more remarkable as nurses completed only an average of eight visits during pregnancy and 25 visits during the child's first two years of life. Visits lasted up to an hour and a half. These short- and long-term gains were accomplished in a very high risk group with the investment of under 50 hours of direct contact between nurses and teenage mothers. In general, the most beneficial effects were found for the families who were at greatest risk. In adapting an efficacious program, there is always a danger that it will not be faithfully applied and that, as corners are cut and important elements are diluted, so too the efficacy of the program can be eroded. The efficacy in preventing depression has not been examined.

The *Incredible Years* training program was originally designed to help children aged 3–8 who had been identified as having conduct problems (Webster-Stratton, 2006). As the program was found to be successful in treating conduct problems, it has been expanded to cover a wider age range and has been offered as a prevention program (Baydar et al., 2003). The program uses group discussion, videotaped modelling, and behavioural rehearsal techniques to promote adult–child interactions that will facilitate children's development of social competence. The primary goal of the *Incredible Years* program is to train parents in skills so that they can effectively play with their child, provide praise for positive behaviours, and set limits on unacceptable behaviours using time-out, ignoring, appropriate consequences, and problem-solving. The basic program is available for different age ranges and includes a minimum of 12 sessions (although additional sessions may be required). In addition an advanced 9–12 session program targets parents' interpersonal difficulties by teaching problem-solving, anger management, communication, emotional regulation skills, and support-seeking skills. A supplementary program *Supporting Your Child's Education* helps parents whose children are experiencing school difficulties. Complementary programs involve training teachers and a 22-week child training program that teaches emotional literacy, perspective-taking, friendship skills, anger management, and problem-solving (Webster-Stratton et al., 2001). The effectiveness of this selective prevention program has been tested with over 1,000 multiethnic, socio-economically disadvantaged families. Results support the effectiveness of the program in promoting good parenting, enhancing children's social competence, and in preventing the development of conduct problems (Gross et al., 2003). The efficacy in preventing depression has not been examined.

Target family functioning in treatment of other disorders

As noted earlier, depression is highly comorbid with a number of disorders that are first evident in childhood, including anxiety disorders, ADHD, and oppositional defiant disorder. As family factors are strongly linked to these disorders, it is likely that family-based interventions to treat these disorders are likely to have positive effects in terms of prevention of the development of later depression (Kessler et al., 2007).

Several small scale studies have reported on efforts to train mothers experiencing post-partum depression to respond sensitively to their infants (e.g., Jung et al., 2007). This early intervention may be a crucial first step in breaking the cycle of risk. Another promising strategy is to target depressive symptoms in mothers of children diagnosed with ADHD (Chronis et al., 2006).

Conclusions

Although there is strong evidence for the role of family factors in the development and maintenance of adolescent depression, the evidence base for family-based prevention is limited. As adolescents negotiate the developmental tasks of separation and individuation, they retain important links with their parents, but are also increasingly affected by peers (Smetana et al., 2006). The family risk factors make successful involvement of the family in prevention efforts at this stage of development a challenge. However, it is important to not abandon family-centred prevention efforts. On the contrary, we argue that many family-based prevention programs work to promote the same relatively simple principles such as promoting positive adult–child relationships; allowing children ample opportunities to be rewarded for appropriate behaviour; providing adequate monitoring and supervision; providing mild corrective feedback for inappropriate behaviour; helping children manage emotions, treat one another with respect, and act assertively rather than aggressively; and facilitating the development of supportive networks (Biglan, 2003; Carr, 2002). Effective prevention programs are usually multi-faceted, involving different modules that operate at the level of the individual, family, school, community, or legal system. This allows the same message to be conveyed by parents, teachers, peers, community leaders, and government (Weissberg et al., 2003). Although the effects of family-based programs may not be evident as quickly as the effects of programs that target children directly, the potential benefits are significant. Furthermore, given the vulnerabilities of families that are prone to depression, attention should also be paid to the need for booster and follow-up sessions. It is likely that many evidence-based parenting programs offered to vulnerable families with young children may have as yet undocumented effectiveness in the prevention of child and adolescent depression.

References

Alpert Gillis, L.J., Pedro-Carroll, J.L., & Cowen, E.L. (1989). The children of divorce intervention program: Development, implementation, and evaluation of a program for young urban children. *Journal of Consulting and Clinical Psychology, 57*, 583–589.

Amato, P.R. (2001). Children of divorce in the 1990s: An update of the Amato and Keith meta-analysis. *Journal of Family Psychology, 15,* 355–370.

Amato, P.R. & Gilbreth, J.G. (1999). Nonresident fathers and children's well-being: A meta-analysis. *Journal of Marriage and the Family, 61,* 557–573.

Amato, P.R. & Keith, B. (1991). Parental divorce and the wellbeing of children: A meta-analysis. *Psychological Bulletin, 110,* 26–46.

Amato, P.R. & Sobolewski, J.M. (2004). The effects of divorce on fathers and children: Nonresidential fathers and step-fathers. In M.E. Lamb (Ed.), *The role of the father in child development* (4th ed., pp. 341–367). New York: Wiley.

Asarnow, J. (this volume). Cognitive–behavioral therapy in a primary care setting.

Asarnow, J.R., Scott, C.V., & Mintz, J. (2002). A combined cognitive–behavioral family education intervention for depressed children: A treatment development study. *Cognitive Therapy and Research, 26,* 221–229.

Barrett, P. & Turner, C. (2004). Prevention of childhood anxiety and depression. In P.M. Barrett & T.H. Ollendick (Eds.), *Interventions that work with children and adolescents: Prevention and Treatment* (pp. 429–474). Chichester UK: Wiley.

Baydar, N., Reid, J., & Webster-Stratton, C. (2003). The role of mental health factors and program engagement in the effectiveness of a preventive parenting program for Head Start mothers. *Journal of Consulting and Clinical Psychology, 74,* 1433–1453.

Beardslee, W.R. & Gladstone, T.R.G. (2001). Prevention of childhood depression: Recent findings and future prospects. *Society of Biological Psychiatry, 49,* 1101–1110.

Beardslee, W.R., Hoke, L., Wheelock, I., Rothberg, P.C., van de Velde, P., & Swatling, S. (1992). Initial findings on preventive interventions for families with parental affective disorder. *American Journal of Psychiatry, 149,* 1335–1340.

Beardslee, W.R., Salt, P., Porterfield, K., Rothberg, P.C., van de Velde, P., Swatling, S., et al. (1993). Comparison of preventive interventions for families with parental affective illness. *Journal of the American Academy of Child and Adolescent Psychiatry, 32,* 254–263,

Beardslee, W.R., Wright, E.J., Salt, P., Drezner, K., Gladstone, T.R.G., Versage, E.M., et al. (1997). Examination of children's responses to two preventive intervention strategies over time. *Journal of the American Academy of Child and Adolescent Psychiatry, 36,* 196–204.

Beardslee, W.R., Versage, E.M., & Gladstone, T.R. (1998). Children of affectively ill parents: A review of the past 10 years. *Journal of the American Academy of Child and Adolescent Psychiatry, 37,* 1134–1141.

Bender, H.L., Allen, J., McElhaney, K.B., Antonishak, J., Moore, C.M., Kelly, H.O., et al. (2007). Use of harsh physical discipline and developmental outcomes in adolescence. *Development and Psychopathology, 19,* 227–242.

Biglan, A. (2003). The generic features of effective childrearing. In A. Biglan, M. Wang. & H.J. Walberg (Eds.), *Preventing youth problems* (pp. 145–162). New York, NY: Kluwer Academic.

Biglan, A., Mrazek, P.K., Carnine, D., & Flay, B.R. (2003). The integration of research and practice in the prevention of youth behavior problems. *American Psychologist, 58,* 433–440.

Birmaher, B., Ryan, N.D., Williamson, D.E., Brent, D.A., Kaufman, J., Dahl, R.E., et al. (1996). Child and adolescent depression: A review of the past 10 years. Part I. *Journal of the American Academy of Child and Adolescent Psychiatry, 121,* 241–258.

Bonanno, G.A. (2004). Loss, trauma, and human resilience. *American Psychologist, 59,* 20–28.

Bosco, G.L., Renk, K., Dinger, T.M., Epstein, M.K., & Phares, V. (2003). The connections between adolescents' perceptions of parents, parental psychological symptoms, and adolescent functioning. *Applied developmental Psychology, 24,* 179–200.

Bouchard, G., Lee, C.M., Asgary, V., & Pelletier, L. (2007). Fathers' motivation for involvement with their children: A self-determination theory perspective. *Fathering, 5*, 23–40.

Boyd, R.C., Diamond, G.S., & Bourjolly, J.N. (2006). Developing a family-based depression prevention program in urban community mental health clinics: A qualitative investigation. *Family Process, 45*, 187–203.

Breland-Noble, A., Bell, C., & Nicolas, G. (2006). Family-first: The development of an evidence-based family intervention for increasing participation in psychiatric clinical care and research in depressed African American adolescents. *Family Process, 45*, 153–169.

Brendgen, M., Wanner, B., Morin, A.J.S., & Vitaro, F. (2005). Relations with parents and with peers, temperament, and trajectories of depressed mood during early adolescence. *Journal of Abnormal Child Psychology, 33*, 579–594.

Brennan, P.A., Hammen, C., Katz, A.R., & Le Brocque, R.M. (2002). Maternal depression, paternal psychopathology, and adolescent diagnostic outcomes. *Journal of Consulting and Clinical Psychology, 70*, 1075–1085.

Brennen, P.A., Le Brocque, R.M., & Hammen, C. (2003). Maternal depression, parent-child relationships, and resilient outcomes in adolescents. *Journal of the American Academy of Child and Adolescent Psychiatry, 42*, 1469–1477.

Brent, D.A., Holder, D., Kolko, D., Birmaher, B., Baugher, M., Roth, C., et al. (1997). A clinical psychotherapy trial for adolescent depression comparing cognitive, family, and supportive therapy. *Archives of General Psychiatry, 54*, 877–885.

Brown, J., Cohen, P., Johnson, J.G., & Smailes, E.M. (1999). Childhood abuse and neglect: Specificity of effects on adolescent and young adult depression and suicidality. *Journal of the American Academy of Child and Adolescent Psychiatry, 38*, 1490–1496.

Brown, G.W. & Harris, T.O. (1978). *Social origins of depression.* London: Free Press.

Buchanan, C., Maccoby, E., & Dornbusch, S. (1991). Caught between parents: Adolescents' experiences in divorced homes. *Child Development, 62*, 1008–1029.

Burt, K.B., Van Dulmen, M., Carlivati, J., Egeland, B., Sroufe, L.A., Forman, D.R., et al. (2005). Mediating links between maternal depression and offspring psychopathology: The importance of independent data. *Journal of Child Psychology and Psychiatry, 46*, 490–499.

Caspi, A., Sugden, K., Moffitt, T.E., Taylor, A., Craig, I.W., et al. (2003). Influence of life stress: Moderation by a polymorphism in the 5-HTT gene. *Science, 301*, 386–389.

Carr, A. (2002). Conclusions. In A. Carr (Ed.). *Prevention: what works with children and adolescents? A critical review of psychological prevention programmes for children, adolescents and their families* (pp. 359–372). Hove, UK: Brunner-Routledge.

Chorpita, B.F., Yim, L.M., Donkervoet, J.C., Arensdorf, A., Amundsen, M.J., McGee, C., et al. (2002). Towards large-scale implementation of empirically supported treatments for children: A review and observations by the Hawaii Empirical Basis to Services Task Force. *Clinical Psychology: Science and Practice, 9*, 165–190.

Chronis, A.M., Gamble, S.A., Roberts, J.E., & Pelham, W.E. (2006). Cognitive–behavioral depression treatment for mothers of children with Attention-Deficit/Hyperactivity disorder. *Behavior Therapy, 37*, 143–158.

Cicchetti, D., Rogosch, F.A., & Toth, S.L. (1994). A developmental psychopathology perspective on depression in children and adolescents. In W.M. Reynolds & H.F. Johnston (Eds.), *Handbook of depression in children and adolescents: Issues in clinical child psychology*, (pp. 123–141). New York: Plenum.

Clarke, G.N., DeBar, L.L., & Lewinsohn, P.M. (2003). Cognitive–behavioural group treatment for adolescent depression. In A.E. Kazdin & J.R. Weisz (Eds.), *Evidence-based psychotherapies for children and adolescents* (pp. 120–134). New York: Guilford.

Clarke, G.N., Hornbrook, M., Lynch, F., Polen, M., Gale, J., Beardslee, W., et al. (2001). A randomized trial of a group cognitive intervention for preventing depression in adolescent offspring of depressed parents. *Archives of General Psychiatry, 58,* 1127–1134.

Clarke, G.N., Rohde, P., Lewinsohn, P.M., Hops, H., & Seeley, J.R. (1999). Cognitive–behavioral treatment of adolescent depression: Efficacy of acute group treatment and booster sessions. *Journal of the American Academy of Child and Adolescent Psychiatry, 38,* 272–279.

Collins, L.M., Murphy, S.A., & Bierman, K.L. (2004). A conceptual framework for adaptive preventive interventions. *Prevention Science, 5,* 185–196.

Compas, B.E., Langrock, A.M., Keller, G., Merchant, M.J., & Copeland, M.E. (2002). Children coping with parental depression: Processes of adaptation to family stress. In S.H. Goodman & I.H. Gotlib (Eds.), *Children of depressed parents: Mechanisms of risk and implications for treatment* (pp. 227–252). Washington, DC: American Psychological Association.

Compton, K., Snyder, J., Schrepferman, L., Bank, L., & Shortt, J.W. (2003). The contribution of parents and siblings to antisocial and depressive behavior in adolescence: A double jeopardy coercion model. *Development and Psychopathology, 15,* 163–182.

Connell, A.M. & Goodman, S.H. (2002). The association between psychopathology in fathers versus mothers and children' internalizing and externalizing behavior problems: A meta-analysis. *Psychological Bulletin, 128,* 746–773.

Coyne, J.C. & Downey, G. (1991). Social factors and psychopathology: Stress, social support, and coping processes. *Annual Review of Psychology, 42,* 401–425.

Cummings, E.M., Goeke-Morey, M., & Raymond, J. (2004). Fathers in family context: Effects of marital quality and marital conflict. In M.E. Lamb (Ed.), *The role of the father in child development* (4th ed., pp. 196–221). New York: Wiley.

Davies, P.T. & Windle, M. (2001). Interparental discord and adolescent adjustment trajectories: The potentiating and protective role of interpersonal attributes. *Child Development, 72,* 1163–1178.

DeGarmo, D.S., Patterson, G.R., & Forgatch, M.S. (2004). How do outcomes in a specified parent training intervention maintain or wane over time? *Prevention Science, 5,* 73–89.

Diamond, G.S., Reis, B.F., Diamond, G.M., Siqueland, L., & Isaac, L. (2002). Attachment based family therapy for depressed adolescents: A treatment development study. *Journal of the American Academy of Child and Adolescent Psychiatry, 41,* 1190–1196.

Diamond, G. & Josephson, A. (2005). Family-based treatment research: A 10-year update. *Journal of the American Academy of Child and Adolescent Psychiatry, 44,* 872–887.

Dozois, D.J.A. (this volume). Risk and protective factors.

Eley, T.C., Liang, H., Plomin, R., Sham, P., Sterne, A., Williamson, R. et al. (2004). Parental familial vulnerability, family environment, and their interactions as predictors of depressive symptoms in adolescents. *Journal of the American Academy of Child and Adolescent Psychiatry, 42,* 1108–1115.

El-Sheikh, M. & Flanagan, E. (2001). Parental problem drinking and children's adjustment: Family conflict and parental depression as mediators and moderators of risk. *Journal of Abnormal Child Psychology, 29,* 417–432.

Essau, C.A. (2004). The association between family factors and depressive disorders in adolescents. *Journal of Youth and Adolescence, 33,* 365–372.

Fergusson, D.M., Horwood, L.J., & Lynskey, M.T. (1995). Maternal depressive symptoms and depressive symptoms in adolescents. *Journal of Child Psychology and Psychiatry, 36,* 1161–1178.

Field, T. (2002). Prenatal effects of maternal depression. In S.H. Goodman & I.H. Gotlib (Eds.), *Children of depressed parents: Mechanisms of risk and implications for treatment* (pp. 59–88). Washington, DC: American Psychological Association.

Focht-Birkerts, L. & Beardslee, W.R. (2000). A child's experience of parental depression: Encouraging relational resilience in families with affective illness. *Family Process, 39,* 417–434.

Foley, D.L., Pickles, A., Simonoff, E., Maes, H., Silberg, J., L., Hewitt, J.K., et al. (2001). Parental concordance and comorbidity for psychiatric disorder and associate risks for concurrent psychiatric symptoms and disorders in a community sample of juvenile twins. *Journal of Child Psychology and Psychiatry, 42*, 381–394.

Forehand, R., Brody, G., Slotkin, J., Fauber, R., McCombs, A., & Long, N. (1988). Young adolescent and maternal depression: Assessment, interrelations, and family predictors. *Journal of Consulting and Clinical Psychology, 56*, 422–426.

Forgatch, M.S. & DeGarmo, D.S. (1999). Parenting through change: An effective prevention program for single mothers. *Journal of Consulting and Clinical Psychology, 67,* 711–724.

Formoso, D., Gonzales, N.A., & Aiken, L.S. (2000). Family conflict and children's internalizing and externalizing behaviour: Protective factors. *American Journal of Community Psychology, 28*, 175–199.

Garber, J. (2006). Depression in children and adolescents: Linking risk research and prevention. *American Journal of Preventive Medicine, 31(6, Suppl 1)*, S104–S125.

Garber, J. & Flynn, C. (2001). Predictors of depressive cognitions in young adolescents. *Cognitive Therapy and Research, 25*, 353–376.

George, C., Herman, K.C., & Ostrander, R. (2006). The family environment and developmental psychopathology: The unique and interactive effects of depression, attention, and conduct problems. *Child Psychiatry and Human Development, 37*, 163–177.

Gillham, J.E., Shatté, A.J., & Freres, D.F. (2000). Preventing depression: A review of cognitive behavioral and family interventions. *Applied and Preventive Psychology, 9,* 63–88.

Goodman, S.H. (2007). Depression in mothers. *Annual Review of Clinical Psychology, 3,* 107–135.

Goodman, S.H. & Gotlib, I.H. (1999). Risk for psychopathology in the children of depressed mothers: A developmental model for understanding mechanisms of transmission. *Psychological Review, 106*, 458–490.

Gotlib, I.H. & Lee, C.M. (1996). The impact of parental depression on young children and infants. In H. Freeman (Ed.), *Interpersonal factors in the origin and course of affective disorders (pp. 218–239)*. London England: Royal College of Psychiatrists Press.

Glover, V. (1997). Maternal stress or anxiety in pregnancy and emotional development of the child. *British Journal of Psychiatry, 171*, 105–106.

Glover, V., Teixeira, J., Gitau, R., & Fisk, N. (1998, April). *Links between antenatal maternal anxiety and the fetus.* Paper presented at the 11th Biennial Conference on Infant Studies, Atlanta, GA.

Gross, D., Fogg, L., Webster-Stratton, C., Garvey, C., Julion, W., & Grady, J. (2003). Parent training with multi-ethnic families of toddlers in day care in low-income urban communities. *Journal of Consulting and Clinical Psychology, 71*, 261–278.

Grych, J.H. & Fincham, F.D. (1992). Interventions for children of divorce: Toward greater integration of research and practice. *Psychological Bulletin, 111*, 434–454.

Gwynn, C.A. & Brantley, H.T. (1987). Effects of a divorce group intervention for elementary school children. *Psychology in the Schools, 24,* 161–164.

Hamilton, E.B., Asarnow, J.R., & Tompson, M.C. (1999). Family interaction styles of children with depressive disorders, schizophrenia-spectrum disorders, and normal controls. *Family Process, 38,* 463–476.

Hammen, C. (2005). Stress and depression. *Annual Review of Clinical Psychology, 1,* 293–319.

Hammen, C., Burge, D., & Adrian, C. (1991). Timing of mother and child depression in a longitudinal study of children at risk. *Journal of Consulting and Clinical Psychology, 59,* 341–345.

Hammen, C., Burge, D., & Stansbury, K. (1990). Relationship of mother and child variables to child outcomes in a high risk sample: A causal modeling analysis. *Developmental Psychology, 26,* 24–30.

Hammen, C., Henry, R., & Daley, S.E. (2000). Depression and sensitization to stressors among young women and a function of childhood adversity. *Journal of Consulting and Clinical Psychology, 68,* 782–787.

Hammen, C., Shih, J., Altmann, T., & Brennan, P.A. (2003). Interpersonal impairment and the prediction of depressive symptoms in the adolescent children of depressed and nondepressed mothers. *Journal of the American Academy of Child and Adolescent Psychiatry, 42,* 571–577.

Hammen, C., Shih, J.H., & Brennan, P.A. (2004). Intergenerational transmission of depression: Test of an interpersonal stress model in a community sample. *Journal of Consulting and Clinical Psychology, 72,* 511–522.

Harkness, K.L., Bruce, A.E., & Lumley, M.N. (2006). The role of childhood abuse and neglect in the sensitization to stressful life events in adolescent depression. *Journal of Abnormal Psychology, 115,* 730–741.

Hawley, K.M. & Weisz, J.R. (2005). Youth versus parent working alliance in usual clinical care: Distinctive associations with retention, satisfaction, and treatment outcome. *Journal of Clinical Child and Adolescent Psychology, 34,* 117–128.

Hilsman, R. (2001). Maternal expressed emotion, child self-cognitions, and psychopathology in children of depressed and nondepressed mothers. *Dissertation Abstracts International Section B: Science and Engineering, 62(2–B),* 1082.

Hjemdal, O., Aune, T., Reinfjell, T., Stiles, T.C., & Friborg, O. (2007). Resilience as a predictor of depressive symptoms: A correlational study with young adolescents. *Clinical Child Psychology and Psychiatry, 12,* 91–104.

Horowitz, J.L., & Garber, J. (2006). The prevention of depressive symptoms in children and adolescents: A meta-analytic review. *Journal of Consulting and Clinical Psychology, 74,* 401–415.

Hughes, H. & Luke, D.A. (1998). Heterogeneity in adjustment among children of battered women. In G.W. Holden, R. Geffner, & E.N. Jouriles (Eds.), *Children exposed to marital violence: Theory, research, and applied issues* (pp. 185–222). Washington, DC: American Psychological Association.

Hunsley, J. & Lee, C.M. (2007). Research-informed benchmarks for psychological treatments: Efficacy studies, effectiveness studies, and beyond. *Professional Psychology: Research and Practice, 38,* 21–33.

Ialongo, N.S., Poduska, J., Werthamer, L., & Kellam, S. (2001). The distal impact of two first-grade preventive interventions on conduct problems and disorder in early adolescence. *Journal of Emotional and Behavioral Dsiorders, 9,* 146–161.

Ialongo, N.S., Werthamer, L., Kellam, S.G., Brown, C.H., Wang, S., & Lin, Y. (1999). Proximal impact of two first-grade preventive interventions for early risk behaviours for later substance abuse, depression, and antisocial behaviour. *American Journal of Community Psychology, 27,* 599–641.

Jaenicke, C., Hammen, C., Zupan, B., Hiroto, D., Gordon, D., Adrian, C., et al. (1987). Cognitive vulnerability in children at risk for depression. *Journal of Abnormal Child Psychology, 15,* 559–572.

Jung, V., Short, R., Letourneau, N., & Andrews, D. (2007). Interventions with depressed mothers and their infants: Modifying interactive behaviours. *Journal of Affective Disorders, 98,* 199–205.

Kane, P. & Garber, J. (2004). The relations among depression in fathers, children's psychopathology, and father-child conflict: A meta-analysis. *Clinical Psychology Review, 24,* 339–360.

Kane, P., Garber, J., & Kaminski, K.M. (2002). Relationship quality as mediators and moderators of the association between fathers' depressive symptoms and adolescents' externalizing and internalizing symptoms (Unpublished manuscript).

Kaplan, S.J., Pelcovitz, D., Salzinger, S., Weiner, M., Mandel, F.S., Lesser, M.L., & Labruna, V.E. (1999). Adolescent physical abuse: Risk for adolescent psychiatric disorders. *American Journal of Psychiatry, 155,* 954–959.

Kazdin, A.E. (2003). Psychotherapy for children and adolescents. *Annual Review of Psychology, 54,* 253–276.

Kazdin, A.E. (2004). Psychotherapy for children and adolescents. In M.L. Lambert (Ed.), *Bergin and Garfield's Handbook of psychotherapy and behavior change* (5th ed., pp. 543–589). New York: Wiley.

Kelly, J.B. & Emery, R.E. (2003). Children's adjustment following divorce: Risk and resilience perspectives. *Family Relations, 52,* 352–362.

Kessler, R.C., Berglund, P., Demler, O., Jin, R., & Walters, E.E. (2005a). Lifetime prevalence and age-of-onset distributions of DSM-IV disorders in the National Comorbidity Survey Replication. *Archives of General Psychiatry, 62,* 593–602.

Kessler, R.C., Chiu, W.T., Demler, O., & Walters, E.E. (2005b). Prevalence, severity, and comorbidity of 12-month DSM-IV disorders in the National Comorbidity Survey replication. *Archive of General Psychiatry, 62,* 617–627.

Kessler, R.C., Merikangas, K.R., & Wang, P.S. (2007). Prevalence, comorbidity, and service utilization for mood disorders in the United States at the beginning of the twenty-first century. *Annual Review of Clinical Psychology, 3,* 137–158.

Kim, S.Y. & Ge, X. (2000). Parenting practices and adolescent depressive symptoms in Chinese American families. *Journal of Family Psychology, 14,* 420–435.

Klein, D.N., Lewinsohn, P.M., Rohde, P., Seeley, J.R., & Durbin, C.E. (2002). Clinical features of Major Depressive Disorder in adolescents and their relatives: Impact on familial aggregation, implications for phenotype definition, and specificity of transmission. *Journal of Abnormal Psychology, 111,* 98–106.

Klerman, G.L., Weissman, M.M., Rounsaville, B.J., & Chevron, E.S. (1984). *Interpersonal psychotherapy of depression.* New York: Basic Books.

Kolko, D.J., Brent, D.A., Baugher, M., Bridge, J., & Birmaher, B. (2000). Cognitive and family therapies for adolescent depression: Treatment specificity, mediation and moderation. *Journal of Consulting and Clinical Psychology, 68,* 603–614.

Kraemer, H.C., Kazdin, A.E., Offord, D.R., Kessler, R.C., Jensen, P.S., & Kupfer, D. J. (1997). Coming to terms with the terms of risk. *Archives of General Psychiatry, 54,* 337–343.

Kraemer, H.C., Lowe, K.K., & Kupfer, D.J. (2005). *To your health: How to understand what research tells us about risk.* New York: Oxford University Press.

Krishnakumar, A. & Buehler, C. (2000). Interparental conflict and parenting beahviors: A meta-analytic review. *Family Relations, 49,* 25–44.

Lamb, M.E. & Tamis-Lemonda, C.S. (2004). The role of the father: An introduction. In M.E. Lamb (Ed.), *The role of the father in child development* (pp. 1–31), 4th ed. New York: Wiley.

Lee, C.M. & Bax, K. (2000). The effects of separation and divorce on children. *Paediatrics and Child Health, 5,* 217–218.

Lee, C.M., Beauregard, C., & Bax, K.A. (2005). Child-related disagreement, verbal aggression, cooperation and child adjustment among families with toddler and preschool age children. *Journal of Family Psychology, 19,* 237–245.

Lee, C.M. & Gotlib, I.H. (1991). Family disruption, parental availability, and child adjustment. In R.J. Prinz (Ed.), *Advances in behavioral assessment of children and families,* (pp. 171–199). London: Jessica Kingsley Press.

Lee, C.M. & Gotlib, I.H. (1994). Mental illness. In L. L'Abate (Ed.). *Handbook of developmental family psychology and psychopathology,* (pp. 243–264). New York: John Wiley & Sons.

Lee, C.M., Picard, M., & Blain, M.D. (1994). A methodological and substantive review of intervention outcome studies for families undergoing divorce. *Journal of Family Psychology, 8,* 3–15.

Leon, K. (2003). Risk and protective factors in young children's adjustment to parental divorce: A review of the research. *Family Relations, 52,* 258–270.

Lewinsohn, P.M. & Clarke, G.N. (1999). Psychosocial treatments for adolescent depression. *Clinical Psychology Review, 19,* 329–342.

Lewinsohn, P.M., Clarke, G.N., Hops, H., & Andrews, J. (1990). Cognitive–behavioral treatment for depressed adolescents. *Behavior Therapy, 212,* 385–401.

Lin, K.K., Sandler, I.N., Ayers, T.S., Wolchik, S.A., & Luecken, L.J. (2004). Resilience in parentally bereaved children and adolescents seeking preventive services. *Journal of Clinical Child and Adolescent Psychology, 33,* 673–683.

Liu, Y. (2003). Parent–child interaction and children's depression: The relationships between parent–child interaction and children's depressive symptoms in Taiwan. *Journal of Adolescence, 26,* 447–457.

Locke, T.F., Newcomb, M.D., Duclos, A., & Goodyear, R.K. (2007). Psychosocial predictors and correlates of dysphoria in adolescent and young adult Latinas. *Journal of Community Psychology, 35,* 135–149.

Lovejoy, M.C., Graczyk, P.A., O'Hare, E., & Neuman, G. (2000). Maternal depression and parenting behavior: A meta-analytic review. *Clinical Psychology Review, 20,* 561–592.

Luppa, M., Heinrich, S., Angermeyer, M.C., König, H., & Riedel-Heller, S.G. (2007). Cost of illness studies of depression: A systematic review. *Journal of Affective Disorders, 98,* 29–43.

Marsiglio, W., Amato, P., Day, R.D., & Lamb, M.E. (2000). Scholarship on fatherhood in the 1990s and beyond. *Journal of Marriage and the Family, 62,* 1173–1191.

Mathews, C.A. & Reus, V.I. (2001). Assortative mating in the affective disorders: A systematic review and meta-analysis. *Comprehensive Psychiatry, 42,* 257–262.

McCarthy, C.A. & McMahon, R.J. (2003). Mediators of the relationship between maternal depressive symptoms and child internalizing and disruptive behavior disorders. *Journal of Family Psychology, 17,* 545–556.

McCauley Ohannessian, C., Hesselbrock, V.M., Kramer, J., Kuperman, S., Bucholz, K.K., Schockit, M. A., et al. (2004). The relationship between parental alcoholism and adolescent psychopathology: A systematic examination of parental comorbid psychopathology. *Journal of Abnormal Child Psychology, 32*, 519–533.

McCloskey, L.A., Figueredo, A.J., & Koss, M.P. (1995). The effects of systemic family violence on children' mental health. *Child Development, 66*, 1239–1261.

Mezulis, A.H., Hyde, J.S., & Clark, R. (2004). Father involvement moderates the effect of maternal depression during a child's infancy on child behavior problems in kindergarten. *Journal of Family Psychology, 18*, 575–588.

Milan, S., Pinderhughes, E.E., & the Conduct Problems Prevention Research Group (2006). Family instability and child maladjustment trajectories during elementary school. *Journal of Abnormal Child Psychology, 34*, 40–53.

Miranda, J., Bernal, G., Lau, A., Kohn, L., Hwang, W.C., & La Frombroise, T. (2005). State of the science on psychosocial interventions for ethnic minorities. *Annual Review of Clinical Psychology, 1*, 113–142.

Monroe, S.M. & Hadjiyannakis, K. (2002). The social environment and depression: Focusing on severe life stress. In I.H. Gotlib & C.L. Hammen (Eds.), *Handbook of Depression* (pp. 314–340). New York: Guildford.

Mrazek, P.J. & Haggerty, R.J. (1994). *Reducing risks for mental disorders: Frontiers for preventive research*. Washington, DC: National Academy Press.

Mufson, L. & Dorta, K.P. (2003). Interpersonal psychotherapy for depressed adolescents. In A.E. Kazdin & J.R. Weisz (Eds), *Evidence-based psychotherapies for children and adolescents* (pp. 148–164). New York: Guilford.

Mufson, L., Dorta, K.P., Wickramaratne, P., Nomura, Y., Olfson, M., & Weissman, M.M. (2004). A randomized effectiveness trial of interpersonal psychotherapy for depressed adolescents. *Archives of General Psychiatry, 61*, 577–584.

Mufson, L., Weissman, M.M., Moreau, D., & Garfinkel, R. (1999). Efficacy of interpersonal psychotherapy for depressed adolescents. *Archives of General Psychiatry, 56*, 573–579.

National Institute for Health and Clinical Excellence. (2005). *Depression in children: identification and management of depression in children and young people in primary, community and secondary care*. Retrieved on February 15th 2005 from http://www.nice.org.uk.

Nation, M., Crusto, C., Wandersman, A., Kumpfer, K.L., Seybolt, D., Morrissey-Kane, E., et al. (2003). What works in prevention: Principles of effective prevention programs. *American Psychologist, 58*, 449–456.

Nicholas, K.B. & Rasmussen, E.H. (2006). Childhood abusive and supportive experiences, inter-parental violence, and parental alcohol use: Prediction of young adult depressive symptoms and aggression. *Journal of Family Violence, 21*, 43–61.

Nomura, Y., Wickramaratne, P.J., Warner, V., & Weissman, M. (2002). Family discord, parental depression and psychopathology in offspring: Ten-year follow-up. *Journal of the American Academy of Child and Adolescent Psychiatry, 41*, 402–409.

Olds, D.L. (2002). Prenatal and infancy home visiting by nurses: From randomized trials to community replication. *Prevention Science, 3*, 153–172.

Olfson, M., Gameroff, M.J., Marcus, S.C., & Waslick, B.D. (2003). Outpatient treatment of child and adolescent depression in the United States. *Archives of General Psychiatry, 60*, 1236–1242.

Olino, T.M., Lewinsohn, P.M., & Klein, D.N. (2006). Sibling similarity for MDD: Evidence for shared familial factors. *Journal of Affective Disorders, 94*, 211–218.

Patterson, G. (1982). *A social learning approach: Coercive family process* (Vol. III). Eugene, OR: Castalia.

Pavlidis, K. & McCauley, E. (2001). Autonomy and relatedness in family interactions with depressed adolescents. *Journal of Abnormal Child Psychology, 29,* 11–21.

Pineda, A.Q., Cole, D.A., & Bruce, A.E. (2007). Mother-adolescent interactions and adolescent depressive symptoms: A sequential analysis. *Journal of Social and Personal Relationships, 24,* 5–19.

Phares, V. & Compas, B.E. (1992). The role of fathers in child and adolescent psychopathology: Make room for daddy. *Psychological Bulletin, 111,* 387–412.

Phares, V. & Lum, J.J. (1997). Clinically referred children and adolescents: Fathers, family constellations, and other demographic factors. *Journal of Clinical Child Psychology, 26,* 216–223.

Phillips, N.K, Hammen, C.L, Brennan, P.A., Najman, J.M., & Bor, W. (2005). Early adversity and the prospective prediction of depressive and anxiety disorders in adolescents. *Journal of Abnormal Child Psychology, 33,* 13–24.

Rapee, R.M., Wignall, A., Sheffield, J., Kowalenko, N., Davis, A., McLoone, J., & Spence, S.H. (2006). Adolescents' reactions to universal and indicated prevention programs for depression: perceived stigma and consumer satisfaction. *Prevention Science, 7,* 167–177.

Rohde, P., Lewinsohn, P.M., Klein, D.N., & Seeley, J.R. (2005). Association of parental depression with psychiatric course from adolescent to youth adulthood among formerly depressed individuals. *Journal of Abnormal Psychology, 114,* 409–420.

Roseby, V. & Deutsch, R. (1985). Children of separation and divorce: Effects of a social role-taking group intervention for fourth and fifth graders. *Journal of Clinical Child Psychology, 14,* 55–60.

Rosello, J. & Bernal, G. (1999). The efficacy of cognitive-behavioral and interpersonal treatments for depression in Puerto Rican adolescents. *Journal of Consulting and Counseling Psychology, 67,* 734–745.

Rudolph, K.D., & Flynn, M. (2007). Childhood adversity and youth depression: Influence of gender and pubertal status. *Development and Psychopathology, 19,* 497–521.

Sanders, J. B. & McCarty, C.A. (2005). Youth depression in the family context: Familial risk factors and models of treatment. *Clinical Child and Family Psychology Review, 8,* 203–219.

Sanders, M.R. (1999). Triple P-Positive parenting program: Towards an empirically validated multilevel parenting and family support strategy for the prevention of behavior and emotional problems in children. *Clinical Child and Family Psychology Review, 2,* 71–90.

Sanders, M.R., Cann, W., & Markie-Dadds, C. (2003). The Triple P-Positive Parenting Programme: A universal population-level approach to the prevention of child abuse. *Child Abuse Review, 12,* 155–171.

Sanders, M.R., Markie-Dadds, C., Turner, K., & Ralph, A. (2004). Using the Triple P system of intervention to prevent behavioural problems in children and adolescents. In P.M. Barrett & T.H. Ollendick (Eds.), *Interventions that work with children and adolescents: Prevention and Treatment* (pp. 489–516). Chichester, UK: Wiley.

Sandler, I.N., West, S.G., Baca, L., Pillow, D.R., Gersten, J.C., Rogosch, F., et al. (1992). Linking empirically based theory and evaluation: The Family Bereavement Program. *American Journal of Community Psychology, 20,* 491–521.

Sanford, M., Byrne, C., Williams, S., Atley, S., Ridley, T., Miller, J., et al. (2003). A pilot study of a parent-education group for families affected by depression. *Canadian Journal of Psychiatry, 48,* 78–86.

Sarigiani, P.A., Heath, P.A., & Camarena, P.M. (2003). The significance of parental depressed mood for young adolescents' emotional and family experiences. *Journal of early Adolescence, 23*, 241–267.

Seligman, L.D., Goza, A.B., & Ollendick, T.H. (2004). Treatment of depression in children and adolescents. In P.M., Barrett & T.H. Ollendick (Eds.), *Interventions that work with children and adolescents: Prevention and treatment* (pp. 301–328). New York: Wiley.

Sheeber, L.B., Davis, B., Leve, C., Hops, H., & Tildesley, E. (2007). Adolescents' relationships with their mothers and fathers: Associations with depressive disorder and subdiagnostic symptomatology. *Journal of Abnormal Psychology, 116*, 144–154.

Sheeber, L., Hops, H., Andrews, J., Alpert, T., & Davis, B. (1998). Interactional processes in families with depressed and nondepressed adolescents: Reinforcement of depressive behavior. *Behaviour research and Therapy, 36*, 417–427.

Sheeber, L., Hops, H., & Davis, B. (2001). Family processes in adolescent depression. *Clinical Child and Family Psychology Review, 4*, 19–35.

Shochet, I. & Dadds, M. (1997). Adolescent depression and the family: A paradox. *Clinical Child psychology and Psychiatry, 2*, 307–312.

Shochet, I.M., Dadds, M.R., Holland, D., Whitefield, K., Harnett, P.H., & Osgarby, S.M. (2001). The efficacy of the universal school-based program to prevent adolescent depression. *Journal of Clinical Child Psychology, 30,* 303–315.

Smetana, J.G., Campione-Barr, N., & Metzger, A. (2006). Adolescent development in interpersonal and societal contexts. *Annual Review of Psychology, 57,* 255–284.

Spoth, R.L., Kavanagh, K.A., & Dishion, T.J. (2002). Family-centered preventive intervention science: Toward benefits to larger populations of children, youth, and families. *Prevention Science, 3,* 145–152.

Stice, E., Ragan, J., & Randall, P. (2004). Prospective relations between social support and depression: Differential direction of effects for parent and peer support. *Journal of Abnormal Psychology, 113*, 155–159.

Stolberg, A.L. & Mahler, J. (1994). Enhancing treatment gains in a school-based intervention for children of divorce through skill training, parental involvement, and transfer procedures. *Journal of Consulting and Clinical Psychology, 62,* 147–156.

Stuewig, J. & McCloskey, L.A. (2005). The relation of child maltreatment to shame and guilt among adolescents: Psychological routes to depression and delinquency. *Child Maltreatment, 10*, 324–336.

Wang, P.S., Berglund, P., Olfson, M., Pincus, H.A.,Wells, K.B., & Kessler, R.C. (2005). Failure and delay in initial treatment contact after first onset of mental disorders in National Comorbidity Survey Replication. *Archives of General Psychiatry, 62*, 603–613.

Wang, P.S., Lane, M., Olfson, M., Pincus, H.A., Wells, K.B., & Kessler, R.C. (2005). Twelve-month use of mental health services in the United States. *Archives of General Psychiatry, 62, 629–640.*

Warner, V., Weissman, M.M., Mufson, L., & Wickramaratne, P.J. (1999). Grandparents, parents, and grandchildren at risk for depression: A three-generation study. *Journal of the American Academy of Child and Adolescent Psychiatry, 38*, 289–296.

Walter, M. (2000). Parental involvement of unwed, nonresident fathers. *Family Matters, 57,* 34–49.

Webster-Stratton, C. (2006). Treating children with early-onset conduct problems: Key ingredients to implementing the Incredible Years Programs with fidelity. In T.K. Neil (Ed.), *Helping others help children: Clinical supervision of child psychotherapy* (pp. 161–175). Washington, DC: American Psychological Association.

Webster-Stratton, C., Reid, M.J., & Hammond, M. (2001). Preventing conduct problems, promoting social competence: A parent and teacher training partnership in Head Start. *Journal of Clinical Child Psychology, 30,* 283–302.

Weissberg, R.P., Kumpfer, K.L., & Seligman, M.E.P. (2003). Prevention that works for children and youth. *American Psychologist, 58,* 425–432.

Weissman, M.M., Gammon, G.D., John, K., Merikangas, K.R., Warner, V., Prusoff, B., et al. (1987). Children of depressed parents: Increased psychopathology and early onset of major depression. *Archives of General Psychiatry, 44,* 847–853.

Weissman, M.M. & Jensen, P. (2002). What research suggests for depressed women with children. *Journal of Clinical Psychiatry, 63,* 641–647.

Weissman, M.M., Wickramaratne, P.J., Nomura, Y., Warner, V., Verdeli, H., Pilowsky, D.J., et al. (2005). Families at high and low risk for depression. *Archives of General Psychiatry, 62,* 29–36.

Weisz, J.R., McCarty, C.A., & Valeri, S.M. (2006). Effects of psychotherapy for depression in children and adolescents: A meta-analysis. *Psychological Bulletin, 132,* 132–149.

Wells, K.C. & Albano, A.M. (2005). Parent involvement in CBT treatment of adolescent depression: Experiences in the Treatment for Adolescents with Depression Study (TADS). *Cognitive and Behavioral Practice, 12,* 209–220.

Whiteside, M.F. & Becker, B.J. (2000). Parental factors and young children's post-divorce adjustment: A meta-analysis with implications for parenting arrangements. *Journal of Family Psychology, 14,* 5–26.

Williamson, D.E., Birmaher, B., Axelson, D.A., Ryan, N.D., & Dahl, R.E. (2004). First episode of depression in children at low and high familial risk for depression. *Journal of the American Academy of Child and Adolescent Psychiatry, 43,* 291–297.

Wolchik, S.A., West, S.G., Sandler, I.N., Tein, J.Y., Coatsworth, D., Lengua, L., et al. (2000). An experimental evaluation of theory-based mother and mother-child programs for children of divorce. *Journal of Consulting and Clinical Psychology, 68,* 843–856.

Wolchik, S.A., West, S.G., Westover, S., Sandler, I.N., Lustig, J., Tein, J.Y., et al. (1993). The Children of Divorce Parenting Intervention: Outcome evaluation of an empirically based program. *American Journal of Community Psychology, 21,* 293–331.

Wolff, J.C. & Ollendick, T.H. (2006). The comorbidity of conduct problems and depression in childhood and adolescence. *Clinical Child and Family Psychology Review, 9,* 201–220.

World Health Organization (2001). *Child and adolescent mental health.* WHO Factsheet (11/01). Retrieved on May 28th 2007 from http://www.who.int/child-adolescent-health.

Zvolensky, M.J., Schmidt, N.B., Bernstein, A., & Keough, M.E. (2006). Risk-factor research and prevention programs for anxiety disorders: A translational research frame. *Behaviour Research and Therapy, 44,* 1219–1239.

Chapter 9

Attachment-based family therapy for depressed adolescents

Guy S. Diamond, Suzanne A. Levy,
Pravin Israel, & Gary M. Diamond

Attachment-based family therapy (ABFT) is a 12–16-week family-based psychotherapy designed to reduce depression, suicidal ideation, and other internalized stress among adolescents. The model has been tested in three clinical trials and shown to be effective in reducing depression, anxiety, suicidal ideation, and family conflict, and in increasing adolescents' attachment to parents. The model is designed around five interrelated treatment tasks that aim to first repair the secure base of family life and then use this refurbished foundation to promote appropriate autonomy and competency. The theoretical rationale and empirical support for each of these tasks, as well as detailed clinical descriptions regarding how to accomplish each task, have been presented in several previously published articles and book chapters. Therefore, in this chapter, we focus on an overview of the clinical process as it unfolds over the course of treatment. After a presentation of some general theoretical ideas, we present a case study that offers practical guidelines for conducting ABFT. To begin, we provide a brief discussion of the overarching principles that guide the work.

A Family-Based Approach. ABFT is a family-focused psychotherapy model. This has several implications (Diamond & Josephson, 2005). First, it means that the family is typically the unit of treatment. When possible and appropriate, all relevant family members participate in the therapy. However, not all family members attend all sessions. Rather individuals, or different constellations of family members (i.e., sub-systems), are invited to specific sessions, depending on the progress of the treatment and the clinical goals at hand. Second, in this treatment, parents, as well as the adolescents, are viewed as clients. Therefore, the therapist invests great effort in building a working alliance with the parent. To accomplish this, the therapist attends to parents' own history of attachment failures, current stressors, and psychiatric problems. This sets the foundation for teaching effective care-giving behaviours. ABFT therapists do not launch a full course of individual or marital therapy, but they do help parents understand how challenges in these adult domains might influence their parenting and the adolescent.

Third, the depression is understood in the context of the family system. In some cases, family processes such as parental rejection, criticism, abuse, as well as family conflict are viewed as causes of the adolescent's depression. In other families, interpersonal dysfunction may not be conceived as the cause of depression, but can certainly exacerbate it. In these families, parents are typically well-meaning and concerned, and adolescents may even feel close to parents. Despite these positive factors, communication may be restricted, problem-solving poorly negotiated, and affect overly regulated. Finally, in other families, the adolescent's depression may cause stress in the family, leading to a breakdown in parenting, family organization, and/or marital support. Such processes then diminish parents' ability to support their adolescent in her/his recovery from depression. Regardless of the mechanism by which negative family process affects adolescent depression, resolving ruptures in family communication, trust, and problem-solving often diffuses family tension and enhances the supportive and organizational functions of the family. This re-establishes the family as an effective and secure base for adolescent development, which can ameliorate depressive symptoms and depressive risk factors.

Empirically Informed Treatment. ABFT is an empirically informed treatment approach. This means we rely on the broad field of developmental psychopathology (Cicchetti & Greenberg, 1991) to identify family processes that have been found to cause, maintain, or exacerbate adolescent depression. When working with families, there are countless themes to address and a myriad of problems to solve. An empirically informed perspective focuses the therapist on processes empirically shown to contribute to depression in adolescence. Targeting these processes should more effectively lead to change. Our core target processes include parental criticism (Expressed Emotion), adolescent apathy and hopelessness, parental stress and psychopathology, negative parenting behaviours, family conflict and disengagement, and adolescent negative self concept and cognitions (see Diamond et al., 2003).

A Treatment Manual. ABFT is written as a manual that provides structure and guidance for the delivery of the model. However, unlike more structured manuals (i.e., psychoeducational or even CBT), ABFT is a more principle driven manual, similar to IPT (Mufson et al., 1993) and Supportive–Expressive psychotherapies (Luborsky, 2001). Rather than providing a structured curriculum, we provide a road map of principles, processes, strategies, and goals that, if executed well, can yield good outcome rapidly. Imagine you are travelling in a new county. Someone gives you a map and tells you to follow this road and see these important sites. You may decide, or need, to take some side roads or a detour, but make sure you get back to these essential landmarks. ABFT identifies essential therapeutic landmarks or tasks that are critical when working with depressed adolescents. Thus, the manual offers a depiction of the moment-by-moment therapist strategies and family responses that would characterize the ideal progress though these treatment tasks. The manual also depicts common pitfalls and barriers toward completing these tasks.

Unfortunately, not every family will cooperate with these proposed processes. Each family is unique, presents with their own history and challenges, and brings to therapy their own set of attributions, affective management skills, intergenerational patterns, and history of successes and failures in dealing with their child's depression. In this regard, ABFT must be applied to each family in a respectful, idiosyncratic, and collaborative manner. However, this is not a 'client centred' approach where each family decides the direction and focus of therapy. Instead, the model guides family members toward and through particular tasks or processes believed to be essential for producing rapid change in the interpersonal environment of the family. The conversation is a give and take, but the therapist's perspective is guided by a scientific understanding of normative and deviant family processes and an understanding of how to heal ruptures in family relationships.

The primary focus of the therapist is not on improving behaviour management or teaching cognitive skills, although we accomplish much of this indirectly. Instead, the ABFT therapist aims to identify core, often longstanding, family conflicts that have damaged trust, communication, and fairness between parents and their adolescent. With great attention to preparation, the therapist then facilitates reparative conversations that can help families clear the ledger of resentment (Boszormenyi-Nagy & Spark, 1973). On the one hand, resolving or at least addressing, often for the first time, these interpersonal problems (divorce, abuse, over control) helps families work through difficult problems. On the other hand, these often emotional problem-solving sequences become a context for teaching new interpersonal skills and emotional regulation. It is proposed that both of these mechanisms will promote a more healthy and resilient family environment.

Self of the Therapist. Although we provide a road map, fundamentally the treatment is a depth psychotherapy. This type of healing process is not simple. It requires tremendous compassion, respect and admiration for all family members. It requires believing that love can be resuscitated. But in order to guide families through conversations that have depth, honesty, and integrity, the therapist must be comfortable with emotional pain and arousal themselves. They must be confident that they can contain and protect each family member. These skills are not easily learned in a treatment manual. Therefore, the self of the therapist is an essential feature of working within the ABFT model. Self development, self growth, and self understanding are the foundational skills of being a good ABFT psychotherapist.

Theory Foundation. The underlying assumption of ABFT is that the quality of interpersonal relationships, social experience, and life events can cause, maintain, or buffer against depression. This view is best articulated in interpersonal theories of depression (Coyne, 1976; Gotlib & Hammen, 1992; Joiner & Coyne, 1999). In this framework, factors such as parental depression (Weissman & Paykel, 1974), marital conflict, ineffective parenting practices (Cummings & Davies, 1994), unmet attachment needs (Greenberg, 1999), loss (Harris et al., 1986), and negative parent–child interaction (Asarnow et al., 1993; Sheeber et al., 2001) are viewed as aetiological and reinforcing factors of depression. This orientation to understanding and treating depression is particularly relevant for children and adolescents for whom the family context has a more potent and inescapable impact than for adults (Macobby & Martin, 1983; Rutter, 1984).

Adolescent Development Research. In the 1950s, psychoanalytic models characterized adolescent development as a time of storm and stress. The central task of adolescence was understood as a push toward independence and autonomy. This view has been challenged by contemporary research, which repeatedly demonstrates that healthy adolescent development depends on an appropriate balance of attachment to and autonomy from parents (Steinberg, 1990). Healthy adolescence is now characterized by (a) continuity in parent child connection, (b) respect for parents' values yet permission to question and negotiate different points of view, and (c) mild to moderate conflicts over daily routines and behavioural organization. Rather than viewing conflict as an upheaval, conflict is viewed as critical for helping adolescents formulate and express ideas and feelings, develop negotiation and problem-solving skills, and forging an independent identity.

Attachment Theory. Adolescent attachment theory and research serves as the primary conceptual framework of ABFT (Allen et al., 1998; Kobak & Sceery, 1988; Lynch & Cicchetti, 1991; Rosenstein & Horowitz, 1996). The importance of appropriate attachment throughout the lifespan has been well-theorized and documented (Ainsworth, 1989; Steinberg, 1990). Several features characterize a secure parent–adolescent relationship. In a secure relationship, the adolescent feels emotionally and physically protected, heard and understood, and parents are available in times of need. Adolescents also feel they can speak to their parents about topics that are embarrassing or difficult without feeling that they will be rejected, abandoned, ridiculed, or controlled. During adolescence, the function of attachment becomes less about protection from physical harm and increasingly about protection from emotional harm (Kobak et al., 1991). When these conditions are met, adolescents are more likely to feel secure, safe, assured, and validated. Secure adolescents display more autonomy seeking, positive peer relations, and higher self-esteem (Allen & Land, 1999). They also freely express negative or vulnerable emotions (e.g., fear, anger, distress) with the expectation of acceptance and comfort, rather than criticism and abandonment. Living in this kind of emotional environment nurtures healthy development.

In contrast, when these family conditions are not met, adolescents are denied this critical developmental context. Many parents of depressed adolescents have experienced depression themselves or other kinds of psychological distress. And many were denied adequate parenting as children and consequently have insecure attachment styles themselves. These parents often feel ambivalent, anxious, or incapable of providing comfort, soothing, and reassurance. Consequently, the expression of negative and vulnerable affect is unwelcome and unsafe. In some families, parents' unavailability and/or unresponsiveness, particularly at critical moments, can also become a source of emotional injury (Kobak & Mandelbaum, 2003). This kind of insecure family environment typically results in adolescents developing more insecure attachment style. Insecure attachment in adolescence has repeatedly been associated with depression and other kinds of functional problems (Kobak & Sceery, 1988; Rosenstein & Horowitz, 1996). Insecure attachment styles are particularly common among adolescents with a history of trauma (Kobak et al., 1991; Rosenstein & Horowitz, 1996).

Clinically, we observe two kinds of insecure attachment strategies. Some adolescents present with a *dismissing* attachment style. They minimize the importance of attachment relationships by devaluing them or negating their influence. These adolescent present as if they no longer need their parents; parents are unimportant and/or ignored. This strategy seems to help protect adolescents from further hurt and disappointment.

Alternatively, some adolescents present with an *anxious* attachment style. They remain intensely focused on and over-involved in their attachment relationships. They vacillate between demanding care and protection and criticizing parents' unavailability. They seem preoccupied with how parents have failed them, but use behavioural conflicts as a means to keep parents engaged (Allen & Land, 1999). Regardless of which insecure strategies they use, these adolescents protect themselves by avoidance, denial, and other maladaptive strategies, instead of learning effective communication and problem-solving skills or developing internal representations of fair and safe relationships.

In fact, depressed adolescents often 'protect' parents from angry or sad feelings, fearing that honesty would overburden their parents or lead to further rejection (Diamond & Siqueland, 1998). Consequently, adolescents express anger about core attachment failures indirectly through conflicts over day-to-day behavioural problems (e.g., chores, curfew, etc). Depressed adolescents also have a tendency to blame themselves for these attachment failures and view themselves as unworthy of love and affection. This can promote a negative schema of self and others, putting them at greater risk for depression (Cicchetti et al., 1995).

Repairing Attachment. The central task of ABFT is to repair attachment ruptures and rekindle or refurbish a secure base that can again support adolescent development. This is accomplished by engineering in-session corrective attachment experiences. These reattachment episodes are essentially sustained conversations about core relational themes that have damaged, or impeded the formation of attachment and felt security. Adolescents are encouraged to share their anger, fear, disappointment, sadness and longing for acknowledgment and closeness, in a regulated, non-aggressive manner. This increases the likelihood of their being heard and understood by their parents. Simultaneously, parents are coached to remain non-defensive, interested, and emotionally engaged in their child's distress and pain. This parenting posture offers safety and comfort, which promotes more adolescent disclosures.

The active mechanism of these corrective attachment experiences can be understood at several levels. First, there is a cathartic experience of finally expressing how one feels in a direct and mature manner. Whether the complaint is that parents are overly controlling or abusive, adolescents feel they are finally being heard and taken seriously (even if it is not the whole truth of the events or dynamics). And in some families, this is the first time they have discussed issues of divorce, marital violence, parent's depression/drug use, or other traumatic events. This can be quite therapeutic.

At another level, the attachment task is about increasing the adolescent capacity for affect regulation. For depressed adolescents who typically vacillate between angry, blaming outburst, and avoidance, such conversations provide an opportunity to learn how to identify and articulate emotionally laden themes in a regulated, direct manner. Such skills are important to the adolescent's cognitive–emotional development and influence the quality of current and future interpersonal relationships with attachment figures (Allen et al., 1996; Kobak & Duemmler, 1994; Kobak & Sceery, 1988). Importantly, the capacity for emotion regulation has been linked with both depression and suicidality (Yap et al., 2007).

For parents, these conversations offer an opportunity to learn and practice effective care giving. Parents learn that encouraging appropriate emotional expression can actually facilitate open and honest communication, and not necessarily lead to escalation and crisis. In this context, parents learn new emotionally focused problem-solving skills (Gottman et al., 1996) that, when appropriate, can help diffuse conflict and strife.

Overall, we have come to think of these corrective attachment episodes as an in vivo exposure to new, more effective, and intimate communication. Typically, exposure treatment focuses on desensitization of negative stimuli. In the reattachment task in ABFT, like other experiential therapeutic modalities such as structural family therapy or Gestalt, the therapist creates sustained exposure experiences to the fear of conflict and rejection. At the same time, the family has an experiential learning moment of interpersonal competency, renewed intimacy, affect regulation, and effective problem-solving.

These in vivo experiences are opportunities to practice newly acquired skills as well as to challenge negative cognitive schemas that discourage this kind of interaction. In addition, being guided through a successful attachment episode promotes confidence in one's own interpersonal skills, trust in others' interpersonal capacity, and a desire for a more satisfying attachment–caregiver relationship. In the long term, it may help revise the adolescent internal working models about safe and satisfying relationships (Fongay et al., 2000; Weinfeld et al., 2000).

Clinical Foundation. ABFT is rooted in the tradition of Structural Family Therapy (SFT; Minuchin, 1974). In this model, therapists pay attention to family structure, work to generate a systemic (rather than intrapersonal) frame for understanding the problem at hand, and utilize enactments—in-session conversations between family members—to promote change. ABFT has also been highly influenced by Multidimensional Family Therapy (MDFT), developed by Howard Liddle (Liddle, 1999; Liddle et al., 2001). A derivative of SFT developed specifically for working with substance abusing adolescence, MDFT systematically—in a sequence of individual and joint sessions—focuses on four modules: the adolescent, the parents, the adolescent–parent interaction, and the family's relationship with the extra-familial world (e.g., school, juvenile justice department, extended family, etc.). The treatment attends to the cognitive, behavioural, and emotional aspects of each individual (Liddle, 1999) and is informed by current research on adolescent development, developmental psychopathology, and parenting. For example, On the basis of research by Baumrind (1991) and others, therapists work to promote authoritative parenting (warmth, acceptance, demanding behaviours, clear expectations, etc.).

ABFT has also been influenced by current research and clinical models addressing the role of emotion in the psychotherapeutic change process. Emotionally Focused Therapy (EFT; Greenberg & Johnson, 1988) uses emotion as the core intervention mechanism. Relying on contemporary research on emotion, EFT therapists assume that while the expression of affect may be cathartic, it is also a primary signalling system that serves a communication function (Greenberg & Safran, 1987). For example, while anger makes others defensive, sadness and pain evoke protection and compassion. Clearly, affect and cognition are linked. Core emotions develop in tandem with cognitions that emerge from strong (positive or negative) experiences. Core traumatic experiences generate a cognitive–affective schema that can organize future behaviour. Creating conversations where these 'hot cognitions' are re-evoked creates a profound learning environment for the inspection, clarification, and modification of these affect-laden, core events.

Clinical Structure of ABFT. ABFT consists of two primary treatment goals: reattachment and autonomy. The first phase of treatment focuses on reattachment: helping the family identify and discuss past and present conflicts that have damaged the attachment bond and violated trust. Once some of these issues have been diffused, if not resolved, the family can serve as a secure base from which to promote adolescent autonomy (e.g., improving school performance and/or attendance, finding a job, developing or returning to social activities). To achieve these goals, five treatment tasks have been developed. A task is a discrete episode with a defined set of therapist procedures for addressing specific patient problem states. Tasks may occur in a single session or, if needed, evolve over several sessions. In ABFT, the full or partial success of each task forms a foundation for future tasks (Diamond & Diamond, 2002). Although the ABFT model provides a recommended order and unique structure for each task, implementation requires constant assessment, judgment, and flexibility by the therapist. We briefly summarize the five tasks and then provide more detail on each (See Figure 9.1).

The Relational Reframe Task (Diamond & Siqueland, 1998) is designed to shift the focus of the therapy away from negative, critical parental attributions of the adolescent (i.e., 'stubborn', 'disobedient', or 'closed down'), which fuel adolescent anger and withdrawal (Fincham & Bradbury, 1988), and onto the quality of the adolescent–parent relationship. An example of a relational reframe would be to ask an adolescent, 'Why do you not go to your parents when you are feeling suicidal?' Again, this type of question shifts the focus of therapy from fixing the adolescent to repairing the relational ruptures that have damaged trust in the family. If trust does not exist, adolescents will not engage in open, honest conversation with their parents about their depression or suicidal feelings and their stressful experiences in general.

The Alliance Building Task with the adolescent focuses on strengthening treatment engagement and building hope for change. With the adolescent alone, the session focuses on strengthening patient–therapist trust, identifying core family dynamics that fuel conflict, and encouraging the adolescent to discuss these issues with a parent. The essential goal of this task is to gain the adolescent's agreement to engage in open, honest conversation with their parent(s) and to prepare the adolescent for such in-session enactments.

The Alliance Building Task with the parent focuses on reducing parental distress and improving parenting practices. This begins with a supportive exploration of stressors affecting the parent (e.g., psychiatric distress, marital problems, and traumatic childhood history). When parents experience empathy for their own vulnerabilities, they become more empathic toward their adolescent's struggles. In this softened state, they become more receptive to learning parenting skills that focus on affective attunement and emotional facilitation (Gottman et al., 1996). The essential goals of this task are for the parent to acknowledge their adolescent's pain and vulnerability,

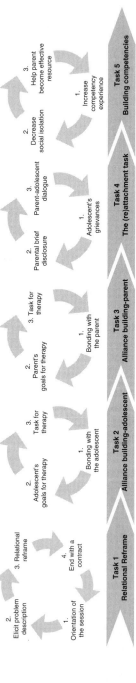

Figure 9.1 Clinical structure of ABFT.

endorse the importance of the adolescent being able to share such pain and vulnerability with his/her parents, learn how to respond to their adolescent in a validating, supportive manner, agree to practice such interactions during in-session enactments, and to prepare the parent for such in-session enactments.

The Reattachment Task culminates the work from the previous three tasks. It involves in-session conversations between adolescent and parent(s), during which the adolescent discloses, often for the first time, past and present experiences, thoughts and feelings that have violated the attachment bond and damaged trust. When reattachment episodes are successful, parents respond to their adolescent's pain, accusations, anger, and hurt in a supportive, understanding, non-defensive manner. In some cases, parents apologize for their role in past attachment failures. Such responses can have a positive influence on the adolescent's cognitions, emotions, and behaviours. Cognitively, the adolescent learns to perceive his/her parent as caring, interested, able to tolerate his/her pain and anger, and able to offer support and validation. This can lead to a restructuring of schemas adolescents have regarding their parent and themselves. More specifically, they begin to see their parents as more caring and themselves as more worthwhile. Feeling cared about, safe and worthwhile is inversely related to depression and suicidal ideation. Furthermore, the opportunity for the adolescents to engage in sustained conversations about his/her negative feelings increases his/her ability to articulate, differentiate, and regulate difficult emotions. Finally, parent's non-defensive, encouraging, and supportive responses reinforce the adolescent's disclosure and sharing, and increase the likelihood that an adolescent will go to his or her parent for help the next time he/she feels stressed, depressed, or suicidal, rather than withdraw or isolate him/herself. In many ways, reattachment episodes are experiential, behavioural interventions that change clients' cognitive and emotional experiences.

The last task, the Competency Promoting Task, is designed to utilize the improved adolescent–parent relationship to facilitate the adolescent's re-involvement and success in extra familial, pro-social contexts (e.g., school, employment, peer relations, sports). Parents are taught to encourage, support, and advocate for their child as she/he navigates the challenges of each of these domains. Adolescents and their parents practice identifying problems, brainstorming, and considering options. Problem-solving training has been a valuable component in other treatment approaches, but is rarely done in a family context where collaboratively resolving problems can also be attachment-building. Furthermore, successful problem-solving and success in school, peer relationships, etc., builds a sense of competency and increases positive experiences, which can buffer against further hopelessness, depression, and suicidal ideation (Cole, 1990; Dumont & Provost, 1999).

Summary of case

Alice* is a 14-year old African American girl who is the youngest of three children. She is in the 8th grade and, until last year, was an A student at a private Catholic school. Alice has many hobbies and skills including dance, music, and theatre, but as is typical with depression, she has lost interest in many of these activities in the last year. Mary, Alice's mother, is currently working as a real-estate agent, but had

---

* Names have been changed to protect participants' identities.

for years worked as a school counsellor. She and her husband, Frank, separated about five years ago over conflicts about money and fidelity. Since her parents were separated, Alice has had sporadic contact with her father, who works as a counsellor for the post office. Alice enjoys talking to her father and feels that she can communicate well with him. However, contact with Frank has steadily decreased over the years as conflicts between mom and dad have increased. This has been more troubling for Alice since entering her adolescence.

Mary learned of Alice's suicidal ideation when she overheard her talking to her friends about a peer who attempted suicide and then later found her crying and upset. Mary immediately took Alice to the emergency room where Frank joined them. Alice was referred to her primary care doctor who referred the family to our study for suicidal adolescents. Mary was surprized to learn of Alice's suicidal feelings, even though she had been depressed off and on for a long time. Alice attributed her sad feelings to anxiety related to school, body image, conflict with her nephew, peer problems, issues with her dad, and difficulty communicating with her mother. Since Alice reported suicidal ideation, her father calls her everyday and meets her regularly. Alice and Mary were the primary participants in therapy. Frank attended 3 sessions, one alone, one with Alice, and one with both Alice and Mary. Suzanne Levy was the therapist.

Task one: The relational reframe

The first session generally focuses on the Relational Reframe tasks. As a first session, this task has many goals. Joining with each family member, getting a good description of the problem behaviours and its impact on the family, and assessing the larger system context of the depression are critical to starting any course of therapy. But the main goal of session one is to develop a contract with the family that the therapy will initially focus on repairing the interpersonal fabric of family trust.

The assumption here is that interpersonal problems have lead to a breakdown in communication, closeness, and trust. Family members overly focus on problem behaviours that, in turn, build up even more resentment and distrust. Consequently, the adolescent begins to recede from parents and withdraw into depression and despair. Unfortunately, the depression reinforces isolation, distrust, indifference, hypersensitivity, and mood states that thwart relationship building. Whether or not it is true, adolescents complain that parents are impatient, controlling, critical, and/or overbearing. In some families, often long-standing interpersonal conflicts and attachment failures have also resulted in deep-seated resentment and disappointment. By the time they get to a therapist, family members are often hopeless, fed up, or feel inadequate to move the relationships forward.

Consequently, many adolescents have given up on having a relationship with their parents, either out of resentment or self-protection. The natural supportive context of the secure base is eroded. But, to protect themselves against further disappointment, both sides have often given up trying to make amends. Given these conditions, the therapists' initial goal is not to necessarily heal the ruptures, but to amplify or resuscitate a desire in the family members to resolve them. Faced with this challenge, the therapist must reactivate a sense of longing, caring, and commitment in the family members in order to help them find the motivation to engage in therapeutic conversations.

As a strategy, the initial play is to the adolescent. As Howard Liddle has so effectively argued, when working with adolescents, they must feel there is something in this therapy for them (Liddle, 1999; Liddle & Diamond, 1991). Although there is the potential to appear overly supportive of the adolescent, the parents know how hard it is to engage a depressed teen. Therefore, they are usually patient when we make the adolescent's concerns the initial focus of treatment. Parents also understand that freedom to express is not freedom to abuse. If they want the opportunity to speak honestly, adolescents have to accept the responsibility of expressing themselves in a mature and modulated fashion.

The transcript below begins in the middle of the first session. The therapist has already spent time building alliance with each family member, getting a description and history of the depression, and its impact on the family. The therapist has also begun to explore some of the interpersonal problems between the adolescent and parent that have ruptured trust and disrupted communication between them. But rather than focuses in detail on the problems themselves, which may evoke more conflict and resentment, the therapist makes a slightly different focus.

> Therapist: (to patients) So it sounds like some things have been upsetting you. And yet you keep them to yourself. You are suffering alone with your problems and mom is suffering alone because she feels she cannot understand you. Why is that? Why don't you talk to your mother about the kinds of things you are saying now?
>
> Daughter: Well …. ah… (mom interrupts)
>
> Mother: Well I didn't know she even felt that way. Um …. until the other week when she said she didn't want to live anymore. I had no idea. Actually none of us had an idea.… OK. so she has been a little depressed at times. But when she said that!.... I called her dad immediately and he dropped everything and came right over. We don't want anything to happen to her, and we both have her interest in heart. But that's why. I didn't know that it as affecting her like that. Cuz she's always so together and strong.

The mother's interruption here is a good example how well-meaning, caring, and concerned parents often push adolescents away. But rather than point that out to the mother now, which might embarrass or insult her, the therapist empathizes with and amplifies her fear of suicide. This deepened emotional state will help make the mother more receptive to seeing and approaching the problem from a new perspective.

> Therapist: … So part of our work here is to make sure she comes to you next time she feels this bad. You would like that right!
>
> Mother: Oh god yes!
>
> Therapist: But this means we need to get some things on the table. We need to better understand why she won't come to you and what makes her afraid of being more honest with you. (Turns to the girl) And it sounds like your mom needs to learn how to listen to you a little better. If she really wants to know what you are feelings, she has to give you a little more time to talk. Does that make sense?
>
> Mother: Absolutely. Especially learning to listen and not react as much. Cuz I'm like 'oh why are you doing that? You just can't do that.'
>
> Therapist: Yes. Your quick to give a suggestion or just react?

Mother: They all tell me that I have a very strong personality. 'You are very critical' they say.

Daughter: She is critical. When I told her I was thinking about suicide, and I'm sitting there crying, she sat there yelling at me. 'Why do you want to do that? What's wrong with you?'

Therapist: I wonder if that's something that gets in the way of going to your mom when you're feeling sad?

Daughter: Yeah, cuz most of the time when I try to talk to my mom, her phone starts to ring and she's telling me to hold on for a minute. And she'll be in a totally other conversation. If she's on the phone for more than ten minutes I forget what I was talking about and she won't remember either.

Therapist: So you get interrupted and that gets in the way of you talking to your mom. How about when you do talk to your mom? Like she just said, do you feel she listens well, or, like she just reacts?

Daughter: (Cautiously nods her head.)

Therapist: Do you think that gets in the way of you talking to her?

Daughter: Yes because some of the things I feel I can't talk to her about because she'll say something that will make me really mad and I feel like she isn't trying to help me, she's just trying to control or criticize me.

Therapist: So the things that are really upsetting you, you keep to yourself. That must make you feel very alone at times.

Daughter: (starts to cry) …. I suppose …..

Therapist: (to Mother) It must pain you to see your child in such distress… (mother nods) and it must disappoint you that you cannot comfort her more …..(mother nods, daughter watches her through the corner of her eye.) You both seem to miss each other. (Mother reaches out and takes daughter's hand. Daughter turns away, but does not remove her hand). I wonder if we could spend the next few weeks helping you two feel a bit closer to each other again. Helping Alice be a bit more honest with you and helping your mom listen a bit more before jumping in. It sounds like she wants to help, but just needs a little help learning from you how she can help…..does that sound right?

Mother: Yes I think that sounds good.

Daughter: I guess (trying to act indifferently).

Therapist: Look, clearly there are many problems I need to help you with. But first, we just need some time to rebuild some safety between the two of you. Without a foundation of love, it is hard to solve day to day problems. Do you think we could just work on getting reconnected first? It is not always easy … and we may need to get some difficult topics on the table. But it is clear to me how much you both love and miss each other. So I think you have the strength to do this. (Both mother and daughter nod in agreement.)

Many themes of the model are apparent from the transcript above. One can see how the focus of the therapy tends to support the adolescent's goals. This is not child saving therapy but an engagement strategy. At the same time, the support for the adolescents' goals becomes leverage when challenging him or her to be more direct, emotionally regulated, and honest. For the mother, although this strategy borders on criticizing her, the therapist clearly respects and believes in the parent, and is interested in promoting her goal: getting closer to the adolescent. In this regard, both family members' feel their needs are taken seriously, but are also challenged to use new interpersonal strategies. This is the delicate therapeutic balance of the reframing task.

Task two: Building alliance with the adolescent

Building on the foundation of the first task, generally the therapist meets alone with the adolescent after the first session. The goals here are multiple. First, we want to continue joining with the adolescent in order to amplify strengths and build up trust. Second the therapist aims to explore the adolescent's depression, its perceived causes, and how it relates to family conflict. Third, the session concludes with helping the adolescent consider discussing these conflicts more directly with his or her parents.

The success of the task hinges on the therapist's ability to identify family conflicts that contribute to depression and persuade the adolescent to discuss these issues with his or her parents. Usually, linking depression to family conflict is easy. Even if family conflict is not the 'cause' of the depression, most depressed adolescent report high conflict with, or detachment from, parents that exacerbate their depression. Helping adolescents see the value of talking with parents about these problems proves to be the harder task. Most adolescents feel that parents will not listen or don't care. Surprisingly many depressed adolescents are protective of their parents and do not want to burden them with honest concerns or problems. Addressing these barriers is central to the success of the task.

> Therapist: So it is pretty clear that you have been unhappy. Some of it is about how your mother treats you and some is about missing your father. But it is less clear why you have not told your parents about this. How come you don't talk to anybody about this?
>
> Daughter: Cuz nobody will really care. Nobody will really pay attention to me. If I tell my mom, all she says is I am being oversensitive, or that she is only trying to help. And if I talk to her about my father … well… that sets off a tirade of things. Then all I hear about for the next few days is about how bad he is and all the things he has done to her. I just can't give her that ammunition.
>
> Therapist: Have you tried to talk to your father about these things?
>
> Daughter: No. I can talk to him about other stuff, school and stuff. But he does not like me to complain. He says I sound like my mother, always busting on him.

So the therapist now has two strong themes or content areas where the adolescent has some legitimate grievances with these parents. But depressed adolescents are conflict avoidant and have low expectations of fair and decent relationships. If this does not change, adolescents are left with their own confusion, fantasies, self blame, and lack of trust in others' ability to honour their feelings. And Alice gives a typical response: parents will not take me seriously or parents will be hurt and abandon me. At this juncture, the therapist must challenge these deeply held beliefs and fears about direct communication. This is a complex conversation that can take many roads, some of which are exemplified in the transcript below.

Therapist: So you are in a bit of a bind here. You lost a lot when your dad left. That must be very painful. And very sad. But you're keeping that all inside, all to yourself. Those are a lot of sad feelings to carry around yourself. (Alice gets a bit teary eyed.) Does it feel that way to you?

Daughter: I suppose. But I just don't think they would understand …..

Therapist: You know, I worry that you underestimate them. That you do not give them enough credit for who they are as people who love you. I wonder … if you were more honest with them … like you are being with me … that maybe they would hear you in a new way.

Daughter: But I have tried before … and it did not work.

Therapist: Well maybe you have, but I hear a different voice in you today; a stronger voice. You are not screaming. You are not pouting. You are not running out the door. You are being honest, direct and insightful …. I bet if they heard that voice … they might respond to you differently.

Daughter: But what if I do. What if I tell them what I think and they still do not listen?

Therapist: Well. I will be there to help you. In fact, I will be meeting with them alone and will help them understand the importance of taking you more seriously. If I think they are not ready for this, I will not let the conversation happen. I am here to protect you. But if you want them to take you seriously, you have to be at your best, like you are here with me.

The above dialogue shows, among other things, how the support for the adolescent's issues can be used to challenge the adolescent to act in a more mature, regulated manner. Of course, many adolescents need education about what this means. This can include role playing, assessing one's cognitive schemas, talking about past events, disclosing unexplored traumatic events, and getting comfortable with affective arousal associated with these topics. But the new or renewed commitment to enter into conversation, the courage to confront problems that have been avoided, and the gained entitlement to fair and just relationships, creates the motivation for change. For many adolescents, it is this perspective shift and decision to enter into these negotiations that brings out their strengths and maturity.

The therapist also says at the end she will support the teen in this process. The therapist's commitment to help the parents be more attentive and protect the adolescent from further harm goes a long way to providing safety and confidence to Alice. In a sense, the therapist serves as the transitional object, the good parent that has listened, supported, empathized, and admired. The therapist provides protection while holding the adolescent to a higher interpersonal standard.

Task three: Building alliance with the parent

The alliance building task with the parent(s) is often the most challenging. Our experience is that, underneath bravado or indifference, depressed adolescents often crave a connection with the parents. For parents, however, the situation is often more complicated. The therapist aims to help the parents resuscitate or amplify a desire for connection with their adolescent and to teach them a new set of parenting skills. But this road is often blocked by layers of intrapersonal, interpersonal, and intergenerational baggage. Many parents we see are themselves depressed or struggling with other kinds of psychopathology. Many parents are embroiled in bad marriages characterized by problems such as alcoholism, divorce, or domestic violence. And many of the parents we see have their own history of attachment disappointments or failures. They have been emotionally abused or abandoned by their parents.

Faced with these stressors, our goal is to first understand and empathize with parents. Raising an adolescent, let alone a depressed one, is hard enough. Add to it these compounding problems, and it is not surprising that parents struggle. ABFT is not a 'blame the parent' strategy. Rather, it involves honouring and respecting what parents struggle with and how that compromises or motivates their emotional availability and caretaking abilities. Remarkably, attending to the parents' own needs and history, even if for a brief time, puts parents in a softened, self-reflective mood, which can open them to a deeper appreciation of how relational failures have negatively impacted their child. With this foundation, the therapist can introduce the goal of the reattachment task and offer parents an opportunity to interrupt the generational pattern of neglect and emotional isolation.

> Therapist: What was it like at your house [growing up]?
>
> Mother: It was nice. My mother was the huggy type. She was the buffer between my dad because he never really spoke to us. He would say good morning and not much more. He never really talked to you unless you did something wrong. You know, but my mom, my aunt, and my grandma, we'd all sit in the kitchen and we'd talk. Or they'd talk and as kids, we'd listen.
>
> Therapist: So you had a lot of warmth and comfort with them?
>
> Mother: Oh yes. I wish my house was like that now.
>
> Therapist: Really?
>
> Mother: Now it is just chaos. Grandma has passed away, and my father is very old. He lives with us too.
>
> Therapist: Not much time for sitting around in the kitchen talking?
>
> Mother: (smiles) No!

Here the therapist, without criticizing the parent, empathizes with the lack of warmth and comfort in the home. The mother remembers what it is like to feel loved and safe, but due to circumstances, it has been unable to replicate that in her own home. Later in the conversation, the mother talks a bit more about herself.

> Mother: I was the middle child, and I was always the one that everyone said, 'If you don't know, ask Mary.' Or, 'If you want the VCR hooked up, ask Mary.' Or, 'If you wanted something done, ask Mary.' Everything was 'ask Mary, ask Mary, ask Mary.'
>
> Therapist: Did you like that or was that something that …
>
> Mom: I thought I liked it at the time, but I didn't realize what it meant …. I was the

one that was responsible … the stable one, the one who didn't fly off the handle and become all emotional. If something happens, I'm like 'lets see what we have to do and do it.' I might be all boo hooey later, but right now we don't have time for that. I kinda still am like that I guess.

Therapist: While on the one hand this is a strength, it sounds like it can be a burden … a lot of pressure on you to be in control.

Mother: YES! Exactly …. And the other day, I realized I was kinda doing the same thing to Alice because she's the one that's responsible. I can count on her to do things. If I tell her to do something, I know she's going to do it without me saying 'figure it out' or 'do it this way or that.' After Friday I realized ok, I'm doing the same thing to her that they did to me. And it is too much for a little girl. And while it is not always like that, I guess to her it seems like all the time.

Therapist: So you have developed some appreciation for the spot she's in.

Mother: Yes. She takes on more than she can manage, like she is trying to save everyone, even me.

Therapist: That's great that you can draw from your own childhood experiences to realize what she is going through. Not a lot of parents can do that. Do you think she feels burdened like you did?

Mother: She must!

The mother is now in a good spot therapeutically. She has developed some empathy for herself as a child and that has given her some insight about her daughter. At this juncture, the goal is to offer her an opportunity to make things different with her daughter; to listen to Alice's concerns with more empathy and patience. Not that all of Alice's complaints are correct, but to give Alice an opportunity to be the vulnerable one, to seek comfort and solace rather than always feel like she has to take care of others.

In the next session, again with the mother alone, this theme is extended. But this time, rather than exploring intrapsychic and intergenerational themes, the therapist provides some psychoeducational training about emotionally focused listening and problem-solving skills. These skills, well articulated in other books (Faber & Mazlish, 1980; Gottman et al., 1996), are used to help facilitate the upcoming reattachment tasks. The skills focus on listening without defending, focusing on vulnerable emotions, helping put feelings into words, and postponing problems-solving until emotional processing is done.

Task four: Reattachment

The reattachment task is the culmination of all previous tasks. The Reframe Task has focused families on relationship building. The Alliance Task with the adolescent has identified core themes or complaints and developed the adolescent's commitment to address these concerns more directly with his/her parents. The Alliance Task with the Parent has emotionally prepared the parent to be more receptive to the adolescent's concerns as a stepping off point for more effective problem-solving. This sort of shuttle diplomacy (e.g., preparing the adolescent, preparing the mother) has positioned the family to have a more productive, honest, and supportive conversation about some important, if not fundamental, problems in the relationship.

The content of these conversations can vary. In some cases adolescents report feeling that their parents are unavailable, don't care about them, and/or care more about other family members. Not infrequently, adolescents complain that their parents are more concerned with controlling their behaviour than listening to how they feel and what they think. In other cases, the attachment relationship has been ruptured or even shattered as the result of maltreatment, neglect, abuse, psychological control, and/or constant parental criticism. These ruptures often stem from chronic and pervasive family disorganization. Although families rarely speak about these issues directly, they often feel relieved to address them in therapy, like the unburdening of a secret that everyone knows but never discusses. In many families, merely identifying and acknowledging these topics help diffuse tension and distrust.

The primary goal for the parent is to encourage the adolescent to continue to express core feelings. This is accomplished by empathic listening, acknowledgement of the adolescent's experiences and some level of self disclosure about their own experience of these events. In some cases, when appropriate, parents may express remorse and apologize for past grievances. When successful, reattachment episodes lead to increased openness, disclosure, vulnerability, and intimacy for both the adolescent and parents. Adolescent and parents often see new sides of each other and consequently become more empathic and understanding. The conversation below demonstrates some of this process. The conversation begins with a focus on mother's criticalness and then moves to conversations about the father.

> Daughter: It makes me feel pressured. I'm supposed to express myself to you, but I feel I'm going to get judged.
>
> Mother: Well, how does the pressure make you feel? I mean, is that something that you can explain?
>
> Daughter: No.
>
> Therapist: It must be really hard to feel like every time you talk to your parents you have to monitor what you say.
>
> Mother: Why do you feel that you have to monitor what you say?
>
> Daughter: Cuz, I know that if I tell you guys certain things that I'm not going to hear what I want to hear. And that's going to make me mad and make me feel like I can't tell you certain things.
>
> Mother: Well …. is it because you want things your way?
>
> Daughter: No.
>
> Mother: Oh. So maybe it is we are giving too much advice instead of listening to you? Rather than just listening and understanding and just being there to hear what you have to say?
>
> Daughter: (nods in agreement). And not judge me!

Here the daughter is struggling to be more direct. The mother does a nice job not getting distracted by what seems immature (wanting it her way). Instead the mother stays focused and moves it a bit deeper. Clearly the mother is now asking more questions than giving advice and focusing more on feelings than behaviours. The daughter begins to discuss feeling judged and criticized by the mother. Regardless of how true these complaints are, it is the first time the daughter has raised it directly and the mother has entered into a civil, respectful conversation about it.

Mother: Well when you come to me with things, what are some of the things you don't like that I do and what are some of the things you do like that I do?

Daughter: I don't like when you interrupt me when I have not finished a sentence and then you don't fully understand what I'm telling you and so you just criticize me and you don't even know what I am talking about. And then I start getting an attitude with you because I feel like you're criticizing. And, um, but I do like that you give me advice.

Mother: You don't like that I give you advice?

Daughter: I DO like the fact that you give me advice. I just want you to understand me better first.

Here the daughter takes a small but important turn. As she feels more heard and understood, she is less defensive and rejecting. She surprizes the mother by saying she actually likes the advice, a clear message of wanting her mother's help. As an emerging young adult, however, she needs to feel more respected and collaborative in the conversation. Although this topic is fairly benign, and not uncommon, depressed adolescents take this issue very seriously. They are sensitive to criticism and will withdraw quickly if they feel attacked or challenged. There is a fine balance to walk between placating and challenging a teen to be more direct and honest. In many families, this is a hard and difficult battle. And, as in many families, other issues are lingering. Latter in the session, this emerges.

Mother: So maybe I can slow down and try to listen to you better. Would you like that?

Daughter: (remains silent. Becomes teary eyed.)

Mother: (To therapist??) What is it … What did I say?

Therapist: Maybe this is not about you. Just focus on your daughter.

Mother: (Takes daughter's hand). What is it baby?

Daughter: I miss daddy (starts to cry). I know you hate him, and I know he had to move out … but he never comes to see me anymore ……

Mother: Alice … I do not hate him ….

Daughter: Yes you do!

Therapist: (to mother) Don't defend …. Just listen.

Mother: (pauses …. a bit confused…) So you miss him?

Daughter: (starts to cry again). Just cause you decided to hate each other …. Doesn't mean that he can't love me …

Mother: (Gets teary.)

Families often have layers of challenges and disappointments. Some layers represent day to day challenges (communicating with mom) and some concern deeper ruptures (divorce and dad's absence). For Alice, she felt safe enough to share these deeper struggles after she felt her mother become more attentive. Alice needed her mother to help and comfort her, but she needed her autonomy to be respected. As she felt she could be close but independent as well, she was able to turn to mom for support, solace, and comfort, something she had not done for years. Several more sessions were held with mother and Alice that helped refine and solidify the kinds of changes that were experienced in this session.

Task five: Promoting autonomy and competency

This task tries to build on the good will that has emerged from the earlier tasks. In many families, the attachment task sets in motion a new desire for closeness, trust, and communication. This new foundation and secure base is then used to help the adolescent move along on the normative track of development. Many depressed teens have given up their social life, hobbies, and sometimes school work and other avocations. Anhedonia can penetrate and destroy an adolescent's life trajectory. Consequently, helping the adolescent turn outward and begin to rebuild his or her life is a critical step in recover from depression and prevention of relapse. Other models describe this as behavioural activation or promoting pleasant activates (Lewinsohn et al., 1996), and we agree with this frame whole heartedly. In ABFT, we usually, although not always, try to resolve relational conflicts at home and then turn to social competency challenges usually out of the home. We also see the parents playing a critical role in promoting the competency and autonomy. Providing a secure base, they can also support, challenge, facilitate, and encourage growth in this domain. In this way, we promote authoritative parenting that gives a balance of warmth and demandingness/expectations (Baumrind, 1991).

In the case we are following above, there were two autonomy domains that were addressed in the latter sessions. The first, related to an attachment tasks, concerned the father. The mother, for the first time, began to understand how distraught the daughter was over the absence of the father. She also began to appreciate how her own anger at her husband had over burdened her daughter and made it more difficult for her husband to remain in contact with Alice. Not only was the mother committed to changing her part in this triangle, but she highly encouraged Alice to invite the father into some sessions to discuss her relationship with him.

Feeling less conflicted regarding loyalty to one parent or the other, the daughter and therapist prepared for a meeting with the father, then met with the father alone and finally met with Alice and her father together. In this joint meeting, Alice expressed her disappointment about his absence. The father was quite receptive to this conversation. He apologized for letting his anger at his ex-wife get in the way of his relationship with Alice. This and a few other meetings were productive for the father and Alice to begin defining a new relationships post the separation and eventual divorce. Throughout these meetings with the father, the mother remained supportive and encouraging without prying into the sessions.

Competency was also promoted in relationships to school performance. During this past year, Alice, usually a straight 'A' student, began missing classes and doing poorly on tests. With her depression, she had lost the motivation and concentration needed to perform to her potential. Throughout the year, the mother had tried to intervene, but this usually resulted in fighting over mothers hopes for Alice to attend college and have the opportunities that she never had. As a new way of discussing problems emerged, mother began backing off the pressure to attend college and began letting her daughter think about other possible career paths. The mother did not give up her dream of Alice attending college, but began to express her willingness to accept whatever work or school plans she chose. This freed Alice to use mother as a sounding board about other possible life ideas: the army, work for a year, travel in Europe, etc. It broke the mother's heart to hear about these alternatives, but the trade-off of being part of Alice's life planning was well worth it. The mother did not hide her joy when Alice eventually asked her to visit some local colleges one weekend, but the expression of joy was done with humour not criticism.

Empirical support

ABFT has garnered empirical support from clinical and process research studies. In the first outcome study (Diamond et al., 2003), funded by the NIMH, 32 adolescents were randomized to 12 weeks of treatment or a six-week waitlist control. Of the 16 treatment cases, 13 (81%) no longer met criteria for MDD post treatment, while only 9 (56%) of the patients on the waiting list no longer met criteria for MDD post-waitlist (X^2 [1] = 4.05, p <04). Clinical improvement was also significantly better in the treatment group where 62% of the adolescents treated with ABFT had a BDI of 9 or less compared to 19% of adolescents in the waitlist condition (BDI < 9, (2 [1] = 6.37, p =.01). Patients treated with ABFT also showed more improvement on anxiety, family conflict, attachment to mothers, hopelessness, and suicidal ideation. Similar results were maintained at 6 months.

Recently, we completed a larger trial funded by the Centre for Disease Control, testing ABFT for adolescents presenting with persistent suicidal ideation (SIQ-JR > 31 for several days) that was not serious enough to warrant hospitalization. In order to be eligible, adolescents also had to report current depressive symptoms (BDI > 20). Sixty-six adolescents were randomized to 14 weeks of ABFT or an enhanced usual care (facilitating referrals to community treatment). The sample included 83% female and 17% male adolescents, ranging in age between 12–18 years (M = 15.20, SD = 1.61). Of the entire sample, 74% identified themselves as African American, 15% as Caucasian, 3% as Hispanic/Latino, 3% as biracial, and 5% chose 'other'. In addition, 73% came from single-parent families. As an indicator of socioeconomic status, 43% of the participants made less than $30,000, 45% made between $30,000 and $80,000, and 12% made over $80,000. Sixty percent of the adolescents reported having made some kinds of suicide attempt in their lifetime, although only 18% reported having ever been hospitalized for emotional or behavioural problems. Although outcome data from this study is not yet in press, we can report that ABFT did better than EUC on reducing suicidal ideation, depression, suicide attempts, and retention.

Other studies have been conducted as well. One study was a small pilot for treating adolescents with Anxiety. ABFT did as well as CBT in remission of diagnosis and better in adolescent report of parent's use of psychological control (Siqueland et al., 2005). We have also conducted several process research studies to further describe or test the proposed mechanism of each task. Many of these studies are reviewed in Diamond et al. (2003). Current projects underway include a randomized clinical trial of ABFT against treatment as usual in a community hospital in Norway and a small pilot study to test ABFT as an aftercare model for adolescents leaving a psychiatric hospital after a suicide attempt.

References

Allen, J.P., Hauser, S.T., & Borman-Spurrell, E. (1996). Attachment theory as a framework for understanding sequelae of severe adolescent psychopathology: An 11-year follow-up study. *Journal of Consulting and Clinical Psychology, 64(2)*, 254–263.

Allen, J.P. & Land, D. (1999). Attachment in adolescence. In P.R. Shaver & J. Cassidy (Eds.), *Handbook of attachment: Theory, research, and clinical applications* (pp. 319–335). New York: Guilford Press.

Allen, J.P., Moore, C., Kuperminc, G. & Hall, K. (1998). Attachment and adolescent psychosocial functioning. *Child Development, 69(5)*, 1406–1419.

Ainsworth, M.D.S. (1989). Attachment beyond infancy. *American Psychologist, 44*, 709–716.

Asarnow, J.R., Goldstein, M.J., Tompson, M., & Guthrie, D. (1993). One-year outcomes of depressive disorders in child psychiatric in-patients: Evaluation of the prognostic power of a brief measure of expressed emotion. *Journal of Child Psychology and Psychiatry, 34(2)*, 129–137.

Baumrind, D. (1991). The influence of parenting style on adolescent competency and substance abuse. *Journal of Early Adolescence, 11*, 56–95.

Boszormenyi-Nagy, I. & Spark, G.M. (1973). *Invisible loyalties: Reciprocity in intergenerational family therapy*. Oxford, England: Harper & Row.

Cicchetti, D. & Greenberg, M.T. (1991). The legacy of John Bowlby. *Development and Psychopathology, 3, 347*–350.

Cicchetti, D., Toth, S.L. & Lynch, M. (1995). Bowlby's dream comes full circle: The application of attachment theory to risk and psychopathology. *Advances in Clinical Child Psychology, 17*, 1–75.

Cole, D.A. (1990). Relation of social and academic competence to depressive symptoms in childhood. *Journal of Abnormal Psychology, 99(4)*, 422–429.

Coyne, J.C. (1976). Toward an interactional description of depression. *Psychiatry, 39*, 28–40.

Cummings, E.M. & Davies, P. (1994). *Children and marital conflict*. New York: Guilford.

Diamond, G.S., & Diamond, G.M. (2002). Studying mechanisms of change: A process research agenda for family-based treatments. In H. Liddle, R. Leant, & J. Bray (Eds.), *Family Psychology Intervention Science*. Washington, DC: American Psychological Association Press.

Diamond, G.S. & Josephson, A.M. (2005). Family-based treatment research: A 10-year update. *Journal of the American Academy of Child and Adolescent Psychiatry, 44(9)*, 872–887.

Diamond, G.S. & Siqueland, L. (1998). Emotions, attachment and the relational reframe. *Journal of Structural and Strategic Therapy, 17*, 36–50.

Diamond, G.S., Siqueland, S., & Diamond, G.M. (2003). Attachment-based family therapy for depressed adolescents: Programmatic treatment development. *Clinical Child and Family Psychology Review, 6(2)*, 107–127.

Dumont, M. & Provost, M.A. (1999). Resilience in adolescents: Protective role of social support, coping strategies, self-esteem, and social activities on experience of stress and depression. *Journal of Youth and Adolescence, 28(3)*, 343–363.

Faber, A. & Mazlish, E. (1980). *How to talk so kids will listen & listen so kids will talk.* New York: Avon Books.

Fincham, F.D., & Bradbury, T.N. (1988). The impact of attributions in marriage: Empirical and conceptional foundations. *British Journal of Clinical Psychology, 27*, 77–90.

Fongay P., Steele, M., Steele, H., Leigh, T., Kennedy, R., Mattoon, G., et al. (2000). Attachment, the reflective self, and borderline states. In S. Goldberg, R. Muir, & J. Kerr (Eds), *Attachment theory: Social, developmental and clinical perspectives* (pp. 233–278). New York: Analytic Press.

Gotlib, I. & Hammen, C. (1992). *Psychological aspects of depression: Towards a cognitive-interpersonal integration.* Chichester, England: Wiley.

Gottman, J.M., Katz, L.F., & Hooven, C. (1996). Parental meta-emotion philosophy and the emotional life of families: Theoretical models and preliminary data. *Journal of Family Psychology, 10(3)*, 243–268.

Greenberg, M.T. (1999). Attachment and psychopathology in childhood. In J. Cassidy & P.R. Shaver (Eds.), *Handbook of attachment* (pp. 469–496). New York: Guilford.

Greenberg, L.S. & Johnson, S.M. (1988). *Emotionally focused therapy for couples.* New York: Guilford Press.

Greenberg, L.S. & Safran, J.D. (1987). *Emotion in psychotherapy: Affect, cognition, and the process of change.* New York: Guilford Press.

Harris, T., Brown, G., & Bifulco, A. (1986). Loss of parent in childhood and adult psychiatric disorder: The lack of adequate parental care. *Psychological Medicine, 16*, 641–659.

Joiner, T. & Coyne, J.C. (1999). *The interactional nature of depression.* Washington, D. C.: American Psychological Association.

Kobak, R. & Duemmler, S. (1994). Attachment and conversation: Toward a discourse analysis of adolescent and adult security. In D. Perlman & K. Bartholomew (Eds.), *Attachment processes in adulthood: Advances in personal relationships*, Vol. 5 (pp. 121–149). Bristol, PA: Jessica Kingsley Publishers, Ltd.

Kobak, R. & Mandelbaum, T. (2003). Caring for the caregiver: An attachment approach to assessment and treatment of problematic child behavior. In S. Johnson (Ed.), *Attachment processes in couples and family therapy* (pp. 144–164). New York: Guilford Press.

Kobak, R. & Sceery, A. (1988). Attachment in late adolescence: Working models, affect regulation, and representations of self and others. *Child Development, 59*, 135–146.

Kobak, R., Sudler, N., & Gamble, W. (1991). Attachment and depressive symptoms during adolescence: A developmental pathways analysis. *Development and Psychopathology, 3(4)*, 461–474.

Lewinsohn, P.M., Clarke, G.N., Rohde, P., Hops, H., & Seeley, J. (1996). A course in coping: A cognitive-behavioral approach to the treatment of adolescent depression. In E.D. Hibbs & P.S. Jensen (Eds.), *Psychosocial treatments for child and adolescent disorders: Empirically based strategies for clinical practice* (pp. 109–135). Washington, DC: American Psychological Association.

Liddle, H.A. (1999). Theory development in a family-based therapy for adolescents' drug abuse. *Journal of Clinical and Child Psychology, 28(4)*, 521–533.

Liddle, H.A., Dakof, G.A., Parker, K., Diamond, G.S., Barrett, K., & Tejada, M. (2001). Multidimensional family therapy for adolescent drug abuse: Results of a randomized clinical trial. *American Journal of Drug and Alcohol Abuse, 27(4)*, 651–687.

Liddle, H.A. & Diamond, G.S. (1991). Adolescent substance abusers in family therapy: The critical initial phase of treatment. *Family Dynamics of Addiction Quarterly*, 1, 55–68.

Luborsky, L. (2001). *Principles of Psychoanalytic Psychotherapy*. New York: Basic Books.

Lynch, M. & Cicchetti, D. (1991). Patterns of relatedness in maltreated and non maltreated children. *Development and Psychopathology, 3*, 207–226.

Maccoby, E.E. & Martin, J.A. (1983). Socialization in the context of the family: Parent–child interaction. In M. Heatherington (Ed.), *Handbook of child psychology, Vol. 4* (pp. 1–10). New York: Wiley.

Minuchin, S. (1974). *Families and family Therapy*. Cambridge, Mass.:Harvard University Press.

Mufson, L., Moreau, D., Weissman, M.M., Wickramaratne, P., Martin, J., & Samoilov, A. (1993). Modification of Interpersonal psychotherapy with depressed adolescents (IPT-A): Phase I and II studies. *Journal of the American Academy of Child and Adolescents Psychiatry, 33(5)*, 695–705.

Rosenstein, D.S. & Horowitz, H.A. (1996). Adolescent attachment and psychopathology. *Journal of Consulting and Clinical Psychology, 64(2)*, 244–253.

Rutter, M. (1984), Family and school influences on behavioral development. *Journal of Child Psychology and Psychiatry, 26*, 349–367.

Sheeber, L., Hops, H., & Davis, B. (2001). Family processes in adolescent depression. *Clinical Child & Family Psychology Review, 4(1)*, 19–35.

Siqueland, L., Rynn, M., & Diamond, G.S. (2005). Cognitive behavioral and attachment-based family therapy for anxious adolescent: Phase I and II studies. *Journal of Anxiety Disorder, 19(4)*, 361–381

Steinberg, L. (1990). Autonomy, conflict and harmony in the family relationships. In S.S. Feldman & G.R. Elliot (Eds.), *At the threshold: The developing adolescent* (pp. 255–276). Cambridge, MA: Harvard University Press.

Yap, M.B.H., Allen, N.B., & Sheeber, L. (2007). Using an emotional regulation framework to understand the role of temperament and family processes in risk for adolescent depressive disorder. *Clinical Child and Family Psychology, 10(2)*, 180–196.

Weinfeld, N.S., Sroufe, L.A., & Egelund, B. (2000). Attachment from infancy to early adulthood: A twenty-year longitudinal study. *Child Development, 71*, 684–689.

Weissman, M.M. & Paykel, E.S. (1974). *The depressed woman: A study of social relationships*. Chicago: University of Chicago Press.

Part 4

Other forms of treatment

Chapter 10

Pharmacotherapy

Dara J. Sakolsky & Boris Birmaher

Approximately 20% of adolescents will experience at least one episode of depression by age 18 (Lewinsohn et al., 1998). If untreated, depression may affect the development of an individual's cognitive, emotional, and social skills and interfere with family relationships (Birmaher et al., 1996, 2002; Lewinsohn et al., 2003). Adolescents with depression are also at high risk for suicide, substance abuse, physical illness, early pregnancy, legal problems, as well as poor academic and psychosocial functioning (American Academy of Child and Adolescent Psychiatry, 2007). Timely identification and successful treatment may diminish the impact of depression on the academic and psychosocial functioning in youth and decrease the risk for suicide, substance abuse, and other sequelae. Evidence-supported treatment interventions have emerged in both psychotherapy and pharmacotherapy. This chapter will focus on medications options for adolescent depression.

The success of pharmacotherapy for adult depression led investigators in the 1970s and 1980s to begin clinical trials of antidepressants in children and adolescents. Initial studies focused on tricyclic antidepressants (TCAs) with mixed results (for review, see Hazell et al., 2002). Treatment of adolescent depression with tricyclic antidepressants was limited by high rates of side effects and concerns about lethal overdoses. When selective serotonin reuptake inhibitors (SSRIs) were showed to be effective for adult depression, studies in children and adolescents soon followed. Two double blind, randomized, placebo-controlled trials with fluoxetine (Emslie et al., 1997, 2002a) demonstrated efficacy and led to its approval by the US Food and Drug Administration for treatment of paediatric depression.

Randomized controlled trials (RCTs) with other SSRIs have shown relatively good response rates, but the placebo response rate has also been high, resulting in many negative studies (for review, see Bridge et al., 2007). Positive trials have been reported for sertraline (Wagner et al., 2003) and citalopram (Wagner et al., 2004), while negative studies have been reported for citalopram (von Knorring et al., 2006), escitalopram (Wagner et al., 2006), and paroxetine (Keller et al., 2001; Berard et al., 2006; Emslie et al., 2006a).

A few RCTs have evaluated the efficacy of other antidepressants. Trials with venlafaxine (Emslie et al., 2007a) and mirtazapine (US Food and Drug Administration NDA 20-415 SE5-011, mirtazapine paediatric supplement, 2004) have shown no difference in effect between drug and placebo. One trial with nefazadone reported a better response to drug than placebo on most clinical measures (Emslie et al., 2002a), but an unpublished study showed no difference (US Food and Drug Administration Review and Evaluation of Clinical Data NDA 20-152 S-032, nefazadone paediatric supplement, 2004).

One measure of treatment efficacy is the number needed to treat (NNT) or the number of patients who must receive the treatment to get one response that is attributable to active treatment. A meta-analysis of published and unpublished RCTs of antidepressants (Bridge et al., 2007) reported the NNT to benefit from an antidepressant was 10 (95% confidence interval, 7–15) for paediatric depression. This meta-analysis also examined the number needed to harm (NNH) or the number of patients who must receive a treatment to get one adverse effect that can be attributed to active treatment. Bridge and colleagues reported the overall NNH for the spontaneous report of suicidal ideation and suicide attempt was 112 for patients with major depressive disorder who were treated with an antidepressant. Despite the limitations of meta-analysis, these numbers suggest a favourable risk-benefit profile for the use of antidepressants as treatment for adolescent depression.

Indications for pharmacotherapy

Many treatment interventions (supportive therapy, cognitive–behavioural therapy, attachment-based family therapy, interpersonal therapy, and pharmacotherapy) can be helpful for adolescents with major depression (American Academy of Child and Adolescent Psychiatry, 2007; National Institute for Health and Clinical Excellence, 2005). When personalizing treatment recommendations for a specific patient, the choice of interventions considered should be based on a variety factors, including depression severity, duration of illness, prior response to treatment, familial and environmental factors, availability of treatment, comorbid disorders, patient, and family preference.

For adolescents with mild or brief depression, little psychosocial impairment, the absence of suicidality, or psychosis, pharmacotherapy is not indicated. In these cases, treatment often begins with education and supportive therapy to target stressors in the family or school. If response is not achieved after 6–8 weeks of supportive therapy, a trial with another type of psychotherapy should be considered.

For adolescents with moderate, chronic, or recurrent depression, significant psychosocial impairment, suicidality, or psychosis, pharmacotherapy is often indicated. Moderate depression may respond to a trial of cognitive–behavioural therapy or interpersonal therapy alone; however, many adolescents will require the combination of psychotherapy and an antidepressant to achieve remission of symptoms (Treatment of Adolescent Depression Study (TADS) Team, 2004). In some cases, the severity of the depressive symptoms (e.g., agitation, poor concentration, sleep disturbance, low motivation, or psychosis) can limit participation in psychotherapy, and so initial treatment with only an antidepressant is recommended. In other cases, comorbid psychiatric disorders (e.g., mental retardation or autism) make participation in cognitive–behavioural therapy or interpersonal therapy difficult, and so treatment with an antidepressant and supportive therapy is indicated. Experienced psychotherapists are not available in all areas, and so pharmacotherapy may be the only option. Even when psychotherapy is available, some adolescents and their families may not wish to participate; thus, treatment with an antidepressant is offered.

For adolescents with severe depression or treatment-resistant depression, pharmacotherapy is needed (American Academy of Child and Adolescent Psychiatry, 2007). Treatment often involves the combination of an antidepressant and psychotherapy, although two large studies in England and in the USA showed that for adolescents with severe MDD, there were no differences between fluoxetine alone and fluoxetine plus CBT (Curry et al., 2006; Goodyer et al., 2007).

Goals of pharmacotherapy

Treatment of depression is generally separated into three phases: acute, continuation, and maintenance (American Academy of Child and Adolescent Psychiatry, 2007). The goal of acute treatment is to attain response, a significant reduction in depressive symptoms for at least 2 weeks, and eventually full remission, no or very few depressive symptoms for at least 2 weeks and less than 2 months. Continuation treatment is needed for all depressed adolescents to sustain benefits achieved during the acute phase and avoid relapses, a major depressive episode that begins during the period of remission. Residual depressive symptoms after acute antidepressant treatment have been associated with higher rates of relapse (Emslie et al., 2004). Thus, the goal of pharmacotherapy is remission rather than response. For some adolescents with severe, chronic, or recurrent major depression, maintenance pharmacotherapy is used to avoid recurrence, a major depressive episode that begins after a patient has been asymptomatic for more than 2 months (American Academy of Child and Adolescent Psychiatry, 2007).

Selective serotonin reuptake inhibitors

Pharmacokinetics of selective serotonin reuptake inhibitors

During the past decade, the efficacy of SSRIs for the treatment of adolescent depression has been tested in many large RCTs; however, few studies have examined the pharmacokinetic properties of these medications in adolescents. Findling et al. (2006a) have recently reviewed this literature and concluded that medication dosing strategies in several RCTs may have contributed not only to the failure of these trials to show a difference in efficacy between medication and placebo, but also to the safety and tolerability of these medications. As adolescents differ from adults in numerous ways, pharmacokinetic studies in adolescents can provide useful information regarding how to dose these medications appropriately in this population.

Some pharmacokinetic studies in adolescents have shown no difference in pharmacokinetic parameters when compared with adult studies, while other studies (citalopram, ecitalopram, paroxetine, and sertraline) have reported shorter half-lives in adolescents and children (for review, see Findling et al., 2006a).

Several pharmacokinetic properties were reported for fluoxetine in a population pharmacokinetic study of children and adolescents (Wilens et al., 2002). Mean steady-state levels of fluoxetine (127 ng/ml) and its primary metabolite, norfluoxetine (151 ng/ml), were achieved after 4 weeks of treatment. Although high intersubject variability was reported, concentrations of fluoxetine and norfluoxetine were approximately two times higher in children than adolescents. When normalized to body weight, fluoxetine and norfluoxetine concentrations were similar for both age groups. Time to steady state, plasma concentration at steady state, intersubject variability, and ratio of drug to metabolite were similar in adolescents when compared to adult studies. On the basis of their findings, Wilens and colleagues (2002) suggested that prepubertal children start fluoxetine at 10 mg/day, whereas initial dosing for adolescents may begin at 20 mg/day.

Pharmacokinetic studies of citalopram, escitalopram, and sertraline suggest that these medications have shorter half-lives in adolescents when used at low doses, but their half-lives are equivalent to adults when given in a higher dose range (for summary of pharmacokinetics studies see Findling et al., 2006a). One pharmacokinetic study in adolescents examined the half life of R-citalopram and S-citalopram after a single 20 mg dose and after 2 weeks of 20 mg/day (Perel et al., 2001). S-citalopram, marketed in the United States as escitalopram, is the therapeutically active isomer of racemic citalopram (Hyttell et al., 1992). The single dose and steady-state half-life of s-citalopram was found to be significantly shorter than previously reported in adults. On the basis of these findings, the authors recommended twice per day dosing when prescribing citalopram 20 mg/day. Similarly, a pharmacokinetic study with a single 10 mg dose of escitalopram found the half-life of escitalopram was shorter in adolescents (19.0 h) than adults (28.9 h). In contrast, a pharmacokinetic study of citalopram 40 mg/day after 3 weeks found pharmacokinetic parameters similar in adolescents (half-life 38 h) and adults (half-life 44 h). The same pattern is also observed in pharmacokinetics studies of sertraline. Pharmacokinetic studies of sertraline in adolescents have reported the mean steady-state half-life is 15.3 h at 50 mg/day, 20.4 h at 100 to 150 mg/day, and 27.1 h at 200 mg/day (Alderman et al., 1998; Axelson et al., 2002). The steady-state half-life of sertraline at 200 mg/day was similar to that previously observed in adults. On the basis of these findings, Axelson and colleagues (2002) suggested an optimal dosing strategy of twice per day at doses of 50mg/day and once daily at 200 mg/day. Therefore, when prescribing citalopram, escitalopram, or sertraline at low dosage range, twice daily dosing should be considered.

The pharmacokinetic properties of paroxetine have been described in two studies using children and adolescents. The first study reported that the half-life of paroxetine after a single 10 mg dose (11.1 h) was significantly shorter than the half-life previously observed in adults (Findling et al., 1999). Other pharmacokinetic parameters (e.g., time to maximum concentration, intersubject variability, cytochrome 2D6 activity highly influenced drug exposure, and nonlinear kinetics) were similar to adults. For individuals who were maintained on 10 mg/day, their paroxetine concentration generally remained stable during treatment; however, an almost 7-fold increase in drug concentration was reported in subjects whose dose was raised to 20 mg/day. On the basis of their findings, Findling and colleagues (1999) concluded that once daily administration of paroxetine was adequate. The second study compared steady-state pharmacokinetic properties after 2 weeks of 10 mg/day, 20 mg/day, and 30 mg/day (Findling et al. 2006a). The nonlinear kinetics of paroxetine was confirmed as supra-proportional increases in drug concentration were seen with increasing dose. Systemic drug exposure at steady state was higher in children than in adolescents at each dose examined. On the basis of their findings, the authors suggested prepubertal children start paroxetine at 5 mg/day or use an extended titration schedule such as 10 mg/day for at least 4 weeks.

In summary, pharmacokinetics studies with SSRIs suggest that optimal dosing strategies may be slightly different for children and adolescents. Fluoxetine and paroxetine may need to be initiated at lower doses in prepubertal children, whereas twice daily dosing should be considered for youths when citalopram, escitalopram, or sertraline is prescribed in the low-dose range.

Although there are some differences, dosing regimens of SSRIs for adolescents are generally similar to adults. It is advisable to start with a low dose and increase until a minimally effective dosage has been achieved. Adolescents should receive an adequate and tolerable dose for a minimum of 4 weeks. If the adolescent has tolerated the SSRI, but remains symptomatic, a dose increase should be considered (Heiligenstein et al. 2006, Hughes et al. 2007). Clinical response should be reassessed every 4 weeks. When a patient fails to show significant improvement after 12 weeks of pharmacotherapy, alternative treatments (e.g., adding psychotherapy, switching to different antidepressant or augmenting with another medication) should be considered.

Efficacy of selective serotonin reuptake inhibitors

Fluoxetine is usually the first choice for pharmacotherapy for adolescent depression since three RCTs (Emslie et al., 1997, 2002b; TADS team, 2004) have demonstrated its efficacy. In their meta-analysis, Bridge and colleagues (2007) pooled the data from all of the RCTs of fluoxetine for paediatric depression. They reported that the NNT to benefit from fluoxetine was 6 (95% CI, 4 to 10), while the NNT to benefit from any antidepressant was 10 (95% CI, 7 to 15). It is unclear if fluoxetine is actually superior to other SSRIs for the treatment of adolescent depression or if the fluoxetine studies were better designed and conducted or recruited more severely depressed patients (for review of methodological issues, see Cheung et al., 2006).

Although fluoxetine is generally the first choice of antidepressants for adolescent depression, there are situations when choosing a different SSRI is rational (e.g., lack of response to an adequate trial of fluoxetine, potential drug interactions, a strong family history of therapeutic response to alternative SSRI, or family resistance).

Both sertraline and citalopram have demonstrated efficacy for adolescent depression in RCTs. Two identical multicentre randomized, double blind, placebo-controlled studies of sertraline were conducted using children and adolescents (Wagner et al., 2003). Patients received a flexible dose of sertraline (50–200 mg/day) or placebo for 10 weeks. Results from the two trials were combined in a prospectively defined data analysis plan. Response rates, defined as 40% decrease in adjusted Children's Depression Rating Scale-Revised (CDRS-R), were 69% for sertraline and 56% for placebo. Mean dose of sertraline was 131 mg/day. On the basis of these studies, Bridge and colleagues (2007) reported that the NNT to benefit from sertraline was 10 (95% CI, 6 to 500).

For citalopram, there is one positive study (Wagner et al., 2004) and one negative study (von Knorring et al., 2006). In the positive trial, patients were randomized to flexible dose citalopram (20–40 mg/day) or placebo for 8 weeks. Response rates, defined as CDRS-R score of less than 28, were 36% for citalopram and 24% for placebo. The mean dose of citalopram was 24 mg/day. In the negative trial, adolescents received citalopram (10–40 mg/day) or placebo for 12 weeks. Unlike other RCTs, participants in this study included both inpatients and outpatients. Some patients received psychotherapy and/or other medications including anticonvulsants, antipsychotics, benzodiapzepines, hypnotics, and stimulants. Response rates, defined as 2 or less on the Schedule for Affective Disorders and Schizophrenia for school-aged children (K-SADS) depression and anhedonia items, were 60% for citalopram and 61% for placebo. Another RCT used flexible dose escitalopram (10–20 mg/day) or placebo for 8 weeks. On the primary outcome measure, change in CDRS-R score from baseline to week 8, there were no significant differences between escitalopram and placebo. However, in a post hoc analysis of adolescents who completed the study, those who received escitalopram had significantly improved scores on all efficacy measures. No difference between escitalopram and placebo was demonstrated with children on any of the outcome measures. The mean dose of escitalopram was 12 mg/day. In their meta-analysis, Bridge and colleagues (2007) pooled the results from the citalopram and escitalopram studies and calculated the NNT to benefit from either medication was 13 (95% CI, 7 to 200). When choosing an alternative to fluoxetine, the data from RCTs supports the use of sertraline, citalopram, or escitalopram for adolescent depression.

The efficacy of paroxetine has been evaluated in three RCTs (Keller et al., 2001; Berard et al., 2006; Emsilie et al., 2006), all of which were negative on the primary efficacy measures. In the first trial (Keller et al., 2001), adolescents received flexible dose of paroxetine (20–40 mg/day) or placebo for 8 weeks. On the two primary outcome measures, Hamilton Rating Scale for Depression (HAM-D) score ≤ 8 or ≥50% reduction in baseline HAM-D and change from baseline HAM-D score, there was no significant difference between paroxetine and placebo. However, four secondary measures of efficacy demonstrated a significant difference between paroxetine and placebo. The mean dose of paroxetine at study endpoint was 28 mg/day. In the second study (Berard et al., 2006), adolescents were randomized to receive a flexible dose of paroxetine (20–40 mg/day) or placebo for 12 weeks. On the two primary efficacy measures, ≥50% reduction of Montgomery-Asberg Depression Rating Scale (MADRS) and change from baseline on the K-SADS depression subscale, there was no significant difference between paroxetine and placebo. The mean dose of paroxetine was 26 mg/day. In the third trial (Emslie et al., 2006b), children and adolescents were randomized to flexible dose paroxetine (10–50 mg/day) or placebo for 8 weeks. On the primary efficacy measure, change from baseline on the CDRS-R, and all secondary measures, there were no significant differences between paroxetine and placebo. The mean dose of paroxetine at study endpoint was 28 mg/day. In their meta-analysis, Bridge and colleagues (2007) were unable to calculate a NNT to benefit from paroxetine as no benefit was demonstrated in these RCTs.

To summarize, evidence from RCTs supports the use of fluoxetine as the first choice of antidepressants for adolescent depression. When choosing an alternative SSRI, data from RCTs suggest that sertraline, citalopram, or escitalopram may also be effective.

Caution must be used when interpreting the results of RCTs for adolescent depression as several factors may moderate the outcomes of these trials. For example, industry sponsored trials are often conducted at a larger number of sites than studies funded by the National Institute of Mental Health. In Bridge and colleagues meta-analysis (2007), the number of trial sites was inversely associated with efficacy, suggesting a reduction in antidepressant effect as the number of study sites is increased. Patient characteristics also moderate the outcome of antidepressant response in RCTs. Longer duration of illness and younger age are associated with poorer outcomes (Bridge et al., 2007). Surprisingly, when Bridge and colleagues limited their analysis to only fluoxetine studies, response was similar for both children and adolescents.

Adverse effects of selective serotonin reuptake inhibitors

In short-term RCTs, SSRIs are generally well-tolerated. Side effects appear to be dose-dependent and often subside with time (Cheung et al., 2005; Emslie et al., 2006a; Safer & Zito, 2006). The most common adverse effects include gastrointestinal symptoms (e.g., nausea, abdominal pain, diarrhea), change in appetite (increase or decrease), headache, dizziness, sleep changes (e.g., insomnia or somnolence, vivid dreams or night mares), dry mouth, restlessness, akathisia, and sexual dysfunction. Impulsivity, silliness, agitation, irritability, or activation can be seen in 3–8% of youth, especially in children. Less common but more severe side effects include serotonin syndrome (Boyer & Shannon, 2005), increased risk of bleeding (e.g., easy bruising, epistaxis, gastrointestinal bleeding, and perioperative bleeding) (Lake et al., 2000; Weinrieb et al., 2005), and increased spontaneous reports of suicidal ideation and behaviour.

In recent years, two meta-analyses have evaluated the risk of suicidal ideation and behaviour in children and adolescents taking antidepressants (Bridge et al., 2007; Hammad et al., 2006). In collaboration with Columbia University, the US Food and Drug Administration assessed the effect of nine antidepressants on suicidality in 24 RCTs of paediatric depression, anxiety disorders, or attention deficit hyperactivity disorder (Hammad et al., 2006). The primary outcome measure was spontaneous reports of suicidal ideation and behaviour termed 'suicidal adverse events'. The overall risk ratio (RR) for suicidality for all the trials and indications was 1.95 (95% Cl, 1.28–2.98). When analyses were limited to depression trials with SSRIs, the overall RR was 1.66 (95% Cl, 1.02–2.68). These results suggest that 1–3 spontaneously reported suicide adverse events occur for every 100 children or adolescents treated with an antidepressant. Hammad et al. also examined worsening or emergence of suicidality using the suicide item scores of depression rating scales from 17 RCTs. These analyses did not reveal any significant RR for worsening of suicidality (0.92; 95% Cl, 0.76–1.1) or for emergence of suicidality (0.93; 95% Cl, 0.75–1.15).

A more recent, comprehensive meta-analysis examined the effect of antidepressants on suicidality in 27 published and unpublished RCTs of paediatric depression and anxiety disorders (Bridge et al., 2007). When using similar statistical methods as the previous study, this meta-analysis found comparable results, a small but significant increase in overall RR for suicidality for all disorders (1.9; 95% Cl, 1.3–3.0) and for depression (1.9; 95% Cl 1.2–2.9). Since RR analysis is limited to trials with at least one event and several trials had no events, Bridge and colleagues also assessed risk difference (RD), which permits inclusion of trials with no events. When using random-effects analysis of RD instead of RR, there was a small but significant overall RD for drug vs. placebo (0.7%; 95% Cl, 0.1–1.3); however, no significant difference was found when analyses were limited to studies with depression (0.9%; 95% Cl, −0.1–1.9). Furthermore, the NNH for depression was 112 (Bridge et al., 2007).

As stated by the US Food and Drug Administration (Hammad et al., 2006), the overall interpretation of these findings and their implications for clinical practice are not clear since there has been a dramatic decline in rate of adolescent suicide in the US during time of increased usage of SSRIs (Olfson et al., 2003). Pharmacoepidemiological studies also suggest a positive relationship between the reduction in adolescent suicide rate and use of SSRIs (Gibbons et al., 2005, 2006; Valuck et al., 2004; Olfson et al., 2003). Since US and European regulators issued warnings on SSRIs, there has been a decrease in the rate of SSRI prescriptions to children and adolescents and an increase in completed suicides rates in the US and Netherlands (Gibbons et al., 2007). Thus, pharmacoepidemiological studies show not only a correlation between increased usage of SSRIs and reduction in suicide rates, but also an association between decreased SSRI usage and elevated youth suicide rates.

In summary, spontaneous reports of suicidal ideation or behaviour are more common in adolescents treated with SSRIs than placebo. However, given the greater number of patients who benefit from SSRIs than who experience serious adverse effects, the reduction in suicidality on depression rating scales with antidepressant treatment, and the lack of any completed suicides in paediatric antidepressant RCTs, the risk-benefit ratio for SSRI use in adolescent depression appears favourable with appropriate monitoring. Trends from pharmachoepidemiological studies highlight the risk of suicide associated with untreated depression and suggest that pharmacotherapy may play a role in diminishing this risk.

Serotonin norepinephrine reuptake inhibitors

Although tricyclic antidepressants (e.g., amitriptyline, clomipramine, despiramine, doxepin, impiramine, and nortripyline) inhibit serotonin and norepinephrine reuptake, these drugs will not be covered in detail as their use in adolescent depression is generally not recommended due to high rates of side effects, risk of lethal overdose, and limited efficacy (for review see Hazell et al., 2002).

Pharmacokinectics of serotonin norepinephrine reuptake inhibitors

To the best of our knowledge, no published studies have examined the pharmacokinetic parameters of venlafaxine extended-release or duloxetine in adolescents. In adult studies, venlafaxine and its active metabolite, O-desmethylvenlafaxine, displays linear pharmacokinetics for doses ranging from 75–450 mg/day (Klamerus et al., 1992). The approximate half-life of venlafaxine is

5 h while the O-desmethylvenlafaxine is 11 h. Given its short half-life, twice daily dosing is recommended for venlafaxine (Troy et al., 1995; Patat et al., 1998). The extended-release formulation of venlafaxine has delayed absorption (e.g., maximum plasma concentration is not achieved until 6 h after administration), resulting in lower peak plasma concentrations and prolonged duration. Once daily dosing is recommended for adults prescribed with extended-release venlafaxine (Patat el., 1998). In a pharmacokinetic study using adult subjects, duloxetine exhibited linear kinetics for doses ranging from 20 mg twice daily to 40 mg twice daily (Sharma et al., 2000). The half-life of duloxetine was 12.5 h (range 9.2–19.1 h) and steady-state plasma concentrations were achieved within 3 days. Once daily dosing of duloxetine is usually recommended for adult depression (Pritchett et al., 2007). Since pharmacokinetics studies in adolescents are lacking for venlafaxine extended-release and duloxetine, physicians generally follow adult dosing guidelines. It is advisable to start with a low dose and increase slowly until a minimally effective dosage is achieved. If an adolescent has tolerated the medication, but remains symptomatic after 4 weeks at a minimally effective dosage, then a dose increase should be considered.

Efficacy of serotonin norepinephrine reuptake inhibitors

The efficacy of venlafaxine extended-release has been evaluated in two identical, randomized, double-blind, placebo-controlled trials using children and adolescents (Emslie et al., 2007a.) Patients received a flexible, weight-based dosage of venlafaxine extended-release (37.5–225 mg/day) or placebo for 8 weeks. Results from both trials were analyzed separately. In both studies, there were no statistically significant differences in response rates based on primary or secondary outcome measures. When the data from the two studies were pooled for post hoc age-subgroup analysis, children showed no differences between velafaxine extended-release and placebo on any outcome measure. In contrast, adolescents demonstrated a significant improvement on venlafaxine versus placebo on the primary outcome measure, change from baseline CDRS-R total score, and several secondary measures. The mean daily dose of venlafaxine was 80 mg/day for children and 109 mg/day for adolescents. On the basis of these RCTs, Bridge and colleagues (2007) reported that the NNT to benefit from venlafaxine extended-release was 10 (95% CI, 5 to 112).

Although several RCTs with adults have shown duloxetine to be effective in the treatment of major depressive disorder (Detke et al., 2002a, b, 2004; Goldstein et al., 2002, 2004), no published RCTs with children or adolescents have been preformed. Meighen (2007) has described the successful treatment of two adolescent females with chronic pain and comorbid major depressive disorder using duloxetine 40 mg/day.

Adverse effects of serotonin norepinephrine reuptake inhibitors

In short-term RCTs of venlafaxine extended-release (Emslie et al., 2007a), the most common treatment emergent adverse effects were abdominal pain (21%) and dizziness (12%). Suicide-related adverse events (e.g., suicidal ideation or behaviour) occurred in 6% of venlafaxine-treated patients and 0.5% of placebo-treated patients. Less frequent but serious adverse effects included hostility, manic switch, agitation, sleep disturbance, convulsion, and hallucinations. In a six month, open-label extension of the RCT of venlafaxine extend-release, 83 of 86 (97%) patients reported treatment emergent adverse events (Emslie et al., 2007b). The most common treatment-emergent adverse events were headache (53%), nausea (26%), infection (24%), abdominal pain (22%), and vomiting (21%). Small but statistically significant increases in blood pressure and heart rate were also reported. Two of 86 patients had clinically important electrocardiogram changes.

Unlike venflaxine extended-release, no large scale studies using duloxetine have been reported in adolescents. In adult RCTs of duloxetine (Perahia et al., 2006), the most common adverse effects include nausea (36%), headache (20%), dry mouth (18%), somnolence (14%), and insomnia (11%). In Meighen's case description of two adolescent females taking duloxetine (2007), the only adverse effect noted was constipation. A case of duloxetine-induced mania has also been reported in an adolescent with bipolar depression (Desarkar et al., 2007).

In summary, venflaxine extended-release has demonstrated some efficacy for the treatment of adolescent depression in RCTs; however, high rates of side effects in long-term use suggest that it should be used only after the failure of other treatment options. The use of duloxetine for the treatment of adolescent depression remains uncertain since it has not been adequately studied in this population.

Other antidepressants

Nefazodone

This antidepressant is both presynaptic serotonin reuptake inhibitor and postsynaptic serotonin receptor antagonist. The pharmacokinetic properties of nefazodone and its active metabolites (hyrdroxynefazadone, triazoledione, and meta-chlorphenylpiperazine) have been examined in children and adolescents (Findling et al., 2000). When compared to published data from adult studies, nefazodone and 2 of its active metabolites have shorter half-lives in children and adolescents. Findling and colleagues (2000) reported the steady-state half-life of nefazodone and metabolites at 100 mg twice daily is 3.9 h for nefazodone, 3.3 h for hydroxynefazodone, and 4.8 h for meta-chlorphenylpiperazine. On the basis of these findings, multiple daily dosing is needed when nefazodone is prescribed to adolescents.

The efficacy of nefazodone has been evaluated in one published (Emslie et al., 2002a) and one unpublished (US Food and Drug Administration Review and Evaluation of Clinical Data NDA 20-152 S-032, nefazadone paediatric supplement) RCT. Both studies were randomized, double blind, placebo-controlled, eight-week trials. In the published study, depressed adolescents received flexible dose nefazodone (100–600 mg/day in equally divided doses twice per day) or placebo. The primary outcome measure, change in CDRS-R score, did not significantly differ from placebo, but several secondary measures demonstrated significantly better response rates for nefazo-done treated patients. Using the response rate data from this trial, Bridge and colleagues (2007) calculated the NNT to benefit from nefazodone was 6 (95 % CI, 3 to 17). In the unpublished study, flexible dose nefazodone was given to children

(100–300 mg/day) and adolescents (200–600 mg/day). On the primary outcome measure, change in CDRS-R score, no difference was seen between nefazodone and placebo. Results of secondary measures or age subgroup analysis were not described. Thus, efficacy data from RCTs with nefazodone for the treatment of adolescent depression have been mixed.

Adverse effects of nefazodone are not well-described in either of the RCTs involving adolescents. The published study (Emsile et al., 2002a) indicated that nefazodone was well-tolerated and the rate of discontinuation for adverse events for nefazodone was equal to placebo (3%). The US Federal Drug Administration review of paediatric nefazodone trials (US Food and Drug Administration Review and Evaluation of Clinical Data NDA 20-152 S-032, nefazadone paediatric supplement) indicates that the safety profile for nefazodone in the paediatric population does not appear to be significantly different from that in adults. Common adverse events in adult studies include headache, somnolence, and nausea (Baldwin et al., 2001). In contrast to the RCTs of nefazodone with adolescents, most subjects in the pharmacokinetic study reported at least one adverse event (Findling et al., 2000). The most common side effects reported by adolescents were headache (46%), fatigue (30%), and sedation (15%). Serious adverse events include hepatotoxicity, orthostatic hypotension, seizure, manic switch, worsening depression, and suicidal ideation. Before starting nefazodone, baseline serum transaminase levels should be obtained and patients should receive education about the signs and symptoms of liver dysfunction as well as instructions to contact their physician if these occur.

In conclusion, nefazodone has demonstrated some efficacy for the treatment of adolescent depression; however, the risk of serious side effects suggest that it should be used only when close monitoring is possible and only after other treatments have failed.

Mirtazapine

This antidepressant is thought to exert its effect by blocking presynaptic noreadrenergic alpha2-autoreceptors which control norepinephrine release directly and alpha2-heteroreceptors which control serotonin release indirectly. Mirtazepine also blocks postsynaptic serotonin receptors. One pharmacokinetic study has examined the pharmacokinetics of mirtazepine in children and adolescents after a single 15 mg dose of mirtazepine (Findling et al., 2001). Results from this study indicate the half-life of mirtazapine varies from 17.8 to 48.4 h. Much of this variability maybe attributable to differences in weight as the half-life of mirtazapine significantly increased with increasing weight.

The efficacy of mirtazapine has been investigated in two unpublished, identical, randomized, double-blind, placebo-controlled trials using children and adolescents (US Food and Drug Administration NDA 20-415 SE5-011, mirtazapine paediatric supplement). Patients received flexible dose mirtazapine (15–45 mg/day) or placebo for 8 weeks. The results of each study were analyzed separately. In both trials, there were no statically significant differences in response rates based on primary or secondary outcome measures. Adverse effects from mirtazapine are not described for either study. In the first study, 6% of subjects treated with mirtazapine and 2% of subjects taking placebo discontinued study participation due to adverse events. In the second study, 5% of mirtazapine-treated subjects and 5% of placebo discontinued study participation because of adverse events.

In summary, mirtazapine has not demonstrated efficacy for adolescent depression in two unpublished, industry sponsored RCTs. Adverse effects from mirtazpine were not well-described in either of these trials. Results from RCTs do not support the use of mirtazapine for adolescent depression.

Buproprion

This antidepressant is both a norepinephrine and dopamine reuptake blocker. Bupropion is available in three different formulations: an immediate release, a sustained release, and an extended release. The pharmacokinetic properties of the sustained-release and extended-release formulations have been evaluated in children and adolescents under steady-state conditions (Daviss et al., 2005, 2006). Bupropion and its metabolites exhibit linear kinetics in the dose ranges (bupropion sustained-release 100–200 mg/day and bupropion extended-release 150–300 mg/day) studied. The half-life of the sustained-release formulation was significantly shorter in youth (12.1 h) when compared to adults (21 h). On the basis of these findings, Daviss and colleagues recommended twice daily dosing for bupropion in children and adolescents. When compared to the sustained-release formulation, the time to maximum concentration and the half-life (16.5 h) for extended-release formulation were prolonged. Thus, Daviss and colleagues confirmed that once daily dosing of buproprion extended-release was appropriate for children and adolescents.

Although several RCTs with adults have shown buproprion to be efficacious for major depressive disorder (Kavoussi et al., 1997; Coleman et al., 1999; Thase et al., 2006), RCTs with children or adolescents have not been performed. Two small open trials of youth with major depression (Glod et al., 2003) or comorbid attention deficit hyperactivity disorder (ADHD) and depression (Daviss et al., 2001) have shown sustained-release buproprion to be effective at reducing depressive symptoms. Both studies used flexible titration schedules with twice daily dosing. The mean dose of sustained-release buproprion was 362 mg/day in the open treatment trial of adolescent major depression (Glod et al., 2003) and mean final doses in the trial of comorbid ADHD and depression were 2.2 mg/kg in the morning and 1.7 mg/kg at 5 PM (Daviss et al., 2001). Both studies reported that sustained-release buproprion was well-tolerated. Adverse effects reported by either study include insomnia, weight loss, dry mouth, irritability, headaches, agitation, light-headedness, diarrhea, tremor, motor tics, or rash. No subjects in either study developed seizures.

In conclusion, open treatment trials have shown sustained-release buproprion to be effective for adolescent depression and generally well-tolerated. RCTs are needed to confirm these preliminary findings. Bupropion may be considered for the treatment of adolescent depression when patients have not responded to trials of other antidepressants.

Comorbid disorders

When treating adolescent depression, it is important to assess and treat comorbid conditions as these disorders may influence the degree of functional impairment, the course of illness, and the probability of achieving symptomatic remission (American Academy of Child and Adolescent Psychiatry, 2007; Birmaher et al., 2002; Curry et al., 2006; Hughes et al., 2007). Only a few studies have examined pharmacotherapy for major depression with comorbid disorders (Cornelius et al., 2001; Daviss et al., 2001). Usually clinicians prioritize the disorder that cause the greatest functional impairment or distress and begin treatment by focusing on that disorder. For a complete discussion of pharmacotherapy for adolescent depression with comorbid disorders, please see either: American Academy of Child and Adolescent Psychiatry, 2007 or Hughes et al., 2007.

Treatment-resistant depression

Treatment-resistant depression is defined as a lack of response to adequate treatment. Only one study has empirically evaluated the treatment of depressed adolescents who have not responded to adequate treatment with a SSRI, Treatment of SSRI-Resistant Depression in Adolescents (TORDIA; Brent et al., 2008). This study defined adequate treatment with medication as at least 8 weeks of antidepressant treatment including 4 weeks of a minimum therapeutic dose and a second 4 weeks at an increased dose (e.g., citalopram 40 mg/day, escitalopram 20 mg/day, fluoxetine 40 mg/day, paroxetine 40 mg/day, sertaline 150 mg/day). In TORDIA, subjects were randomized to treatment with a different SSRI, a different SSRI plus CBT, venlafaxine, or venlafaxine plus CBT. The combination of CBT plus either medication resulted in higher rates of response than medication alone. There was no difference in clinical response between switching to a different SSRI and venlafaxine. However, venlafaxine produced more side effects (e.g., minimal increase in diastolic blood pressure and pulse and more frequent skin problems, rash). Thus, the combination of CBT and switch to an alternative SSRI is as effective as CBT plus venlafaxine, and results in fewer adverse effects (Brent et al., 2008).

Consensus opinion recommends switching to another class of medication (e.g., venlafaxine, buproprion, mirtazapine, or duloxetine (Hughes et al., 2007)) if an adolescent does not to respond to two adequate trials of SSRIs. When a patient has achieved partial response to a SSRI, the clinician may consider increasing the dose, continuing the current dose for a longer duration, augmenting with another medication (e.g., lithium, thyroxine, buproprion, lamotrigine, or an atypical antipsychotic (Carpenter et al., 2002; Hughes, et al., 2007; Ryan et al., 1988; Strober et al., 1992; Trivedi et al., 2006)) or adding psychotherapy. These recommendations are based on results from studies of adult depression since similar studies have not been performed with adolescents (for review, see Hughes et al., 2007).

When a patient is considered a nonresponder to treatment with an SSRI, the clinician should document the lack of improvement and attempt to identify factors contributing to inadequate treatment response. Although these factors are often interrelated, they can be divided into four general categories: clinician, patient, environmental, and family. Clinician factors include misdiagnoses, overlooked comorbid disorders, inappropriate pharmacotherapy and/or psychotherapy, failure to recognize adverse effects leading to poor adherence, limited rapport with adolescent, and clinician unavailability. To identify possible misdiagnosis, the clinician should review all current medications to exclude the possibility of a substance-induced mood disorder, explore physical complaints indicative of an underlying medical illness that may be causing the depressive symptomatology, and assess for symptoms of hypomania or mania suggestive of bipolar disorder. As the symptoms of unipolar and bipolar depression are very similar, it can be complicated to determine whether a patient needs only an antidepressant or may benefit from concomitant use of a mood stabilizer. Patient factors include early age of illness onset, severity of depression, low motivation and negative cognitive style, poor compliance with treatment, comorbid disorders, and pharmacokinetic or pharmacodynamic variability. Environmental factors include negative stressors (e.g., bullying at school, sexual or physical abuse), lack of quality friendships and other supportive relationships, as well as cultural and racial issues. Lastly, family factors include limited parental cooperation in keeping appointments or following though with treatment recommendations, family psychopathology, and ongoing conflicts or violence. In conclusion, effective management of treatment-resistant depression requires the identification of contributing factors and implementation of appropriate education, psychotherapy, and pharmacotherapy.

Conclusions

Treatment of all youth with depression should include psychoeducation, supportive management, family, and school involvement. For adolescents with moderate depression, evidence suggests that specific forms of psychotherapy are equally as effective as antidepressants. For youth with severe depression, pharmacotherapy with or without psychotherapy is needed. The goal of treatment should always be complete remission of symptoms. Until further studies are available, current evidence from RCTs supports the use of fluoxetine as the first choice of antidepressants for adolescent depression. When choosing an alternative SSRI, data from RCTs suggest that sertaline, citalopram or escitalopram may also be effective. Spontaneous reports of suicidal ideation or behaviour are more common in adolescents treated with SSRIs than placebo. However, given the greater number of patients who benefit from SSRIs than who experience serious adverse effects, the risk-benefit ratio for SSRI use in adolescent depression appears favourable with appropriate monitoring. When adolescents do not respond to SSRIs or are unable to tolerate them, clinicians should consider other medications including venlafaxine, buproprion, mirtazapine, nefazadone, or duloxetine together with psychotherapy.

Acknowledgement

Dr. Sakolsky was supported by T32 MH18951 from the National Institute of Mental Health. The content of this chapter is solely the responsibility of the authors and does not necessarily represent the official views of the National Institute of Mental Health or the National Institutes of Health.

References

Alderman, J., Wolkow, R., Chung, M., & Johnston, H.F. (1998). Sertraline treatment of children and adolescents with obsessive-compulsive disorder or depression: pharmacokinetics, tolerability, and efficacy. *Journal of the American Academy of Child and Adolescent Psychiatry, 37*, 386–394.

American Academy of Child and Adolescent Psychiatry (2007). Practice parameter for the assessment and treatment of children and adolescents with depressive disorders. *Journal of the American Academy of Child and Adolescent Psychiatry, 46(11)*, 1503–1526.

Axelson, D.A., Perel, J.M., Birmaher, B., Rudolph, G.R., Nuss, S., Bridge, J., et al. (2002). Sertraline pharmacokinetics and dynamics in adolescents. *Journal of the American Academy of Child and Adolescent Psychiatry, 41(9)*, 1037–1044.

Baldwin, D.S., Hawley, C.J., Mellors, K., & CN104-070 Study Group. (2001). A randomized, double-blind controlled comparison of nefazodone and paroxetine in the treatment of depression: Safety, tolerability and efficacy in continuation phase treatment. *Journal of Psychopharmacology, 15(3)*, 161–5.

Berard, R., Fong, R., Carpenter, D.J., Thomason, C., & Wilkinson, C. (2006). An international, multicenter, placebo-controlled trial of paroxetine in adolescents with major depressive disorder. *Journal of Child and Adolescent Psychopharmacology, 16(1–2)*, 59–75.

Birmaher, B., Arbelaez, C., & Brent, D. (2002). Course and outcome of child and adolescent major depressive disorder. *Child and Adolescent Psychiatry Clinics of North America, 11(3)*, 619–637.

Birmaher, B., Ryan, N.D., Williamson, D.E., Brent, D.A., Kaufman, J., Dahl, R.E., et al. (1996). Childhood and adolescent depression: A review of the past ten years. Part I. *Journal of American Academy of Child and Adolescent Psychiatry, 35(11)*, 1427–1439.

Boyer, E.W. & Shannon, M. (2005). The serotonin syndrome. *New England Journal of Medicine, 352*, 1112–1120.

Brent, D., Emslie, G., Clarke, G., Wagner, K.D., Asarnow, J., Keller, M.K., et al. (2008). Switching to venlafaxine or another SSRI with or without cognitive behavioral therapy for adolescents with SSRI-resistant depression: The TORIDA randomized control trial. *Journal of the American Medical Association, 299(8)*, 901–913.

Bridge, J.A., Iyengar, S., Salary, C.B., Barbe, R.P., Birmaher, B., & Pincus H.A. (2007). Clinical response and risk for reported suicidal ideation and suicide attempts in pediatric antidepressant treatment: A meta-analysis of randomized controlled trials. *Journal of the American Medical Association, 297*, 1683–1696.

Carpenter, L.L., Yasmin, S., & Price, L.H. (2002). A double-blind, placebo-controlled study of antidepressant augmentation with mirtazapine. *Biological Psychiatry, 51(2)*, 183–188.

Cheung, A.H., Emslie, G.J., & Mayes, T.L. (2005). Review of the efficacy and safety of antidepressants in youth depression. *Journal of Child Psychology and Psychiatry, 46(7)*, 735–754.

Cheung, A.H., Emslie, G.J., & Mayes, T.L. (2006). The use of antidepressants to treat depression in children and adolescents. *Canadian Medical Association Journal, 174(2)*, 193–200.

Coleman, C.C., Cunningham, L.A., Foster, V.J., Batey, S.R., Donahue, R.M., Houser, T.L. et al. (1999). Sexual dysfunction associated with the treatment of depression: a placebo-controlled comparison of bupropion sustained release and sertraline treatment. *Annals of Clinical Psychiatry, 11(4)*, 205–215.

Cornelius, J.R., Bukstein, O.G., Birmaher, B., Salloum, I.M., Lynch, K., Pollock, N.K., et al. (2001). Fluoxetine in adolescents with major depression and an alcohol use disorder: an open-label trial. *Addictive Behaviors, 26(5)*, 735–739.

Curry, J., Rohde, P., Simons, A., Silva, S., Vitiello, B., Kratochvil, C., et al. (2006). Predictors and moderators of acute outcome in the Treatment for Adolescents with Depression Study (TADS). *Journal of the American Academy of Child and Adolescent Psychiatry, 45(12)*, 1427–1439.

Daviss, W.B., Bentivoglio, P., Racusin, R., Brown, K.M., Bostic, J.Q., & Wiley, L. (2001). Bupropion sustained release in adolescents with comorbid attention-deficit/hyperactivity disorder and depression. *Journal of the American Academy of Child and Adolescent Psychiatry, 40(3)*, 307–314.

Daviss, W.B., Perel, J.M., Birmaher, B., Rudolph, G.R., Melhem, I., Axelson, D.A., et al. (2006). Steady-state clinical pharmacokinetics of bupropion extended-release in youths. *Journal of the American Academy of Child and Adolescent Psychiatry, 45(12)*, 1503–1509.

Daviss, W.B., Perel, J.M., Rudolph, G.R., Axelson, D.A., Gilchrist, R., Nuss, S., et al. (2005). Steady-state pharmacokinetics of bupropion SR in juvenile patients. *Journal of the American Academy of Child and Adolescent Psychiatry, 44(4)*, 349–357.

Desarkar, P., Bakhla, A., & Sinha, V.K. (2007). Duloxetine-induced ultrarapid cycling in an adolescent with bipolar depression. *Journal of Clinical Psychopharmacology, 27(1)*, 115–116.

Detke, M.J., Lu, Y., Goldstein, D.J., Hayes, J.R., & Demitrack, M.A. (2002a). Duloxetine, 60 mg once daily, for major depressive disorder: a randomized double-blind placebo-controlled trial. *Journal of Clinical Psychiatry, 63(4)*, 308–315.

Detke, M.J., Lu Y., Goldstein, D.J., McNamara, R.K., & Demitrack, M.A. (2002b). Duloxetine 60 mg once daily dosing versus placebo in the acute treatment of major depression. *Journal of Psychiatric Research, 36(6)*, 383–390.

Detke, M.J., Wiltse, C.G., Mallinckrodt, C.H., McNamara, R.K., Demitrack, M.A., & Bitter, I. (2004). Duloxetine in the acute and long-term treatment of major depressive disorder: a placebo- and paroxetine-controlled trial. *European Neuropsychopharmacology, 14(6)*, 457–470.

Emslie, G.J., Fingling, R.L., Rynn, M.A., & Marcus, R.N. (2002a). Efficacy and safety of nefazodone in the treatment of adolescents with major depressive disorder [Abstract]. *Journal of Child and Adolescent Psychopharmacology, 12(4)*, 299.

Emslie, G.J., Findling, R.L., Yeung, P.P., Kunz, N.R., & Li, Y. (2007a). Venlafaxine ER for the treatment of pediatric subjects with depression: results of two placebo-controlled trials. *Journal of the American Academy of Child and Adolescent Psychiatry, 46(4)*, 479–488.

Emslie, G.J., Heiligenstein, J.H., Hoog, S.L., Wagner, K.D., Findling, R.L., McCracken, J.T., et al. (2004). Fluoxetine treatment for prevention of relapse of depression in children and adolescents: a double-blind, placebo-controlled study. *Journal of the American Academy of Child and Adolescent Psychiatry, 43(11)*, 1397–1405.

Emslie, G.J., Heiligenstein, J.H., Wagner, K.D., Hoog, S.L., Ernest, D.E., Brown, E., et al. (2002b). Fluoxetine for acute treatment of depression in children and adolescents: a placebo-controlled, randomized clinical trial. *Journal of the American Academy of Child and Adolescent Psychiatry, 41(10)*, 1205–1215.

Emslie, G., Kratochvil, C., Vitiello, B., Silva, S., Mayes, T., McNulty, S., et al. (2006a). Treatment for Adolescents with Depression Study (TADS): Safety results. *Journal of the American Academy of Child and Adolescent Psychiatry, 45(12)*, 1440–1455.

Emslie, G.J., Rush, A.J., Weinberg, W.A., Kowatch, R.A., Hughes, C.W., Carmody, T., et al. (1997). A double-blind, randomized, placebo-controlled trial of fluoxetine in children and adolescents with depression. *Archives of General Psychiatry, 54*, 1031–1037.

Emslie, G.J., Wagner, K.D., Kutcher, S., Krulewicz,S., Fong, R., Carpenter, D.J., et al. (2006b). Paroxetine treatment in children and adolescents with major depressive disorder: a randomized, multicenter, double-blind, placebo-controlled trial. *Journal of the American Academy of Child and Adolescent Psychiatry, 45(6)*, 709–719.

Emslie, G.J., Yeung, P.P., & Kunz, N. R. (2007b). Long-term, open-label venlafaxine extended-release treatment in children and adolescents. *CNS Spectrums, 12(3)*, 223–233.

Findling, R.L., McNamara, N.K., Stansbrey, R.J., Feeny, N.C., Young, C.M., Peric, F.V., et al. (2006a). The relevance of pharmacokinetic studies in designing efficacy trials in juvenile major depression. *Journal of Child and Adolescent Psychopharmacology,16(1–2)*, 131–145.

Findling, R.L., Nucci, G., Piergies, A.A., Gomeni, R., Bartolic, E.I., Fong, R., et al. (2006b). Multiple dose pharmacokinetics of paroxetine in children and adolescents with major depressive disorder or obsessive-compulsive disorder. *Neuropsychopharmacology, 31(6)*, 1274–1285.

Findling, R.L., Preskorn, S.H., Marcus, R.N., Magnus, R.D., D'Amico, F., Marathe, P., et al. (2000). Nefazodone pharmacokinetics in depressed children and adolescents. *Journal of the American Academy of Child and Adolescent Psychiatry, 39(8)*, 1008–1016.

Findling, R.L., Reed, M.D., Blumer, J.L., Boyle, K.R., & van den Heuvel, M.W. (2001). Mirtazapine pharmacokinetics in depressed children and adolescents [Abstract]. Annual Meeting of the American Academy of Child and Adolescent Psychiatry.

Findling, R.L., Reed, M.D., Myers, C., O'Riordan, M.A., Fiala, S., Branicky, L., et al. (1999). Paroxetine pharmacokinetics in depressed children and adolescents. *Journal of the American Academy of Child and Adolescent Psychiatry, 38(8)*, 952–959.

Gibbons, R.D., Brown, C.H., Hur, K., Marcus, S.M., Bhaumik, D.K., & Erkens, J.A. (2007). Early evidence on the effects of regulators' suicidality warnings on SSRI prescriptions and suicide in children and adolescents. *American Journal of Psychiatry, 164(9)*, 1356–1363.

Gibbons, R.D., Hur, K., Bhaumik, D.K., & Mann, J.J. (2005). The relationship between antidepressant medication use and rate of suicide. *Archives of General Psychiatry, 62*, 165–172.

Gibbons, R.D., Hur, K., Bhaumik, D.K., & Mann, J.J. (2006). The relationship between antidepressant prescription rates and rate of early adolescent suicide. *American Journal of Psychiatry, 163*, 1898–1904.

Glod, C.A., Lynch, A., Flynn, E., Berkowitz, C., & Baldessarini, R.J. (2003). Open trial of bupropion SR in adolescent major depression. *Journal of Child and Adolescent Psychiatric Nursing, 16(3)*, 123–130.

Goodyer, I., Dubicka, B., Wilkinson, P., Kelvin, R., Roberts, C., Byford, S., et al. (2007). Selective serotonin reuptake inhibitors (SSRIs) and routine specialist care with and without cognitive behaviour therapy in adolescents with major depression: Randomised controlled trial. *British Medical Journal, 335(7611)*, 142–150.

Goldstein, D.J., Lu, Y., Detke, M.J., Wiltse, C., Mallinckrodt, C., & Demitrack, M.A. (2004). Duloxetine in the treatment of depression: A double-blind placebo-controlled comparison with paroxetine. *Journal of Clinical Psychopharmacology, 24(4)*, 389–99.

Goldstein, D.J., Mallinckrodt, C., Lu, Y., & Demitrack, M.A. (2002). Duloxetine in the treatment of major depressive disorder: A double-blind clinical trial. *Journal of Clinical Psychiatry, 63(3)*, 225–231.

Hammad, T.A., Laughren, T., & Racoosin, J. (2006). Suicidality in pediatric patients treated with antidepressant drugs. *Archives of General Psychiatry, 63*, 332–339.

Hazell, P., O'Connell, D., Heathcote, D., & Henry, D. (2002). Tricyclic drugs for depression in children and adolescents. *Cochrane Database of Systematic Reviews, 2*, CD002317.

Heiligenstein, J.H., Hoog, S.L., Wagner, K.D., Findling, R.L., Galil, N., Kaplan, S., et al. (2006). Fluoxetine 40–60 mg versus fluoxetine 20 mg in the treatment of children and adolescents with a less-than-complete response to nine-week treatment with fluoxetine 10–20 mg: A pilot study. *Journal of Child and Adolescent Psychopharmacology, 16(1–2)*, 207–217.

Hughes, C.W., Emslie, G.J., Crismon, M.L., Posner, K., Birmaher, B., Ryan, N., et al. (2007). Texas Consensus Conference Panel on Medication Treatment of Childhood Major Depressive Disorder. Texas Children's Medication Algorithm Project: update from Texas Consensus Conference Panel on Medication Treatment of Childhood Major Depressive Disorder. *Journal of the American Academy of Child and Adolescent Psychiatry, 46(6)*, 667–686.

Hyttell, J., Bogeso, K.P., Perregaard, J., & Sanchez, C. (1992). The pharmacological effect of citalopram resides in the (S)-(+)-enantiomer. *Journal of Neural Transmission General Section, 88*, 157–160.

Keller, M.B., Ryan, N.D., Strober, M., Klein, R.G., Kutcher, S.P., Birmaher, B., et al. (2001). Efficacy of paroxetine in the treatment of adolescent major depression: A randomized, controlled trial. *Journal of the American Academy of Child and Adolescent Psychiatry, 40(7)*, 762–772.

Kavoussi, R.J., Segraves, R.T., Hughes, A.R., Ascher, J.A., & Johnston, J.A. (1997). Double-blind comparison of bupropion sustained release and sertraline in depressed out-patients. *Journal of Clinical Psychiatry, 58(12)*, 532–537.

Klamerus, K.J., Maloney, K., Rudolph, R.L., Sisenwine, S.F., Jusko, W.J., & Chiang, S.T. (1992). Introduction of a composite parameter to the pharmacokinetics of venlafaxine and its active O-desmethyl metabolite. *Journal of Clinical Pharmacology, 32*, 716–724.

Lake, M.B., Birmaher, B., Wassick, S., Mathos, K., & Yelovich, A.K. (2000). Bleeding and selective serotonin reuptake inhibitors in childhood and adolescence. *Journal of Child and Adolescent Psychopharmacology, 10*, 35–38.

Lewinsohn, P.M., Rohde, P., & Seeley, J.R. (1998). Major depressive disorder in older adolescents: prevalence, risk factors, and clinical implications. *Clinical Psychology Review, 18*, 765–794.

Lewinsohn, P.M., Rohde, P., Seeley, J.R., Klein, D.N., & Gotlib, I.H. (2003). Psychosocial functioning of young adults who have experienced and recovered from major depressive disorder during adolescence. *Journal of Abnormal Psychology, 112*, 353–363.

Meighen, K.G. (2007). Duloxetine treatment of pediatric chronic pain and co-morbid major depressive disorder. *Journal of Child and Adolescent Psychopharmacology, 17(1)*, 121–127.

National Institute for Health and Clinical Excellence. (2005). *Depression in children and young people identification and management in primary, community and secondary care, National clinical practice guideline number 28.* Available at *http://www.nice.org.uk/CG028.*

Olfson, M., Shaffer, D., Marcus, S.C., & Greenberg, T. (2003). Relationship between antidepressant medication treatment and suicide in adolescents. *Archives of General Psychiatry, 60*, 978–982.

Perel, J.M., Axelson, D.A., Rudolph, G., & Birmaher, B. (2001). Stereoselective pharmacokinetic/pharmacodynamic (PK/PD) of ± citalopram in adolescents, comparisons with adult findings [Abstract]. *Clinical Pharmacology and Therapeutics, 69*, 30.

Patat, A., Troy, S., Burke, J., Trocherie, S., Danjou, P., LeCoz, F., et al. (1998). Absolute bioavailability and electroencephalographic effects of conventional and extended-release formulations of venlafaxine in healthy subjects. *Journal of Clinical Pharmacology, 38*, 256–267.

Perahia, D.G., Gilaberte, I., Wang, F., Wiltse, C.G., Huckins, S.A., Clemens, J.W., et al. (2006). Duloxetine in the prevention of relapse of major depressive disorder: Double-blind placebo-controlled study. *British Journal of Psychiatry, 188*, 346–353.

Pritchett, Y.L., Marciniak, M.D., Corey-Lisle, P.K., Berzon, R.A., Desaiah, D., & Detke, M.J. (2007). Use of effect size to determine optimal dose of duloxetine in major depressive disorder. *Journal of Psychiatric Research, 41(3–4)*, 311–318.

Ryan, N.D., Meyer, V., Dachille, S., Mazzie, D., & Puig-Antich, J. (1988). Lithium antidepressant augmentation in TCA-refractory depression in adolescents. *Journal of the American Academy of Child and Adolescent Psychiatry, 27(3)*, 371–376.

Safer, D.J. & Zito, JM (2006). Treatment-emergent adverse events from selective serotonin reuptake inhibitors by age group: Children versus adolescents. *Journal of Child and Adolescent Psychopharmacology, 16*, 159–169.

Sharma, A., Goldberg, M.J., & Cerimele, B.J. (2000). Pharmacokinetics and safety of duloxetine, a dual-serotonin and norepinephrine reuptake inhibitor. *Journal of Clinical Pharmacology, 40*, 161–167.

Strober, M., Freeman, R., Rigali, J., Schmidt, S., & Diamond, R. (1992). The pharmacotherapy of depressive illness in adolescence: II. Effects of lithium augmentation in nonresponders to imipramine. *Journal of the American Academy of Child and Adolescent Psychiatry, 31(1)*, 16–20.

Thase, M.E., Clayton, A.H., Haight, B.R., Thompson, A.H., Modell, J.G., & Johnston, J.A., (2006). A double-blind comparison between bupropion XL and venlafaxine XR: sexual functioning, antidepressant efficacy, and tolerability. *Journal of Clinical Psychopharmacology, 26(5)*, 482–488.

Treatment of Adolescent Depression Study (TADS) Team (2004). Fluoxetine, cognitive-behavioral therapy, and their combination for adolescents with depression: Treatment for Adolescents with Depression Study (TADS) randomized controlled trial. *Journal of the American Medical Association, 292*, 807–820.

Troy, S., Parker, V.P., Fruncillo, R.J., & Chiang, S.T. (1995). The pharmacokinetics of venlafaxine given in twice-daily regimen. *Journal of Clinical Pharmacology, 35*, 404–409.

Trivedi, M.H., Fava, M., Wisniewski, S.R., Thase, M.E., Quitkin, F., Warden, D., et al. (2006). STAR*D Study Team. Medication augmentation after the failure of SSRIs for depression. *New England Journal of Medicine, 354(12)*, 1243–1252.

US Food and Drug Administration, NDA 20-415 SE5-011, mirtazapine pediatric supplement (2004). http://www.fda.gov/CDER/foi/esum/2004/20415SE5_011_Mirtazapine%20O%20ReviewFIN.pdf. Accessibility verified January 29, 2008.

US Food and Drug Administration, Review and Evaluation of Clinical Data ND 20-152 S-032, nefazadone pediatric supplement (2004). http://www.fda.gov/cder/foi/esum/2004/20152s032_Serzone_clinical_BPCA_FIN.pdf. Accessibility verified January 29, 2008.

Valuck, R.J., Libby, A.M., Sills, M.R., Giese, A.A., & Allen, R.R. (2004). Antidepressant treatment and risk of suicide attempt by adolescents with major depressive disorder: a propensity-adjusted retrospective cohort study. *CNS Drugs, 18*, 1119–1132.

von Knorring, A.L., Olsson, G.I., Thomsen, P.H., Lemming, O.M., & Hulten, A. (2006). A randomized, double-blind, placebo-controlled study of citalopram in adolescents with major depressive disorder. *Journal of Clinical Psychopharmacology, 26(3)*, 311–315.

Wagner, K.D., Ambrosini, P., Rynn, M., Wohlberg, C., Yang, R., Greenbaum, M.S., et al. (2003). Efficacy of sertraline in the treatment of children and adolescents with major depressive disorder two randomized controlled trials. *Journal of the American Medical Association, 290*, 1033–1041.

Wagner, K.D., Jonas, J., Findling, R.L., Ventura, D., & Saikali, K. (2006). A double-blind, randomized, placebo-controlled trial of escitalopram in the treatment of pediatric depression. *Journal of the American Academy of Child and Adolescent Psychiatry, 45(3)*, 280–288.

Wagner, K.D., Robb, A.S., Findling, R.L., Jin, J., Gutierrez, M.M., & Heydorn, W.E. (2004). A randomized, placebo-controlled trial of citalopram for the treatment of major depression in children and adolescents. *American Journal of Psychiatry, 161(6)*, 1079–83.

Weinrieb, R.M., Auriacombe, M., Lynch, K.G., & Lewis, J.D. (2005). Selective serotonin re-uptake inhibitors and the risk of bleeding. *Expert Opinion on Drug Safety, 4*, 337–344.

Wilens, T.E., Cohen, L., Biederman, J., Abrams, A., Neft, D., Faird, N., et al. (2002). Fluoxetine pharmacokinetics in pediatric patients. *Journal of Clinical Psychopharmacology, 22(6)*, 568–575.

Chapter 11

Interpersonal psychotherapy for adolescents

Jami F. Young & Laura Mufson

Interpersonal psychotherapy (IPT) is a brief outpatient treatment that was developed for the treatment of depressed, nonbipolar, nonpsychotic adults (Weissman et al., 2000). IPT is based on the premise that depression occurs in the context of one's relationships. Regardless of the aetiology, depression affects our relationships and our relationships affect our mood. As such, IPT views the patient's depressive symptoms and the interpersonal context in which these symptoms occur as targets for intervention that will lead to recovery. IPT is informed by interpersonal theorists such as Sullivan (1953) and Meyer (1957) who believed that interpersonal interactions form the basis of personality and that good relationships are the foundation for good mental health. Sullivan (1953) argued that psychiatric problems develop from and are perpetuated by poor communication with others and therefore treatment needs to address the individual's interpersonal interactions, as well as his behaviours and symptoms. Similarly, Meyer (1957) believed that one needed to understand the individual's current interpersonal experiences to understand his psychiatric illness.

There is a building literature to support an interpersonal framework for the conceptualization and treatment of depression (Hammen, 1999; Joiner et al., 1999). In both community and clinical samples, depression is associated with significant interpersonal problems in people of all ages (e.g., Lewinsohn et al., 1994; Puig-Antich et al., 1993; Sheeber et al., 1997; Stader & Hokanson, 1998). Interpersonal events or experiences often precipitate the onset of depression (Hammen, 1999) and once someone is depressed he engages with others in ways that can lead to a loss of or difficulty in relationships. These relationship difficulties further exacerbate the depression (Coyne, 1976; Weissman & Paykel, 1974). These research findings highlight the importance of focusing on interpersonal events and interpersonal skills when treating depression. This is supported by a large number of studies that have demonstrated the efficacy of IPT with depressed adults (e.g., Elkin et al., 1989; Frank et al., 1991; Sloane et al., 1985; Weissman et al., 1979).

According to IPT, depression is composed of three elements: symptom formation, social functioning, and personality. Given its brief treatment duration, IPT focuses on symptom formation and social functioning with the central goal being an improvement in both depressive symptoms and interpersonal functioning. Intervening and altering personality is believed to take longer than a 3–4 month intervention. To improve symptoms and relationships, the therapist and patient identify a specific interpersonal problem for the treatment focus (one of four interpersonal problem areas), discuss relevant communication and problem-solving techniques, practice these skills in session, and then have the patient apply these techniques in interactions occurring outside of session in the context of his relationships.

On the basis of the success of IPT with adults, the similarities between depressive symptoms in adults and adolescents (Ryan et al., 1987), and the interpersonal literature discussed above, IPT was adapted for the treatment of depressed adolescents by Mufson and colleagues. Interpersonal psychotherapy for depressed adolescents (IPT-A) was initially outlined in a book (Mufson et al., 1993), which has been subsequently revised (Mufson et al., 2004a). An adolescent version of IPT seemed particularly relevant given adolescents' focus on interpersonal relationships and the developmental changes that occur in relationships during adolescence, such as separation from parents and the increasing importance of peer and romantic relationships. IPT-A helps adolescents increase their independence while negotiating their interdependence on others.

Therapeutic goals and methods

IPT-A identifies and targets interpersonal problems that are causing or contributing to the adolescent's depression. Because IPT posits that improving the interpersonal context will lead to an improvement in depressive symptoms, both the assessment and intervention phases focus on the individual's interpersonal interactions and how these interactions are affecting the adolescent's mood and other depressive symptoms. As is true with adult IPT, adolescents' interpersonal problems generally fall into one of four categories: grief, inter-personal disputes, role transitions, and interpersonal deficits. During treatment, the therapist identifies the appropriate interpersonal problem area and helps the adolescent become aware of and alter his maladaptive interpersonal patterns (Kiesler, 1991). By addressing the interpersonal problem, the adolescent is likely to get more positive feed-back from significant others, thereby breaking the negative interpersonal cycle often seen in depressed individuals (e.g., Coyne, 1976; Weissman & Paykel, 1974). As a result, the adolescent develops a sense of agency in relationships and begins to feel better.

A number of alterations have been made to the IPT manual to increase the model's appropriateness for the treatment of adolescent depression. First, a parent component has been added to the treatment protocol. Although IPT-A is an individual treatment, some degree of involvement on the part of the parent or guardian is recommended. The frequency and timing of parent sessions will be discussed in more detail in the ensuing sections outlining specific phases of the treatment. Second, the techniques used to decrease depressive symptoms and improve interpersonal functioning have been geared toward adolescents. Techniques employed specifically with adolescents include using a 1–10 mood rating scale to monitor improvement, doing more basic social skills work, increasing perspective-taking skills to counteract adolescent black and white thinking, and learning how to negotiate parent–child tensions. Finally, strategies were developed for dealing with specific issues that may arise in the course of treating adolescents, including school refusal, abuse, and suicidality.

IPT-A may be viewed as consisting of three main components: psychoeducation, affective training, and interpersonal skills training. The psychoeducational aspect of IPT-A is manifest in all three phases of treatment. In the initial phase, it is the primary task of the first two sessions in which the therapist educates the adolescent and parent about the nature of depression, treatment options, the notion of the limited sick role, and the adolescent's and parent's roles in the treatment. It also is a part of the remaining sessions in the therapist's education of the patient and sometimes other significant people about helpful communication and problem-solving techniques. The second major component of the treatment is its focus on affect. The therapist will assist the adolescent to more accurately identify his feelings as well as the interpersonal events that trigger these feelings. A significant task is to help the adolescent clarify these feelings so that communication can occur more effectively, which will improve mood. Finally, the third component is that of interpersonal skills training. The therapist devotes the middle phase of treatment to helping the adolescent develop new communication strategies and problem-solving skills to improve his relationships. To assist in this training, the therapist engages with the adolescent using communication analysis, decision analysis, role-playing, and interpersonal experiments to be tried outside of the therapy sessions. These techniques will be further described in the session-by-session outline.

As stated above, each individual is conceptualized as having a primary and possibly secondary interpersonal problem area: grief, interpersonal disputes, role transitions, and interpersonal deficits. In the sections that follow, we briefly discuss each problem area. A more detailed discussion of each problem area can be found in the IPT-A manual (Mufson et al., 2004a).

Grief: Many adolescents who experience the death of a loved one report some depressive symptoms including dysphoria, anhedonia, sleep difficulties, and appetite disturbance. IPT-A is appropriate when the adolescent's grief is prolonged and results in significant depressive symptoms and impairment in functioning. It is particularly useful for those adolescents who have experienced a significant disruption in their support network as a result of the death or who had a conflictual relationship with the deceased, two situations that are associated with more complicated bereavement (Clark et al., 1994). IPT-A helps the adolescent mourn the loss of a loved one, while developing and strengthening other relationships that can provide support to the adolescent.

Interpersonal disputes: A dispute involving interpersonal roles exists when two or more people have nonreciprocal expectations about the relationship (Klerman et al., 1984). Adolescents frequently have disputes with their parents or guardians about sexuality, authority, money, and the adolescent's increasing independence. Although disputes between adolescents and parents are often the focus of treatment, adolescents may also present with disputes with peers or other people in their lives that can be addressed in treatment. Individual disputes do not necessarily lead to adolescent depression. However, when these disputes become chronic and unmanageable to the point where they are significantly impairing the relationship, they may act as a trigger for depression. Once an adolescent is depressed, he may become more irritable or have other symptoms that make it even more difficult to manage interpersonal conflict. In such cases, the dispute may exacerbate the adolescent's depression. The goal of treatment is to help resolve the dispute if possible, and if not, to help the adolescent develop strategies to better cope with the limitations or stresses inherent in the relationship.

Role transitions: Role transitions are changes that occur in a person's life that cause him to take on a new social role. Role transitions may occur developmentally at different stages in adolescence, such as the transition to high school. There are also non-normative or unexpected role transitions such as the divorce of parents or moving to a new city. Certain adolescents may have a difficult time meeting the demands of the new role, resulting in depression and impaired interpersonal functioning. Transitions are especially difficult when they occur too rapidly, are experienced as a loss by the individual, are associated with unwanted or unexpected secondary changes, or are met by inflexibility on the part of the adolescent or significant others in his life. Treatment is focused on helping the adolescent mourn the loss of the old role and develop the skills needed to manage the new role more successfully. A specific subset of role transitions that can trigger depression are those changes associated with changes in family structure due to divorce, remarriage, or a change in parenting in the adolescent's life. Oftentimes, these transitions result in some conflict with the new parenting situation. To help the adolescent negotiate this type of transition, the adolescent must mourn the loss of the old role, while learning to communicate more effectively and to negotiate new relationships within the changed familial structure. As such, the therapeutic work is a combination of strategies focused on role transitions and role disputes.

Interpersonal deficits: This is the identified problem area when an adolescent lacks the social skills needed to have positive relationships with family members and friends. Adolescents with this problem area often experience loneliness and low self-worth, which can lead to or exacerbate feelings of depression. The depression can result in further social withdrawal and isolation, leading to further deficits in interpersonal skills. IPT-A is best suited to adolescents who have a history of satisfactory relationships in the past and whose interpersonal deficits are less pervasive or are a consequence of the depression. The goal of treatment is to help the adolescent develop the skills needed to have more satisfying interpersonal relationships.

Session-by-session delivery of the program

IPT-A is a time-limited treatment. It is designed as a once weekly, 12-session treatment. Treatment can be extended to 16 sessions if it is clinically indicated, but typically should not be extended beyond this point to maintain its time-limited structure. If the treatment is going to be longer than 12 weeks, it is important to determine this before initiating the middle phase of treatment. This helps maintain the structured nature of the treatment and gives the adolescent a clear sense of when treatment will end. If needed, IPT-A can be delivered more flexibly than once weekly treatment, such as in the school effectiveness study conducted by Mufson and colleagues (Mufson et al., 2004b). To address the demands of the school environment, the first 8 sessions were delivered over 8 consecutive weeks and the remaining 4 sessions were more flexible, depending on the individual student's need or school schedule, and were conducted over an additional 8-week time period.

IPT-A is divided into three phases: (1) the initial phase, (2) the middle phase, and (3) the termination phase. At the beginning of each session, regardless of the phase of treatment, the clinician assesses the adolescent's depressive symptoms, noting any changes that occurred over the course of the week and linking changes in symptoms to interpersonal events. Following the review of symptoms, the session progresses to the tasks particular to that phase of treatment, for instance conducting the interpersonal inventory, role-playing an interpersonal interaction, or discussing the adolescent's warning signs of depression. This structure helps focus the treatment on issues related to the identified interpersonal problem.

Throughout treatment, both the therapist and adolescent play an active role in the sessions. The therapist assesses depressive symptoms, inquires about interpersonal relationships, links depression symptoms to interpersonal functioning, and guides the work on the interpersonal problem area. The adolescent is expected to discuss his interpersonal relationships, work to find solutions to the interpersonal problem, and practice new interpersonal techniques both in session and at home. The important element is that the therapist and patient are working collaboratively to identify interpersonal difficulties as well as the strategies that might be helpful for improving their targeted interpersonal problem.

Initial phase of treatment

The initial phase of treatment does not begin until after the completion of a psychosocial and psychiatric evaluation, which rules out any possible medical conditions that could be contributing to the adolescent's symptoms of depression. Therefore, when treatment is initiated, the therapist already has some developmental and family history as well as information about the onset of the depression symptoms and psychosocial stressors. The initial phase of treatment consists of sessions 1 through 4. The main goals of the initial phase are to educate the adolescent and parent about depression and IPT, to assign the patient the limited sick role, and to conduct a detailed inventory of the adolescent's relationships to determine the focus of treatment.

Session 1: The first session in IPT-A ideally involves both the adolescent and his parents, although it is not uncommon to only have the adolescent present. The session typically begins with the adolescent alone to conduct a comprehensive review of his depression symptoms. Although patients have already had a complete diagnostic assessment, it is important for the clinician to review the adolescent's depression symptoms in the first session to establish a baseline. The clinician should assess the patient's current depressive symptoms, history of depressive symptoms, as well as other symptoms, such as mania, substance abuse, or suicidality, which might make IPT-A an inappropriate treatment. In research projects, a tool such as the Hamilton Depression Rating Scale is used to conduct this symptom review but any comprehensive assessment of symptoms will suffice. The checklists ensure that the clinician does not skip particular depression symptoms in the review based on the adolescent's presentation that may not accurately reflect his level of depression. Subsequent IPT-A sessions begin with a briefer review of the adolescent's depression symptoms over the past week, including any suicidal thoughts or behaviours.

After reviewing the depression symptoms and confirming a depression diagnosis, the therapist invites the parents into the session to join the adolescent. The therapist provides the family with education about the symptoms of depression, rates of depression in adolescents, the medical model of depression, and various treatment options. This education is important for several reasons. First, informing the adolescent and parents that depression is a common illness normalizes the adolescent's and family's experience. Second, this discussion familiarizes the family with the symptoms of depression and provides a potential explanation for seemingly unconnected behaviours. Parents often come in complaining about their adolescent's recent behaviour without realizing that much of this behaviour can be attributed to the irritability associated with depression. Similarly, they may not know that depression impairs concentration and that this impaired concentration may be the explanation for recent academic difficulties. Third, informing families that depression is a medical illness that can be treated decreases the stigma associated with depression, takes the blame off the individual for causing the depression, and provides hope that the adolescent will improve. Lastly, by outlining the different treatment options, it gives the family hope that there are different approaches to treating depression and that these other treatments will be considered if IPT is not helpful.

In IPT-A, an important part of psychoeducation is assigning the adolescent the limited sick role. This involves discussing with the adolescent and his parents that similar to someone with a medical illness, an adolescent with symptoms of depression may not be able to do things as well as before the depression. However, despite it being more difficult to do certain things such as concentrate in school or play on sports teams, it is important for the patient to do as much of his normal routine as possible. For instance, the therapist might say, 'Depression is a medical illness. Similar to when you have the flu, you may not feel like doing your schoolwork or playing basketball with your friends. But it is important for you to do as many of your regular activities as possible. Staying active will help you feel better'.

This differs from adult IPT where the patient is given the sick role (i.e., not the limited sick role) and is encouraged to scale back on activities until he or she feels better. Because it is very important developmentally for an adolescent to be in school, the goal is to get the adolescent back to a regular school schedule and attendance as soon as possible. The parent is advised to be supportive rather than punitive and to encourage the adolescent to engage in as many normal activities as possible, while recognizing that it may be difficult for the adolescent.

At the end of session one, the therapist defines the structure and context of the treatment, including the brief, time-limited nature of IPT-A, the roles of the therapist, adolescent, and parents, the limits of confidentiality, and the theory behind IPT-A. The adolescent and family are told that IPT-A is based on the premise that depression occurs in an interpersonal context. Regardless of the cause of the depression, depression affects our relationships and our relationships affect our mood. Thus, the focus of treatment will be on improving the adolescent's relationships with the hope that this will lead to improvements in mood. This discussion helps explain why the treatment focuses on the patient's relationships, as opposed to other parts of the patient's life.

The therapist also clarifies the nature of the confidentiality of the therapy sessions, specifically that the therapist will share information with the parent if the patient may be a danger to himself or others. If there are other topics discussed by the teen that the therapist feels would be important to share with the parent, the therapist will discuss this with the teen and together they will decide if and how to communicate this information with the other person. However, if the therapist meets with the parents alone, he or she will share the general discussion with the adolescent so that the adolescent will not feel that the therapist is holding secrets with the parent. This is important so as not to jeopardize the therapeutic relationship with the adolescent. Finally, the therapist outlines the course of treatment including the number of sessions and future involvement of parents. This discussion makes the course of treatment more predictable and decreases the likelihood of dropout and also helps enlist the parents as collaborators in the treatment.

Session 2: In the beginning of session 2, as is the case with all of the remaining sessions, the therapists begins the session by checking in with the adolescent about the past week and evaluates his current depression symptoms. In addition to assessing specific symptoms, the therapist teaches the adolescent to rate his mood on a 1–10 scale over the past week. This mood rating becomes a useful tool later in treatment to monitor changes in the adolescent's mood and to link these changes to interpersonal events that occurred in the previous week. In addition to asking the patient to rate his average mood for the past week, it is helpful for the therapist to ask whether there has been any time in the past week when the adolescent felt better or worse than that average rating. If the adolescent can identify such times, the therapist should probe for what was happening on the day the adolescent felt worse and the day he felt better, which will help the adolescent begin to make connections between his feelings and events happening in his interpersonal relationships.

In session 2, the therapist and adolescent begin the interpersonal inventory, which is the main focus point of the initial phase of treatment. The interpersonal inventory is an assessment of important relationships that helps the therapist to gain a better understanding of the adolescent's social realm. The goal of the inventory is to identify those interpersonal issues that are most closely related to the onset or persistence of the depression. Although the primary informant for the interpersonal inventory is the adolescent, parents can also provide information about the adolescent's relationships in the first session or in subsequent sessions if they are present.

To conduct the inventory, it is helpful for the therapist to draw a closeness circle, which is a series of circles one within the other, resembling a bulls-eye. The closeness circle is presented as the means by which the adolescent will begin to tell the story about his current life and depression. The circle provides a way for the adolescent to depict the main characters in his story and the closeness and importance of these relationships for his emotional well-being. The adolescent's name is placed in the middle of these circles and then he is asked to identify the people in his life that are of varying levels of importance and to place them in the appropriate spot on the circles (the closest relationships go on the inner most circle, followed by slightly less close relationships, etc.). The result is a picture of the significant people in the adolescent's life. The closeness circle provides the therapist with a visual depiction of the interpersonal context of the depression as it may reveal a paucity of relationships, a bounty of acquaintances but few close relationships, or the adolescent's estrangement from significant people such as a mother, father, or sibling. It provides early clues as to which relationships may need the most exploration during the course of the interpersonal inventory.

Once the circle has been completed, the adolescent is asked to choose the person he would like to talk about first, but the therapist usually selects the ensuing people to discuss based on his or her growing hypothesis of the problem area. The therapist then asks detailed questions about that relationship, followed by the other relationships depicted on the closeness circle. Examples of questions from the inventory are: 'What are the positive and negative aspects of your relationship with your dad? Are there things you would like to change about this relationship? What types of things do you argue about with your dad? How do these arguments begin and end?' The therapist uses these questions to help the adolescent tell the story of his relationship, focusing in particular on how the relationship may be impacting his depression symptoms and how the depression may have impacted the relationship. This type of questioning helps develop an understanding of the interpersonal context of the depression.

The amount of time spent on each person in the inventory will vary depending on the frequency of interaction, level of conflict, physical proximity, etc., but generally, the therapist spends about 10–15 minutes on each relationship trying to get a sense of how this relationship may have contributed, exacerbated, or been affected by the adolescent's depression. If the therapist believes that a particular relationship is closely related to the adolescent's depression, he or she would spend more time on that relationship. As such, session 2 is spent discussing 2–3 relationships that the adolescent has placed on his closeness circle.

Session 3: After a brief symptom check-in and mood rating, session 3 continues the interpersonal inventory. While the adolescent may have been uncomfortable with the questioning initially, by session 3 he knows the types of information that the therapist is interested in gathering, and so the inventory becomes less of a question and answer session and more of an open dialogue about his relationships. It is important when conducting the interpersonal inventory for the therapist to obtain information about relationships that illustrate interpersonal strengths as well as those that illustrate areas of difficulty and to ask for specific examples of conversations or conflicts. This allows the therapist to learn which communication and problem-solving strategies have or haven't been tried within the relationship. The focus of treatment in the middle phase will involve addressing the areas of difficulty, as well as increasing the frequency of interactions that positively impact the adolescent's mood. As the inventory progresses, the therapist should look for patterns that occur across relationships, such as the adolescent not talking about his problems with people because he wants to protect their feelings, the inability to see another person's perspective that would allow for negotiation and compromise, or an adolescent who has withdrawn from relationships and stopped communicating since becoming depressed.

Session 4: In session 4, the therapist and adolescent complete the interpersonal inventory. On the basis of the inventory, the adolescent and therapist choose one of the four interpersonal problem areas that will be the focus of treatment: grief, role disputes, role transitions, or interpersonal deficits. The therapist should explain to the adolescent the connection between the depressive symptoms and his interpersonal difficulties and how this fits into the framework of the identified problem area. The therapist's formulation might be, 'We have been reviewing your important relationships and it sounds like you feel most depressed after your arguments with your mother. These arguments seem to focus on the different views you and your mother have about where you should be and what you should be doing after school and on the weekends. It seems like you and Mom haven't been able to talk about what kinds of things you want to do and with whom as well as Mom's concerns for your safety when you are outside your house. You feel that Mom hasn't recognized that you are growing up and can do more things. When you two argue, you feel very sad and you withdraw into your room and many of your other symptoms increase as well. I think it would be helpful for us to focus on your relationship with Mom, helping you learn to communicate better with her, and learn better ways to solve your differences. Does that sound like the current issue that most affects your mood? Do you think you could explain it back to me in your own words?'

It is very important to have the adolescent explain the problem formulation to the therapist to ensure that he really understands it so that the therapist and adolescent can work on the problem most effectively. If the adolescent cannot explain the formulation to the therapist, then it is likely he doesn't fully understand it and therefore will not be able to address the issues as effectively. In this case, the therapist should spend more time discussing the formulation until the adolescent understands it. While it is most common to identify one interpersonal problem area to address in treatment, there are times when two problem areas are identified. In this case, the therapist and adolescent should discuss how the two problem areas will be addressed during the remainder of treatment. Typically, the therapist will focus on the primary area, that is the area causing the most difficulties at the moment and then address the secondary area when some resolutions to the immediate problem have been attained.

Following the identification of the interpersonal problem area, the adolescent and therapist establish a verbal treatment contract. In this contract, the adolescent's and parents' roles in treatment are specified and the identified problem area is highlighted. The therapist emphasizes that as the treatment moves to the middle phase, the adolescent will need to bring in information about interactions that occurred in his relationships. In addition, the adolescent is informed that his parents might be invited into sessions, particularly if the identified problem is conflict with parents. During this session, the therapist also reviews the structure of treatment, highlighting the number of sessions that have elapsed and the number of sessions that remain. The therapist emphasizes the importance of the adolescent coming to treatment on time and calling to cancel if necessary. For instance, the therapist might say, 'We have met 4 times over the past several weeks. This means that we have 8 sessions left. During these sessions we will talk about what is happening in your relationships and how this is related to your depression. We may invite your parents in for a session or two if we feel like that will be helpful, but we can discuss this more as treatment progresses'. Finally, the goals of the treatment for the individual teen are explained. These goals should be attainable and should emphasize reduction of depressive symptoms and improvement of interpersonal functioning. This contract is helpful for the treatment and serves as a model of clear communication.

Middle phase of treatment

The middle phase of IPT-A consists of sessions five through nine. The main goals of the middle phase of treatment are to clarify the interpersonal problem and then identify and implement techniques and strategies to deal with the problem. The hope is this will lead to an improvement in interpersonal relationships and depression symptoms. It is difficult to break down the middle phase into a session-by-session outline because the content of the sessions is largely determined by the interpersonal problem area and the interactions that the adolescent brings in for discussion each week. As such, we have grouped these sessions together and where appropriate indicate specific topics that should be addressed during a particular session.

During the middle phase sessions, the therapist should guide the discussion so that the focus remains on the problem area, helping the adolescent to link his feelings to interpersonal events and to express these feelings appropriately. The therapist educates the adolescent about interpersonal strategies and encourages the adolescent to identify strategies on his own. The therapist and adolescent practice these strategies in session using role-plays and the adolescent is asked to apply these techniques outside of session. In addition, as the adolescent shares and discusses interpersonal difficulties and improvements, the therapist helps elucidate the connection between the adolescent's mood or symptom level and the interpersonal events. When addressing interpersonal problems in the middle phase, it is best to start with a topic that is manageable and has a high likelihood of success. This will generate hope in the adolescent that these strategies can help facilitate change in his relationships. So as much as possible, we recommend that the therapist begin the middle phase by working on smaller issues and then moving to more difficult issues in later sessions.

Sessions 5–9: As is the case in the initial phase, each session begins with the therapist reviewing the adolescent's depression symptoms and obtaining a mood rating for the week, including the best and worst ratings for the week. This allows the therapist to monitor changes in mood and to link these changes to interpersonal events that may be useful to discuss in the remainder of the session. If an adolescent comes in and reports a worsening of symptoms, the therapist should review the week in detail to help determine what interpersonal event or events may have been responsible for the change in mood. The remainder of the session would then be spent discussing this event or interaction in greater detail. If nothing specific emerges from the depression review, the therapist might ask the adolescent whether anything happened in his relationships this week related to the interpersonal problem area that he might want to discuss.

If an adolescent reports an interpersonal event that occurred during the week, the next step would be to analyze the communication, which is known in IPT-A as communication analysis. This involves getting detailed information about the conversation such as 'How did the discussion start? When did the conversation take place? Where did it happen? What exactly did the adolescent say? What did the person say back? How did that make the adolescent feel? What happened next? Is that the outcome the adolescent wanted?' It is very important to spend time getting a detailed description of the conversation as it occurred, as this helps determine the best course of action.

The goals of communication analysis are to help the adolescent recognize the impact of his words and nonverbal behaviours on others and the feelings generated by the communication. As the adolescent reveals what was specifically said, the therapist should also pay attention to nonverbal behaviours such as eye contact, body posture, tone of voice, and other nonverbal communications. It is helpful to educate adolescents that often it is not what they say that is the problem, but rather how it is said that leads to conflict or anger in the communication. Once the therapist has a clear understanding of the communication, it is useful to discuss how altering the communication at various points might have led to a different outcome, beginning with any ideas the adolescent may have about what he could have done or said differently. For instance, starting the conversation by letting the other person know that he understands her point of view may lead to a calmer discussion or postponing the discussion of a solution until everyone has calmed down instead of trying to negotiate when irritable and angry may lead to a better outcome.

Once the communication analysis is complete, the session can go in a number of different ways. If an adolescent comes in with an argument with his mother about going out with friends and he repeatedly has these arguments, it may be helpful to role-play the argument using new interpersonal techniques and strategies. This way the adolescent is prepared to handle the situation differently the next time the argument arises. Other times, it is more helpful to move the session towards a discussion of ways to proactively have a conversation with the other person about what is upsetting the adolescent and ideas about how to resolve the problem. This would involve talking to the adolescent's mother about his feelings about being able to go out with friends before an argument happens. Or in the case of a role transition where a student has started a new school away from old friends, this might involve thinking about having a conversation with a friend about how they can continue to see each other and maintain the friendship.

It may be helpful to conduct a decision analysis to determine the best course of action. Decision analysis in IPT-A closely resembles problem-solving techniques used in other therapies, but in IPT-A it is specifically focused on addressing interpersonal problems. Decision analysis includes selecting an interpersonal situation, encouraging the adolescent to generate possible solutions, evaluating the pros and cons of each solution, and selecting a solution to try first.

Role-playing follows directly from the communication analysis and decision analysis. In both instances, it is helpful for the adolescent and therapist to role-play the interpersonal interaction to help the adolescent feel more comfortable utilizing the skills or strategies in real life. For instance, following a decision analysis, if an adolescent decides to talk to his mother about going out with friends, the therapist and adolescent would role-play this discussion. In the case of a role transition discussed earlier, the therapist and adolescent would role-play the teenager talking to his friend about finding ways to spend time together despite the change in schools. It is helpful to introduce the adolescent to the concept of a role-play. 'Do you know what a role-play is? Role-playing is kind of like acting. One person plays one part and another person plays a different part. We are going to be doing a lot of role-playing as a way of practicing some of the new communication techniques we talk about in treatment. It is going to feel funny at first, but it really helps you think about what you want to say and the best way to say it'.

When doing a role-play, it is important to act out the conversation, not just talk about it. Adolescents may be initially uncomfortable with the role-plays. To make the adolescent more comfortable, it is important that the role-play is structured so that the adolescent knows what to expect. If an adolescent is really anxious, it may be helpful to write out a script with him before role-playing. It is helpful to liken the exercise to what actors and actresses do in preparation for a show: have a script, read through the script to tweak the lines, do many practices, have a dress rehearsal, and then put on the final show. The final show for the adolescent may be going home to try the interaction on his own or if that seems too difficult because of the unpredictability of the parent, bringing the parent into the session so that the therapist can coach both the parent and adolescent to ensure the interaction goes smoothly.

Before the role-play, the therapist and adolescent can discuss how the adolescent could start the conversation and how the other person might respond. This way the adolescent is prepared with potential responses. For instance, in the case of a mother not letting the adolescent go out with friends, the discussion might start by the adolescent telling his mom that he is feeling left out from his friends because he isn't permitted to socialize with them outside of school. If the adolescent anticipates that his mom would respond by saying that she isn't comfortable with him being out until 10:00 p.m., the adolescent might respond with a potential solution of seeing friends during the day on the weekends or staying out until 9:00 p.m. Once the conversation has been discussed in this level of detail, the actual role-play can begin. The role-play is a dress rehearsal for the actual interaction and the closer it resembles a real conversation, the more helpful it will be. As such, it is important to role-play ideal outcomes as well as less successful interactions to prepare the adolescent for real life interactions.

If the adolescent and therapist are able to identify an interpersonal event, conduct a communication analysis, and decision analysis when appropriate, and practice the new communication techniques, the session might end with a work at home assignment to try the interpersonal techniques outside of the session. Interpersonal work at home is an extension of the work done in the session that allows the adolescent to address difficulties in outside relationships by practicing skills in between sessions. In the examples used so far, an assignment might involve having the adolescent talk to his mom about spending time with friends or the adolescent approaching his friend about his desire to maintain contact.

When explaining the work at home assignment, it is helpful to characterize the assignment as an interpersonal experiment that will help the teenager determine the best combination of techniques for dealing with important people in his life. The experiments give the adolescent the opportunity to try out new strategies and to collect data and tweak the experiment more than once to find useful strategies for the identified problem. The metaphor of a lab experiment may help address any resistance the adolescent may have about trying these techniques outside of the session. The message conveyed is that the experiments outside the session are opportunities to collect more data about how to improve the relationship and to identify which strategies will be most useful. Difficulties are viewed not as failures but as an opportunity to gather information about why the interaction couldn't occur or why it didn't occur the way that the adolescent had planned. This message helps prepare the adolescent for the possibility that the interaction may not be successful, but that the experience will help guide later decisions about the best way to handle the interpersonal problem.

The following session, the therapist and adolescent should review the work at home assignment, examining possible reasons for its success or difficulties. This will likely involve conducting a detailed communication analysis of the conversation to help determine which techniques the adolescent used, their level of success, the outcome of the conversation, and possible modifications to work on in the session. Once previous homework has been reviewed (or in the case when an interpersonal experiment is not assigned), the session progresses to discuss any interpersonal events from the previous week and their impact on the adolescent's mood and symptoms.

Parent–adolescent session: During the middle phase of treatment, it is often helpful to invite parents in for a combined session. The timing of this session will vary but typically occurs during session 7 or 8. This allows time for the therapist and adolescent to work on the interpersonal problem individually for the first couple of middle phase sessions and then permits time after the dyadic session to process the session and continue the middle phase work. The purpose of inviting a parent in during the middle phase differs somewhat depending on the identified problem area. For all teenagers, this session is a good opportunity to review how the teenager is doing and to discuss areas that still need to be addressed. In addition, it is useful to involve the parents again to get their perspective on whether or not there have been noticeable changes in the adolescent and to identify continued problematic areas. For adolescents whose identified problem area involves the parent, this session provides an opportunity for the teenager to practice new communication techniques with the parent in the safety of the therapeutic environment.

Typically, the therapist would begin this session by meeting with the adolescent alone to conduct a brief depression review. If the adolescent would benefit from practicing communication with the parent, he and the therapist would identify a mildly hot topic to discuss with a high likelihood for resolution (if they have not already done so in the previous session). The goal is to pick a topic that can easily be discussed so that the focus can be on the process of the interaction and communication more than on the content of the discussion. The goal is to have the parent and adolescent experience an interaction differently and more positively than they have in the past to motivate them to continue to practice new ways of interacting. For example, the parent and adolescent might discuss his desire to go to a friend's house after school. The therapist can help decrease the adolescent's anxiety about the conversation by helping him identify a good way to begin the conversation and by discussing key communication techniques. The therapist should assure the teenager that he or she is there to help everything go as smoothly as possible.

Once the parent joins the session, it is helpful for the therapist to begin by briefly reviewing the adolescent's progress in treatment and areas in need of further work. The therapist should ask the parent to discuss his or her observation of the adolescent's progress since attending treatment. In this discussion, it is important to maintain a positive outlook on the teenager's experience by highlighting progress that has been made. It is also necessary to listen and acknowledge the parent's continued areas of concern. This should lead to a discussion with the adolescent and parent about how best to approach these issues in the remaining sessions.

The therapist should inform the parent that the adolescent has been working on new ways of communicating with important people in his life and that during the remainder of the session he would like to practice the communication skills that he has been working on in treatment. 'Mrs. Smith, Bill has been working really hard in treatment. He has been learning new ways of expressing himself. This is hard work and needs a lot of practice. I am hoping that Bill can practice some of these skills with you in here today'. The therapist should then encourage the adolescent to start the conversation as he practiced. The therapist is there primarily as an observer and to help coach the adolescent as needed. The therapist can intervene when necessary, for instance if the conversation gets too heated or the adolescent returns to using maladaptive communication patterns.

After the adolescent and parent have had the opportunity to discuss the identified issue for ten or fifteen minutes, the therapist should highlight for the family how this conversation is different from previous conversations they have had. This may involve identifying strategies that made the conversation more successful. The therapist would also want to discuss with the family how they can continue this conversation outside of the session. Before the end of the session, the therapist may choose to meet with the adolescent alone for a few minutes to debrief about the session, particularly if it has been a difficult one.

If the therapist is concerned that the parent will not be receptive or helpful to have in the session with the adolescent due to the parent's own difficulties, it is recommended that the therapist meet alone with the parent. This allows the therapist to provide further needed psychoeducation for the parent and assess the workability of the parent. The therapist might conclude that the parent will not be able to alter her behaviour and that the focus should be on helping the adolescent learn how to cope with the parent's particular challenges.

Problem area specific session structure: The section above describes generally what occurs in the middle phase of treatment. However, session structure and format vary depending on the assigned interpersonal problem area. Below we will briefly discuss problem area specific topics that are addressed in the middle sessions.

Grief: If the assigned problem area is grief, it is important for the adolescent to discuss the loss in significant detail, including the adolescent's relationship with the deceased. This includes discussing the sequence of events prior to, during, and after the death. During this process, the therapist encourages the adolescent to identify and express feelings associated with the relationship and the loss, both positive and negative. For instance, the therapist might say, 'Most people have both good and bad times in their relationships. Can you tell me about some of the times that were more difficult with your father? What happened during those times? How did you feel?' The purpose of this review is to help the adolescent develop a better understanding of the complexity of the previous relationship so that he can have a more realistic memory of the deceased person and the relationship. This allows for a more normal grieving process. In addition, the therapist helps the adolescent find a way to honour the memory of the deceased while engaging in other relationships.

As the middle phase progresses, the therapist encourages the adolescent to develop new relationships and/or further develop established relationships to help replace the support that was lost. This involves exploring the adolescent's fears about developing new relationships and rehearsing skills needed to develop relationships or to engage in new activities. The therapist will often utilize role-plays and work at home assignments to practice the skills and techniques that are necessary to encourage the development of relationships and to help the adolescent resume more normal social interactions.

Interpersonal role disputes: When an adolescent presents with an interpersonal dispute, the therapist should help the adolescent clarify the dispute and any differences in expectations that may be contributing to the disagreement. Helpful questions include 'What do you and your mother fight about? How do the fights begin and end? How do they make you feel? What expectations do you have for your relationship with your mom? Are these expectations met? What if your mom can't change, how might you handle it?' It is helpful in the beginning of the middle phase of treatment to clarify the stage of the dispute: renegotiation, impasse, and dissolution (Klerman et al., 1984). During renegotiation, the adolescent and significant other are communicating with each other and are attempting to resolve the dispute. During an impasse, the two people have stopped trying to discuss or resolve the conflict but still have a desire to mend the relationship. During dissolution, the adolescent and significant other have decided that the dispute cannot be resolved and have chosen to end the relationship. Typically with adolescents, this stage is encountered solely in conflict with peers or in romantic relationships, not in familial relationships.

Next the therapist and adolescent assess and then modify maladaptive communication patterns that may be contributing to the conflict. Additionally, more adaptive interpersonal techniques are taught, such as the art of negotiation. For example, if the adolescent is fighting with his mother about spending time with friends, the therapist might say, 'You and your mom are fighting a lot about your time spent with friends. It seems to me that one of the main reasons for this argument is because you and your mom have different opinions about appropriate times to spend with friends. I'd like to help you find new ways of talking with your mom about how you feel. This will probably include thinking about your mom's perspective and concerns, your expectations, and some possible compromises that would make your mom feel more comfortable and you less lonely and depressed'.

When a conflict involves a parent, he or she is invited into treatment to help address the problem. However, this problem area can be addressed with an adolescent alone when necessary. If a resolution seems impossible, the therapist works with the adolescent to develop strategies for coping with a relationship that cannot be changed. For instance, the therapist points out that decreasing the frequency of conflict can result in improved mood, even if the relationship cannot be changed completely. The therapist also encourages the adolescent to seek out other relationships that may address the adolescent's emotional needs more effectively.

Role transition: For a role transition, the middle phase of treatment begins with a discussion about what the transition means to the adolescent, demands associated with this change, and gains and losses associated with the transition. It is important to encourage the adolescent to explore his feelings related to each of these areas. In particular, it is helpful to identify what makes the new role difficult for the adolescent and what skills may be needed to help the adolescent manage the new role. The following is a list of helpful questions: 'What was it like for you to start high school? Was high school different than what you expected? How did you feel? How did your relationships with friends change? How did these changes make you feel?'

If the role transition involves the adolescent's parents, they should be involved in some of the middle phase sessions whenever possible. For instance, if the role transition is the normative transition into adolescence and the adolescent's parents are having a difficult time with the adolescent's attempts to individuate, then a parent–adolescent session might directly address the adolescent's and parents differing expectations about what are normal adolescent developmental tasks. The therapist might explain to the parent, 'Your child has become an adolescent and is experiencing new things. It can sometimes be hard for parents to see their child change, especially when it feels like your child is growing away from you. These changes don't mean that your son doesn't love you. It is normal for adolescents to want to spend more time with friends and less time with family. I understand that this is difficult but it is important that your child feels that you support the changes that he is going through'. The middle phase work would likely also involve communication analysis to review how the adolescent has communicated to significant others about the changes in his life, decision analysis about the best strategies to handle the role transition, and role-plays and work at home to implement new ways of communicating to help him better cope with the transition.

Interpersonal deficits: The middle phase of treatment involves reviewing past significant relationships, with a focus on problematic patterns in these relationships. The therapist helps the adolescent recognize the link between these interpersonal problems and the depression. For instance, when working with an adolescent who has difficulty talking to family members about his feelings, the therapist might point out that the adolescent's social isolation leads to an increase in depressive symptoms, which in turn leads to an increase in social isolation. 'As we talked about your relationship with your mom and brothers, I noticed some similarities. You talk to them about your day, but you haven't really talked to them directly about your feelings. As a result, your family may not know how you are feeling or what you need to feel supported by them. You end up feeling isolated from your mom and brothers and this makes you feel more depressed. It seems like one of the things we need to work on is helping you to communicate more about your feelings'.

Following this, the therapist introduces new strategies for handling interpersonal relationships and the adolescent and therapist practice these strategies in role-plays. For example, a middle session might involve having the adolescent practice asking a friend to do some activity with him or trying to initiate a conversation with a new person in school. The therapist might say, 'Let's pretend that you ask a friend to go to the movies. When might you ask your friend? What could you say? What if he says he has other plans? How would you feel? What might you say to him?' Once the adolescent has a basic sense of how the conversation might go, he and the therapist can role-play the interaction. The adolescent is encouraged to try these strategies outside of the session in a work at home assignment and to report on how it went the following week. In this follow-up session, the therapist would conduct a communication analysis of the interaction.

In interpersonal deficits, more than in the other problem areas, it may be useful to utilize the relationship between the therapist and the adolescent to help the adolescent recognize his patterns of interacting. The therapist can be helpful by giving the adolescent feedback about how his interpersonal style is impacting the therapist and can assist the adolescent in identifying new ways of interacting in the session. A therapist might say 'I get the sense that you are upset about something although you haven't told me that. I can tell from your posture and tone of voice when you are speaking to me today. Have I said something to upset you? If so, I would like you to tell me so I can understand how you are feeling. It is important for me to know how you feel so I can better help you'. The hope is that pointing out the interpersonal patterns occurring in the session will help elucidate patterns in outside relationships. Specific interpersonal techniques and strategies that are applied to the therapeutic relationship can be generalized to outside relationships, particularly with the help of work at home assignments.

Termination phase The termination phase of IPT-A involves sessions 10 through 12. The tasks of the termination phase include discussion of successful strategies identified in therapy, generalization of skills to future situations, clarification of the adolescent's warning symptoms of depression, and discussion of the need for further treatment. A session-by-session outline of the termination phase is provided below but this should be used only as a rough guideline. The tasks of the termination phase can be accomplished in whatever order seems most appropriate for the adolescent or for a given discussion.

Session 10: Session 10 begins with a brief review of symptoms and a mood rating. This session acts as a transition between the middle phase of treatment and the termination phase. Often there is remaining interpersonal work that needs to be addressed in this session before moving to the tasks of termination. For instance, if the therapist assigned interpersonal work at home in session 9, it is important to review how the discussion or interaction went, in particular highlighting strategies that were successful. Other times, an adolescent may come in to session 10 with a pressing interpersonal issue and the therapist may make the decision to do a more typical middle phase session. If this decision is made, it is important to emphasize how the techniques being discussed generalize to other situations since generalization is an important task of the remaining sessions. If the adolescent is ready to move to termination phase work, then the therapist would proceed to the tasks outlined in sessions 11 and 12.

Sessions 11 and 12: The therapist begins each session with a review of the adolescent's symptoms for the past week. The therapist and adolescent should discuss how the adolescent's symptoms and mood ratings have changed over the course of the treatment. This discussion is helpful because it makes explicit the changes that have occurred over the past few months. These improvements in symptoms and mood are linked to changes in interpersonal relationships, especially those that are related to the identified problem area. Changes in interpersonal functioning and relationships are linked to improved mood and decreased symptoms. The therapist might say, 'Bill thinking back over the past 12 weeks, there are a number of changes in your symptoms. Your irritability and social withdrawal have really improved, as have your weekly mood ratings. I noticed that these improvements really started around session 6 when you started communicating more with your mom about how you have been feeling'.

Because depression is a recurrent illness, it is important to discuss the adolescent's warning signs of depression and what he can do to address these symptoms if they return. This discussion can occur in either session 11 or 12 and flows nicely from the symptom review. At this point in treatment, the adolescent is very knowledgeable about the symptoms of depression and with the help of the therapist should identify which symptom or symptoms would be an indication that his depression might be returning. It is also important for the therapist to educate the adolescent that depression can re-occur and that this does not mean that the adolescent is a failure or that the treatment wasn't successful. The hope is that preparing the adolescent for the possibility of recurrence and identifying specific warning signs will help the adolescent seek treatment sooner if needed.

During the termination phase, the therapist should identify the changes that he or she observes in the adolescent such as improved communication, increased awareness about his own feelings associated with a relationship, or the successful establishment of new relationships. The therapist and adolescent together highlight how specific strategies have enabled him to make improvements within his identified problem area, in specific relationships, and most importantly in his mood. 'Over the past couple of months, you have tried out new ways of speaking with your mom about spending time with friends. As a result, you were able to find a compromise allowing you to spend Friday evenings doing something with your friends. Do you have a sense of what specific strategies were useful with your mom?' The therapist and adolescent should discuss the importance of continuing to implement these strategies after termination, as well as highlight areas that still need improvement or might benefit from additional treatment.

Terminating treatment with an adolescent also means terminating treatment with the family. Depending on the situation and the wishes of the adolescent, the therapist might meet with the parents separately or have a session with the adolescent and parents together. It is important for parents to hear progress made, the skills and strategies that were learned, and warning signs of a possible relapse. It is also helpful to discuss any changes in family interactions and functioning that occurred as a result of the treatment. The termination phase enables both the adolescent and parent to participate in the review of accomplishments and the identification of areas that would benefit from further treatment. As is the case with the adolescent, it is important for the family to know about the possible recurrence of mild symptoms shortly after termination and the possibility of future episodes of depression. This should lead to a discussion about how to manage future depression symptoms or episodes.

There are adolescents for whom there has been some improvement, but who continue to be moderately symptomatic at the conclusion of treatment. Further treatment may be necessary under certain circumstances when the symptoms may not have fully remitted or when there are other more chronic problems contributing to the adolescent's impairment. If the therapist believes this is the case, he or she should discuss the possibility of continuing treatment with the adolescent and parents and what treatment options they might consider.

Recent empirical findings

IPT-A meets four conditions that permit its inclusion as an efficacious treatment: (1) the treatment is manual-based (Weissman et al., 2000; Mufson et al., 2004a), (2) the sample characteristics are detailed, (3) the treatment has been tested in randomized clinical trials (Mufson et al., 1999; Rosselló & Bernal, 1999; Mufson et al., 2004b), and (4) at least two different investigator teams have demonstrated the intervention's effects (Chambless & Hollon, 1998; Chorpita, 2003). In an open clinical trial, 12–18 year olds with depressive symptoms who were referred to a hospital outpatient clinic were treated with IPT-A. After treatment, none of the subjects met DSM-III-R criteria for depression. The subjects were functioning at a higher level in school and at home and showed a significant decrease in psychological distress and depressive symptoms (Mufson et al., 1994).

In a controlled trial, conducted by Dr. Mufson and colleagues (Mufson et al., 1999), depressed adolescents who had been referred to a hospital-based clinic were randomized to receive either IPT-A ($N = 24$) or clinical monitoring ($N = 24$) for 12 weeks. At the end of treatment, significantly more adolescents in the IPT-A condition met recovery criteria for major depression than adolescents receiving clinical monitoring. Adolescents receiving IPT-A also had a significant decrease in depressive symptoms and increased social functioning and problem-solving skills.

Rosselló and Bernal (1999) compared a different adaptation of IPT designed specifically for depressed adolescents in Puerto Rico to cognitive–behaviour therapy (CBT) and wait list condition. They showed that depressed adolescents receiving IPT ($N = 23$) or CBT ($N = 25$) experienced a greater reduction in symptoms, greater increase in self-esteem, and more improvement in social functioning than those subjects in the wait list condition ($N = 25$). Furthermore, 52% of subjects receiving CBT versus 82% of those receiving IPT met recovery criteria.

Dr. Mufson and colleagues recently investigated the effectiveness of IPT-A in school-based health clinics in impoverished neighbourhoods in New York City (Mufson et al., 2004b). Clinicians employed in several school-based health clinics were trained to deliver IPT-A. Adolescents with major depression, dysthymia, depression disorder not otherwise specified, or adjustment disorder with depressed mood were randomized to receive either treatment as usual (supportive, individual counselling) or IPT-A. School-based clinicians delivered both treatments. Adolescents with comorbid anxiety disorders, ADHD, and oppositional defiant disorder were allowed to participate in the study. Adolescents receiving IPT-A ($N = 34$) compared to treatment as usual ($N = 29$) demonstrated a greater decrease in depression symptoms and depression severity, greater overall functioning, and significantly better social functioning. These findings support IPT-A as an effective treatment when delivered by community clinicians.

New adaptations

Over the past several years, there have been a number of adaptations to the IPT-A model. Dr. Mufson and colleagues (Mufson et al., 2004c) developed a group model of IPT-A (IPT-AG). In IPT-AG, adolescents are seen for 2 or 3 individual pre-group sessions to conduct the interpersonal inventory and then participate in 12 weekly hour and a half group sessions with both a middle and end of group individual session to track the adolescent's specific progress. A pilot-controlled clinical trial of this group adaptation was conducted in a mental health specialty clinic comparing IPT-A to IPT-AG in depressed adolescents. Data from this preliminary study found no significant differences between the treatment conditions, indicating that IPT-AG may be an efficacious treatment for depression in adolescents.

Dr. Young and Mufson developed Interpersonal Psychotherapy-Adolescent Skills Training (IPT-AST), a group preventive intervention for adolescents with subthreshold symptoms of depression (Young & Mufson, 2003). IPT-AST has 2 pre-group sessions and 8 weekly hour and a half group sessions. The focus on the group is teaching adolescents specific interpersonal and communication skills that can be applied to their current relationships. A randomized controlled trial compared IPT-AST to usual school counselling as provided by school guidance counsellors or social workers. Adolescents who received IPT-AST reported significantly fewer depression symptoms and better overall functioning than adolescents in school counselling post-intervention and up to 6 months following the intervention (Young et al., 2006).

Dr. Verdeli and colleagues have developed an IPT-based preventive intervention for adolescent children of parents with bipolar disorder (IPT-PA) who themselves have subsyndromal mood symptoms. The intervention is conducted over 12 sessions, 4 of which are 90 minutes in length and include family members. IPT-PA involves 3 components: family psychoeducation, individual interpersonal psychotherapy, and a social rhythm component as needed. In an open clinical trial of 7 adolescents with subsyndromal affective symptoms, IPT-PA was associated with an improvement in symptoms and functioning. Furthermore, families and adolescents reported a high level of satisfaction with the intervention (Verdeli et al., 2007).

Other adaptations are currently underway, including using IPT-A to treat depressed adolescents who engage in non-suicidal self-injury and to treat prepubertal children ages 9 through 12 years of age. In addition, an open trial is currently being conducted in which another model of IPT, Interpersonal and Social Rhythm Therapy, is being adapted and used as an adjunctive treatment with medication for bipolar adolescents. Finally, a small study is being conducted examining models for training therapists in IPT-A, comparing the intensity of supervision and use of audiotapes in long distance training of community-based clinicians.

Conclusions

IPT is an evidence-based psychotherapy that is based on the theory that depression occurs in an interpersonal context. The goals of treatment are to improve the patient's interpersonal relationships and his depression symptoms. The adolescent version, IPT-A, was adapted to address the developmental needs of adolescents and their families in a time-limited manualized treatment (Mufson et al., 2004a). IPT-A has been demonstrated to be effective both in university and community settings and when delivered by both expert and community clinicians (Mufson et al., 1999; 2004b; Rossello & Bernal, 1999). These research studies, and clinical experience working with depressed adolescents, suggest that IPT-A is a treatment of choice for adolescent depression given its effectiveness and the ease of training clinicians in this treatment modality.

References

Chambless, D.L. & Hollon, S.D. (1998). Defining empirically supported therapies. *Journal of Consulting and Clinical Psychology, 66*, 7–18.

Chorpita, B.F. (2003). The frontier of evidence-based practice. In A.E. Kazdin & J.R. Weisz (Eds.), *Evidence-based psychotherapies for children and adolescents* (pp. 42–59). New York, New York: Guilford Press.

Clark, D., Pynoos, R., & Goebel, A. (1994). Mechanisms and processes of adolescent bereavement. In R. Haggerty (Ed.), *Stress, risk, and resilience in children and adolescents: Processes, mechanisms, and interventions* (pp. 100–145). Cambridge, England: Cambridge University Press.

Coyne, J. (1976). Toward an interactional description of depression. *Psychiatry, 39*, 28–40.

Elkin, I., Shea, M.T., Watkins, J.T., Imber, S.D., Sotsky, S.M., Collins, et al. (1989). National Institute of Mental Health Treatment of Depression Collaborative Research Program: General effectiveness of treatments. *Archives of General Psychiatry, 46*, 971–983.

Frank, E., Kupfer, D.J., Wagner, E.E., McEachran, A.B., & Cornes, C. (1991). Efficacy of interpersonal psychotherapy as a maintenance treatment of recurrent depression: Contributing factors. *Archives of General Psychiatry, 48*, 1053–1059.

Hammen, C. (1999). The emergence of an interpersonal approach to depression. In T. Joiner & J. Coyne (Eds.), *The interactional nature of depression: Advances in interpersonal approaches* (pp. 22–36). Washington, DC: American Psychological Association.

Joiner, T., Coyne, J., & Blalock, J. (1999). On the interpersonal nature of depression: Overview and synthesis. In T. Joiner & J. Coyne (Eds.), *The interactional nature of depression: Advances in interpersonal approaches* (pp. 3–20). Washington, DC: American Psychological Association.

Kiesler, D. (1991). Interpersonal methods of assessment and diagnosis. In C.R. Snyder & D.R. Forsyth (Eds.), *Handbook of social and clinical psychology: The health perspective* (pp. 438–468). Elmsford, NY: Pergamon Press.

Klerman, G.L., Weissman, M.M., Rounsaville, B.J., & Chevron, E.S. (1984). *Interpersonal psychotherapy of depression.* New York: Basic Books.

Lewinsohn, P.M., Roberts, R.E., Seeley, J.R., Rohde, P., Gotlib, I.H., & Hops, H. (1994). Adolescent psychopathology: II. Psychosocial risk factors for depression. *Journal of Abnormal Psychology, 103*, 302–315.

Meyer, A. (1957). *Psychobiology: A science of man.* Springfield, IL: Charles C. Thomas.

Mufson, L., Dorta, K.P., Moreau, D., & Weissman, M.M. (2004a). *Interpersonal psychotherapy for depressed adolescents* (2nd Ed.). New York: Guilford Press.

Mufson, L., Dorta, K.P., Wickramaratne, P., Nomura, Y., Olfson, M., & Weissman, M.M. (2004b). A randomized effectiveness trial of interpersonal psychotherapy for depressed adolescents. *Archives of General Psychiatry, 63*, 577–584.

Mufson, L., Gallagher T., Dorta K.P., & Young J.F. (2004c). Interpersonal Psychotherapy for Adolescent Depression: Adaptation for group therapy. *American Journal of Psychotherapy, 58*, 220–237.

Mufson, L., Moreau, D., Weissman, M.M., & Klerman, G.L. (1993). *Interpersonal psychotherapy for depressed adolescents.* New York: Guilford Press.

Mufson, L., Moreau, D., Weissman, M.M., Wickramaratne, P., Martin J., & Samoilov, A. (1994). The modification of interpersonal psychotherapy with depressed adolescents IPT-A: Phase I and Phase II studies. *Journal of the American Academy of Child and Adolescent Psychiatry, 33*, 695–705.

Mufson, L., Weissman, M.M., Moreau, D., & Garfinkel, R. (1999). Efficacy of interpersonal psychotherapy for depressed adolescents. *Archives of General Psychiatry, 56*, 573–579.

Puig-Antich, J., Kaufman, J., Ryan, N.D., Williamson, D.E., Dahl, R.E., Lukens, E., et al. (1993). The psychosocial functioning and family environment of depressed adolescents. *Journal of the American Academy of Child and Adolescent Psychiatry, 32*, 244–253.

Rosselló, J. & Bernal, G. (1999). The efficacy of cognitive-behavioral and interpersonal treatments for depression in Puerto Rican adolescents. *Journal of Consulting and Clinical Psychology, 67*, 734–745.

Ryan, N.D., Puig-Antich, J., Ambrosini, P., Rabinovich, H., Robinson, D., Nelson, B., et al. (1987). The clinical picture of major depression in children and adolescents. *Archives of General Psychiatry, 44*, 854–861.

Sheeber, L., Hops, H., Alpert, A., Davis, B., & Andrews, J. (1997). Family support and conflict: Prospective relations to adolescent Depression. *Journal of Abnormal Child Psychology, 25*, 333–344.

Sloane, R.B., Stapes, F.R., & Schneider, L.S. (1985). Interpersonal therapy versus nortriptyline for depression in the elderly. In G.D. Burrow, T.R. Norman, & L. Dennerstein (Eds.), *Clinical and pharmacological studies in psychiatric disorders* (pp. 344–346). London: Libbey.

Stader, S. & Hokanson, J. (1998). Psychological antecedents of depressive symptoms: An evaluation using daily experiences methodology. *Journal of Abnormal Psychology, 107*, 17–26.

Sullivan, H.S. (1953). *The interpersonal theory of psychiatry*. New York: W.W. Norton.

Verdeli, H., Weissman, M.M., & Mufson, L. (2007). IPT for symptomatic children of bipolar parents. Poster presented at the NIMH workshop on Pediatric Bipolar Disorder, Washington, DC

Weissman, M.M., Markowitz, J.C., & Klerman, G.L. (2000). *Comprehensive guide to interpersonal psychotherapy*. New York: Basic Books.

Weissman, M.M., & Paykel, E.S. (1974). *The depressed woman: A study of social relationships*. Oxford: University of Chicago Press.

Weissman, M.M., Prusoff, B.A., DiMascio, A., Neu, C., Goklaney, M., & Klerman, G.L. (1979). The efficacy of drug and psychotherapy in the treatment of acute depressive episodes. *American Journal of Psychiatry, 136*, 555–558.

Young, J.F. & Mufson, L. (2003). *Manual for interpersonal psychotherapy—adolescent skills training (IPT-AST)*. Columbia University, New York, NY.

Young, J.F., Mufson, L., & Davies, M. (2006). Efficacy of Interpersonal Psychotherapy—Adolescent Skills Training: An indicated preventive intervention for depression. *Journal of Child Psychology and Psychiatry, 47*, 1254–1262.

Chapter 12

'Working Things Out'—a therapeutic resource for professionals working with young people

Carol Fitzpatrick, Eileen Brosnan, & John Sharry

'Working Things Out' (WTO) is an interactive CD-ROM/DVD, which contains the personal stories of eleven adolescents who have managed difficult problems in their lives such as depression, bullying, eating problems, suicidal behaviour, and self-harm. With the help of therapists, the young people narrated their personal stories, which are illustrated by animation, graphics, and music, and are presented as a collection of ten mini-movies and one recorded song.

The 'Working Things Out' resource pack includes

1. The CD ROM/DVD,
2. A manual with the scripts of the stories and ideas about how they may be used by professionals working with young people,
3. Handouts, which may be photocopied, on a variety of mental health difficulties, and
4. Lists of resources and link sites for young people.

Background to development of 'Working Things Out'

The idea for the Working Things Out project emerged during the 'Challenging Times' study (Lynch et al., 2004, 2006), which looked at the prevalence of depressive disorders and other mental health difficulties amongst 12–15 year olds in secondary schools in Dublin, Ireland. This study, which used the KSADS-PL (Kaufman et al., 1997) found that 4.5% of the young people studied had a current depressive disorder, while 8.4% had a history of a past depressive disorder. Many of those with past depressive disorders had recovered without professional input of any kind. This group of young people were of particular interest to the research team, who wondered how they had managed to get over their depression. This lead to a qualitative study in which these young people, along with an age-matched sample of young people who had attended mental health services for treatment of depression and other mental health problems, were invited to take part in individual interviews and focus groups about how they coped with depression and other difficult life experiences (Fitzpatrick & Sharry, 2004). The main theme to emerge from this study was the importance placed by the young people of telling someone how they were feeling, which they identified as being the start of 'getting better'. From this project emerged the idea of making something, which might help other young people who were going through 'a tough time'.

Making 'Working Things Out'

The 'Working Things Out' project grew out of a desire to create a tool that could be used for multiple purposes: to help engage young people referred to mental health services; as an accessible means of providing mental health information; and as a means of demonstrating how young people used cognitive behavioural therapy ideas to overcome problems in their everyday lives. To ensure that the tool would be relevant and appealing to young people, participants from the above study were involved in the making of the CD-ROM/DVD in which they shared their personal stories of dealing with a difficult life experience during adolescence. A group of multi-media professionals worked with the research and clinical team to develop the CD-ROM/DVD and the young people became involved in the creative and technical aspects of the production. The inclusion of real young people's experiences in a story format makes the material much more real and relevant.

To develop a 'script' for the stories, each young person attended a series of individual meetings with a therapist (E.B.) who, through a process of listening and clarifying, helped each person to tell their story in a structured format. This structure focused on their experience of having a problem, how they coped and what supports and resources helped them. The final scripts for the short movies were co-authored by the therapist and the young person. Some young people were able to write the majority of the script themselves and others needed more support (e.g., the therapist would transcribe the main points from a recorded interview and re-read to the young person for approval). The stories were then recorded, using the young peoples' own voices.

The young people were also involved in the creative aspects of the animations and soundtracks to accompany the script. They became involved in creating images, in the storyboarding of scenes, choosing the graphic style, developing soundtrack material, and recording voiceovers. Alongside the individual sessions, workshops were conducted with the young people on animation, photography, and digital audio. This helped the young person take ownership of his/her story, both in its script and in how it would be represented. A key aspect of this project was to ensure that the stories were personal and meaningful to the participating adolescents and their families. The introduction to the stories was written in conjunction with the young people and is as follows:

Welcome to 'Working Things Out' the stories of 11 young people who have gone through some difficult life experiences. By sharing our stories, our feelings and our ways of coping with our problems, we hope that others who might be going through a similar hard time will be reminded that they are not alone and that there are many different things you can do to make things better.

Telling our stories definitely made us feel better, it was good to get stuff off our chests. We hope that the very real experiences you hear will be a source of support and learning for you. Our stories are ongoing and not all our problems have gone away but the way we understand and deal with them has changed. While we don't have all the answers, we might have some useful messages and information.

Treatment for adolescent depression in the 'real world'

'Working Things Out' was developed in the context of a busy, under-resourced community-based Child and Adolescent Mental Health Service (CAMHS), where the gap between the evidence-based treatments for depression with which we were familiar (Clarke et al., 1990, 1992, 1999; Curry, 2000; March et al., 2006) and the 'real world' seemed at times very great. Most members of the research team were also clinicians who often struggled to engage the most troubled adolescents in any form of conversation, let alone structured therapeutic interventions, such as cognitive behavioural therapy or interpersonal psychotherapy. Adolescents referred to mental health services usually have comorbid disorders, and those with depressive disorders often also have oppositional defiant disorder, attention deficit disorder, or conduct disorder (Verhulst & van der Ende, 1997). Language disorders, developmental and communication difficulties, and stressful family backgrounds are also common (Gunther et al., 2003), along with specific learning difficulties. Such young people are often angry and frightened, and may either deny that they have any problems, or feel that nothing can be done to help them. It can be very difficult to engage these young people, who may find it hard to remain in an office with an authority figure, let alone to talk about their problems! The most important 'first step' with such young people is to develop a therapeutic relationship. There is evidence that a positive therapeutic relationship is strongly related to positive outcome across a variety of mental health interventions (Krupnick et al., 1996; Diamond et al., 2006; McKay et al., 1998), although this is a relatively under-researched area. Using 'Working Things Out' with a young person can facilitate the development of a therapeutic relationship, particularly with those who are difficult to engage.

'Real world' child and adolescent mental health service (CAMHS) provision is also characterized by difficulty in engaging clients in attending for regular and repeated sessions. Many adolescents refuse to attend at all, and it is not uncommon for young people and their parents to attend for assessment, but not to attend for follow-up treatment (Hoare et al., 1996), or to miss appointments regularly (Conduit et al., 2004). Those who attend fewer appointments tend to have greater levels of dysfunction (Kazdin, 1996). It is important to make early sessions as positive and productive as possible, bearing in mind that these may be the only sessions attended. 'Working Things Out' provides a tool to help with this.

Can technology assist therapeutic engagement and motivation?

There is no doubt that most young people enjoy using computers. Seymour Papert suggests that it is timely for '*child therapists to bridge the digital generation gap and innovate with computers in their work with children of the digital age*' (Papert, 1996). Integrating the use of computers into a therapeutic intervention could be key to positively engaging and motivating adolescents. In the development of the 'Working Things Out' CD-ROM/DVD, practitioners worked closely with the adolescent participants, keeping them central to the process of producing the resource. This experience showed that by asking young people what worked for them, a wealth of important information and personal stories of coping was uncovered. Essentially the participants became engaged. This engagement was further enhanced by the use of multimedia in working with them to tell their stories. This raised an important question of how to make the use of multimedia and computer technology accessible to a wider range of practitioners as a tool for engaging and working therapeutically with young people (Brosnan et al., 2005). 'Transforming Stories' multimedia story-building software was developed in response to this growing need for creative computer-based tools to use with young people in the therapeutic context. The programme allows users to create story sequences using a database of customizable 2D characters, story props, and background environments (school, home, community settings). It can be accessed at www.transformingstories.com. See Figures 12.1 and 12.2 for examples of story graphics and the character palette.

In almost all genres of counselling and psychotherapy, there is an important 'joining stage' where the counsellor seeks to establish connections with their clients. Mental health practitioners working with adolescents often use conversation, questions about likes and dislikes, hobbies, etc., to create points of connection. This part of the process of establishing a trusting relationship with the young person can significantly contribute to the positive outcomes of the therapy (Monk & Winsdale, 1997). Therapists use media such as art and clay, and techniques such as journal writing and work sheets as a way of helping the young person to express their ideas and feelings. In a similar way, computer technology and multimedia can provide a new and novel means of

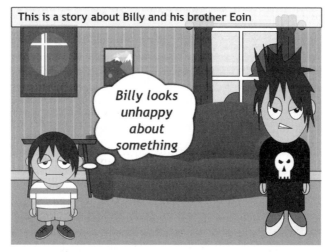

Figure 12.1 Story interface.

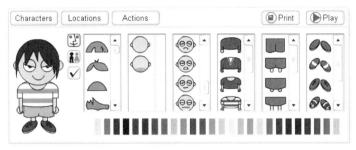

Figure 12.2 Character customisation palette.

establishing a connection with the young person and offer them a medium to express themselves creatively. In the field of education, the use of technology can enhance student learning and bring a subject matter to life (Heppel, 1994). Using a multimedia story building application such as 'Transforming Stories' in a psychotherapy session can similarly enhance the young person's therapeutic learning experience. They are helped to plan and structure the narrative by creating and linking scenes. This 'linking' of material can give the young person another way of processing often difficult emotional content. It is important that these possibilities are researched and developed further, as it will contribute to the development of innovative new approaches to adolescent mental health work.

Adolescents have grown up in a computer age and are generally comfortable with multimedia applications. Many of them will be familiar with interactive multimedia from using computer games, the Internet, and a range of educational packages. It is our experience that the initial 'resistance' at coming to therapy often expressed by adolescents dissipates when the computer is used as an engagement tool. The traditional face-to-face question and answer format of therapist/client interaction may be very daunting for an adolescent. This can be avoided by the young person and therapist sitting side by side, focussing on the computer screen, using a medium with which the young person is often more comfortable than the therapist! Technology is now an integral part of the human communication system and the therapeutic arena provides a diversity of new contexts in which it can be applied.

Overview of content of 'Working Things Out'

The 'Working Things Out' Resource Pack includes a CD ROM and a DVD, a manual with the scripts of the stories and ideas about how they may be used by professionals working with young people, handouts which may be photocopied on a variety of mental health difficulties, and lists of resources and link sites for young people. The CD ROM and DVD contain the ten mini-movies of the young peoples' stories and one recorded song written by one participant who preferred to share his experiences in lyrics and music. The mini-movies may be run straight through, or may be stopped at any point. Clicking on icons brings up points for discussion, which the professional may wish to use with the young person.

Summary of each story and selected examples of story graphics

Jack

'Knocking down the wall: Overcoming my depression'

Jack describes how he felt when he was depressed, and how life became very difficult for him. Telling his mother about how he was feeling was the turning point for him. Through talking things over he began to understand his feelings better, and his parents were better able to understand him. Things began to improve for him, and he is fine now.

Ciara

'Scaredy-Cat, Mad Woman: Stopping my fears ruling my life'

Ciara talks about how she developed a big problem with fears and anger, which almost overwhelmed her and her family at times, leading her to feel she was going mad. Making the move to get professional help was the start of her recovery. She talks about her mixed feelings about having to take medication. And though the medication helped, she still had to do the work herself and learn ways of beating her fears.

Louise

'OCD: Managing my obsessions'

Louise talks about how obsessive compulsive disorder was taking over her life, how she learned ways of dealing with it through working with a therapist, and how now she feels much more in control. Figures 12.3 and 12.4 are examples of the artwork from Louise's story.

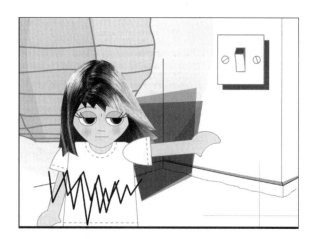

Figure 12.3 Light switch compulsion.

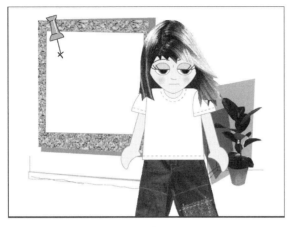

Figure 12.4 Learning to deal with OCD.

Sam

'About bullying: Not letting things get out of control'

Sam talks about his experience of being bullied in primary school, and again when he moved to secondary school. He talks about the bullying which has now eased off, but still happens from time to time, and how he has learned to cope with this. Figures 12.5 and 12.6 are examples of the artwork from Sam's story.

The full text of Sam's story is reproduced in Box 12.1 below.

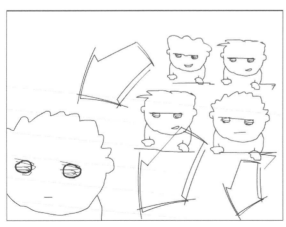

Figure 12.5 Sam feels picked on by peers.

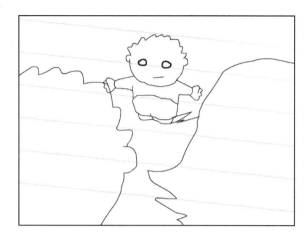

Figure 12.6 Getting support from parents.

Kevin

'Beating bullying: being bullied can really affect you'

Kevin is very clear in advising other young people who are being bullied to talk to someone about it. His view is that talking things over helps, and he has found some solutions to the problem of bullying. These have helped him to feel better and to have a positive attitude now.

Susan

'A sad story: It took time, but I learned to live with my brother's death'

Susan tells a very moving story about how she and her family were affected by her brother's death by suicide. At times, Susan felt so low that she felt suicidal herself. She confided in a friend who told her mother, who then got her help. Through counselling Susan was able to talk through her feelings about her brother and this helped her cope better. Though she still misses her brother, she can also recall happy memories about him. Figures 12.7 and 12.8 are examples of the artwork from Susan's story.

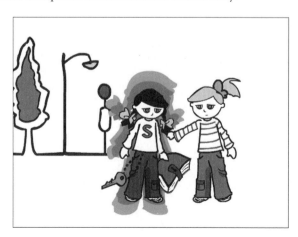

Figure 12.7 Susan feels depressed.

Box 12.1 Sam's story

'About Bullying—Not letting things get out of control'

Using Sam's story

Sam's story would be suitable for any young person who has been or is being bullied. There is a definite link between depression and being bullied in young people,
and many victims of bullying do not tell anyone about it, and so it may be worth
showing this story to anyone who may be at risk of being bullied, and asking their
views about it. This may help them open up and talk about their experience and
with discussion it could also help them generate strategies to deal with actual or
potential bullying. This is also a useful story to show to a class or youth group as a
part of a wider programme for tackling or preventing bullying.

Complete story script

*'When I was going into fifth class in primary school I moved to a new school and for
the first few months I was happy. It was a big change but I thought my classmates
seemed like nice guys and I thought that I'd get used to it. After a couple of months they
turned nasty for no reason. The name-calling, the verbal abuse was the worst, but
sometimes it got physical too—you know. The thing with bullies is that they go for
people who either seem very quiet or very forward, forward as in they see you as a
threat, and quiet as in you're an easy victim. If you're in the middle they won't really
go for you.*

*It started off very light, just the odd comment, but it got worse and worse. They'd
always be looking for a fight. They thought they were hard men. They used to set
people up to fight against each other. They did that to me. That was the only way
to get their respect, was to take on one of the big guys in the class and win. Someone
would come up to me and say I heard what you said about me and I wouldn't have
said anything. Or they'd try to get me in trouble with the teachers. I think they
might have bullied me because I was probably cleverer than they were. You had
to act stupid; you had to act stupid, to be accepted cause if you were clever they'd
see you as an outsider. I had a different background too and I didn't fit in with
their way of thinking. I felt anxious, stressed and uptight about going to school. I'd
do anything to get out of going. I pretended to be sick, I even made myself sick
sometimes.*

*Eventually I got angry with what was going on. I told the principal first and then my
parents. My parents were shocked but they really helped me to move on and deal with
it all. At the time they had this programme called—The Stay Safe Programme—going
on at school. It encouraged people to go and tell if they were being bullied. The principal gave the bullies a warning and it went okay for a while but it never really stopped
completely. Sometimes, it worked out worse when you told cause they'd see you as a rat
and no one would trust you.*

Box 12.1 Sam's story *(continued)*

Myself and my Mom, started looking into other secondary schools because I didn't want to go to the one that the primary school was linked up to.

My first year in secondary went fine, but in second year I started getting rebellious. Well, I got into fights with other guys and I was in trouble with teachers too. I'd give cheeky answers and wouldn't do my homework. I probably lost respect for their authority because the teachers in my old school didn't help me and I tarred them all with the same brush. If they said white I'd say black, just for an argument. It was like I was taking out my frustration over what happened in primary school.

I'd take the frustration home with me too and take it out on my family. I'd be moody and would shout at them over small things. They'd react and it would erupt into one big row. Later when things calmed down we'd talk about it and it would get sorted.

Then over the summer before the Junior Cert. year I just decided that I wasn't going to go back to school with that attitude. I didn't like how I was behaving myself. I asked my parents if I could see a counsellor. It really helped having someone to listen. He never really told me what to do or anything, it was just very relaxed and I got a lot of things off my chest. When I went back to school I was feeling a lot better and that year went well for me. I did well in my Junior Cert. and this year in school hasn't been a bother.

If I hadn't got help and dealt with the problem I'd say I'd still be the same guy I was in second year, and I'm glad I'm not that person any more. It was mainly me that got me through, but with support from my family and friends. I feel my experiences have made me more street-wise and more independent. I look back now and think what was I so upset about—they were all just idiots. My advice is get help early on, and don't let things get too out of control'.

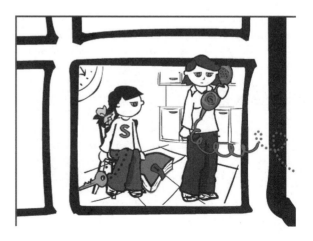

Figure 12.8 Getting help.

John

'?' (Question Mark): My feelings in song

John expresses his experience with music and lyrics.

Brian

'My Story: Coming back after being at rock bottom'

Brian had a lot of bad experiences. He was sexually abused, suffered bullying, and was so depressed that he attempted suicide. He talks about how things were for him when he felt suicidal, and how he slowly got his life back on track, with help from other people. He now feels good about himself, and has a strong message of hope for other young people who may feel despair.

Michelle

'Shocked into reality: Other kids at school were calling me fat'

Michelle talks about when she had an eating disorder and how distorted her view of herself was at that time. Fear of having to go into hospital was what made her start to deal with her eating disorder, and with the support of her mother she began to manage better.

Linda

'The terrors: Managing my anger and my stress'

Linda describes how her anger and stress made things very difficult for her in her family, and how that made her more angry. Being able to talk about things helped, as did finding new ways of expressing her anger, and dealing with her stress.

Amy

'A last resort: Harming myself was not the answer'

Amy talks about how she got into the habit of cutting herself as a way of dealing with the unbearable feelings she was experiencing, and how she came to realize that cutting herself was not the answer. She found different ways of coping, in particular avoiding time alone ruminating, and spending more time with people.

Who can use 'Working Things Out'?

'Working Things Out' can be used by professionals working with individual young people or with groups, in mental health services, in counselling, youth work, or school settings. It can be used by the full range of professionals who work with young adolescents in these settings, including psychologists, psychiatrists, psychotherapists, social workers, counsellors, teachers, community workers, and youth leaders.

Some of the stories deal with issues such as bullying (Sam's story, Kevin's story), depression (Jack's story), problems with parents, and peers (Linda's story), which are relevant to a wide range of adolescents, while others are more suited for use in mental health clinical settings, as they deal with more serious mental health issues such as eating disorders (Michelle's story), obsessive compulsive disorder (Louise's story), self-harm (Amy's story), and suicidality (Brian's story).

Working Things Out is not designed as a self-help guide for young people to use on their own. It is designed as a tool to facilitate communication between a young person and the professional working with them.

Limitations to the use of 'Working Things Out'

The 'Working Things Out' stories were told by white Irish young people with Irish accents. This may or may not limit its usefulness with young people from different cultures. It is assumed that young people are more likely to identify with those who are most similar to them in terms of gender, colour, ethnic background, and socio-economic group, but there has been little research in this area, and what has been done has shown that attribute similarity does not automatically enhance identification or modelling (Schunk, 1987).

Many of the stories in 'Working Things Out' describe family conflict, but also much support from parents. This may limit their use with young people who do not have family support, or who are in the care of the state because their families are unable to care for them. We have used the stories with such young people, focussing on helping them to identify who might be 'support people' in their lives.

None of the 'Working Things Out' stories describe extreme behavioural difficulties, such as may occur in conduct disorder. Young people with such difficulties are often the most difficult to engage, and future plans for 'Working Things Out' include additional stories by young people who have overcome such behaviours, and stories by young people from a variety of ethnic backgrounds.

Uses for 'Working Things Out'

'Working Things Out' may be used in a variety of situations and settings:

1. As a tool for engagement in clinical or community mental health settings

2. As a tool to illustrate cognitive–behavioural therapy concepts

3. In group work with adolescents

4. To help parents understand mental health difficulties from the young person's perspective

5. As a mental health resource in classroom settings.

As a tool for engagement in clinical or community mental health settings

'Working Things Out' can be used with young people aged 11 years and over referred to clinical or community mental health services with a range of emotional and/or behavioural problems. It is used to facilitate communication between a young person and a therapist and in particular to help a young person open up and to begin to tell their story. It is particularly useful for 'reluctant attenders' who are often there because they have been put under some pressure to attend by their teachers, parents, or carers. Such young people are often fearful and angry. They may feel that nothing can be done to help in their particular situation, or that no-one else has ever felt the way they do. Many feel that they are 'going mad'. The stories in 'Working Things Out' may help to allay some of these fears. 'Working Things Out' provides a useful way of engaging young people who might find it initially hard to express themselves or to put words on their experience. Hearing the experience of a peer who has overcome a similar difficulty is reassuring, and helps the young people to develop insight into their own situation. Viewing the stories often helps a young person to 'get going' and to open up and describe their own experiences.

Which story to use in clinical settings?

Deciding which stories to use will depend on the clinical presentation of the young person. The referral information and initial assessment interview will give an overview of the young person's problem areas, strengths, and level of engagement. This will help the professional to decide which stories to use in subsequent sessions. The key to using 'Working Things Out' successfully is to have a thorough knowledge of the content of the young people's stories on the CD-ROM/DVD, so that it is possible to match as closely as possible the story/stories to be used with the difficulties being faced by the referred young person. There will never be a perfect match, but choosing a story with which the young person can identify at some level is important. Matching for gender is important in early sessions, but from clinical experience, seems less so once the young person has become engaged.

As part of the engagement process, it is important to remember to clarify issues of confidentiality with the young person, and with the parents/carers. This is an important and complex area, and practice will be governed by legislation, the policy of the agency in which the work is taking place, and individual factors relating to the young person.

Young people with suicidal behaviour

Suicidal ideation is relatively common in adolescents in general. Several community-based studies have shown rates varying from 4% to 20% (Garrison et al., 1991; Grunbaum et al., 2002). Young people with depressive disorders are at particular risk (Mann et al., 2005; Tuisku et al., 2006). A study by Liu et al. (2006) of a sample of over 500 young people with major depressive disorders attending mental health facilities showed that almost half had suicidal ideation, 30% had a suicide plan, and 12% had attempted suicide.

Two of the 'Working Things Out' stories (Brian's and Susan's) refer to suicidal behaviour, while a third (Amy's) describes the use of self cutting as a means of relieving unbearable feelings. In all three stories, the young people describe their suicidal or self-harming behaviour in the context of how they were feeling when they were at 'rock bottom' and talk in some detail about how they coped and moved on from those most difficult times. Using these stories with young people who have engaged in suicidal behaviour can be very useful, helping to reduce their feelings of isolation and showing them how other young people have managed to get their lives 'back on track' after a suicide attempt.

We recommend only using Brian's, Susan's, or Amy's stories in young people who have engaged in suicidal behaviour. Because of concerns about 'copycat' suicidal behaviour, we would not use them with young people who have not engaged in suicidal behaviour.

Introducing 'Working Things Out' to a young person

We find it works best to introduce 'Working Things Out' to the young person as something that we are interested in getting their views on, rather than necessarily suggesting that they might find it useful. Using this approach helps to establish a collaborative way of working, which often helps circumvent the understandable 'resistance' of young people to engaging in therapy. We explain that 'Working Things Out' was made by a group of young people who had come through difficult times in their lives, and that they made it in order to share their experiences with other young people. We invite them to look at the story we have selected, and to give us their views on what the young person in the story has experienced and what helped them to get through. The process of the therapist and the young person jointly engaging with the computer, rather than directly with each other, is reassuring for many young people who find direct face to face interaction too daunting.

It is best to show the story in full initially, and then, depending on the response of the young person, to go over it again, pausing to highlight certain points and to open discussion. The control buttons can be used to pause, rewind, and fast forward at any point in the story.

It can be best to initially use a 'third person' approach, focusing on the young person in the story rather than asking the client directly about their own experiences, as this is less threatening especially for young people who find expressing themselves difficult.

Examples of third party questions:

- What do you think of what Sam in the story was going through?
- How do you think he was feeling? What was his family feeling?
- What made the difference in helping him cope?
- If you were a friend of Sam, how would you help him?

In practice, most young people quickly identify with the young people in the stories, and spontaneously relate the content of the stories to their own experience. Once some trust is established, it can be useful to explore this with them with questions such as

- Have you gone through anything similar?
- How would you cope with a similar situation?
- Was there a time when you felt a bit like Sam?
- How did you deal with this?

Each story includes some Professional's Comments, which give ideas and questions that may help to open up communication with the young person.

As a tool to illustrate cognitive behavioural therapy concepts

The evidence base for cognitive behavioural therapy (CBT) in the treatment of mild to moderate depressive disorders in young people has been established (Brent et al., 1997; Weisz et al., 1997; Clarke et al., 1999, 2002; Compton et al., 2004; March et al., 2006; Kennard et al., 2006). In the more severe disorders, where antidepressant medication may be necessary to help lift the young person's mood to a level where they can engage in therapy, cognitive behaviour therapy may also have a role to play (National

Institute for Health and Clinical Excellence Guidelines, 2005; Murray & Cartwright-Hatton, 2006). There are a number of manualized CBT treatment programmes for adolescent depression available (Clarke et al., 1990; Lewinsohn et al., 1996; Curry et al., 2000), but many young people attending mental health services have comorbid psychiatric disorders, language, communication, and learning difficulties that may make it hard for them to grasp CBT concepts. This is where 'Working Things Out' can be used to great effect. The visual, 'real life', personalized, peer delivered messages can be used to bring CBT concepts to life. In Box 12.2 and in Box 12.3, we give the scripts

Box 12.2 Linda's story

'The terrors—Managing my anger and my stress'

Using the story

The opening of this story focuses on 'bad moods', rows, and conflict with parents and then goes on to explore the reasons for this (bullying, pressure in school, etc). It would be a good story to show a young person who is experiencing 'angry moods' and/or conflict with their parents in order to help them express and understand their feelings and to begin to understand underlying reasons. The story could also be used with a young person dealing with parental separation.

Complete story script

'I'm always fighting with my Mam. They are usually over stupid things like not tidying my room, or not feeding the cat. Or like if I come home from school and I'm in a bad mood after a hard day. I lash out at her over stupid small things. I'd say something and like she'd just say something back and I'd just give her loads of cheek, and I'd shout, "I hate you" and run up to my room and if anybody came near me it's like walking into a death zone.

The whole family knows to keep away from me when I'm in a mood. They're like, they're like, "oh, steer clear of her, she's in her mood again, she's in The Terrors . . . again."

The last year at school has been really difficult. I was coming home upset and I wasn't eating as much and my Mam was really worried about me. The girls in the class were really really mean to me. I was paranoid going in to school every morning about what would happen that day. It was kind of bullying, except I wasn't hit or anything, mostly just being mean. I'd try not to listen to them, like I'd ignore them completely. My Mam helped me a lot through that year; though I sometimes lashed out at her, she was always there for me.

I was getting stressed with what was happening in school and with study and with my Mam, so I went to see a psychiatrist. My Mam set it up. It was easier to talk to someone outside the family about the family, getting tips on how to relax and cope. I could talk about my problems with my Mam, it was kinda like bitching about her to someone else. I had a chance to get it all out. It was scary the first time to go in, I'm shy when I meet someone new. Then after I opened up, I got to know the routine and I liked going. I just went with the flow.

Box 12.2 Linda's story *(continued)*

The older I get, things seem to get better, it was worse last year. I am getting out of that school and going to another new school next year. I'm looking forward to making a new start.

In the family I've taken more responsibility, I'm the eldest and I feel I should be setting an example for the other three. I'm trying to 'cop on' and make more of an effort. I try not to let things bother me as much.

There have been other times when I have had to deal with stuff as well. When my Dad and my Mam split up, I was real upset over that. I was only 6. After my Dad left, it was only the three of us, me, my brother and my Mam, so we had to stick by each other. They were always fighting before they split up—they tried to not let us hear. I was so young I didn't really understand. My Mam married again, and when she first got her new boyfriend I was really upset because I wasn't giving up on my Dad coming back. I don't mind about it now. I get on great with my stepfather, and I have a new stepbrother and stepsister. They are really young, and I love them. My brother waddles around like a penguin around the house—he's lovely and my sister is a real drama queen. It's great there's always something to laugh about with them.'

of Linda's and Brian's stories respectively and describe how they could be used as tool to illustrate cognitive–behavioural techniques.

Discussion of Linda's story could be used to illustrate CBT concepts:

Show the link between thoughts, feelings, and behaviour

> *'I'm always fighting with my Mam. They are usually over small things like not tidying my room, or not feeding the cat. Or like if I come home from school and I'm in a bad mood after a hard day. I lash out at her over stupid small things . . .'.*

Identify all the different thoughts, feelings, and behaviours that Linda described

Illustrate automatic negative thoughts

> *'I was paranoid going in to school every morning about what would happen that day'.*

Demonstrate and discuss coping strategies:

> *'I'd try not to listen to them, like I'd ignore them completely'.*

Give an example of externalizing the problem:

> *'. . .she's in The Terrors again'.*

Show how being able to talk about the difficulties can be helpful

> *'. . .then after I opened up, I got to know the routine and I liked going',*

Introduce the concept of taking control

> *'In the family I've taken more responsibility . . .I'm trying to cop on and make more of an effort'.*

Box 12.3 Brian's story

'Coming back after being at rock bottom'

Using the Story

Brian takes a relatively long-term view in this story, saying that though he suffered a lot and was at rock bottom, he was eventually able to come through it all and not only cope but also to learn how to be happy. His message of hope could be useful to many young people who are in despair and might be able to help them take a long-term view. The story particularly deals with attempted suicide and might be helpful to young people who have got to this point in their lives.

Complete story script

'*When I was younger I went through a lot. I was at school, maybe in 1st or 2nd class, when things started to get bad. I hadn't really planned it or anything, but one day my Mum asked me, "how are you?" and everything just came out. My granddad was sexually abusing me.*

I had a pretty good relationship with my Mum, so maybe that was why I was able to tell her.

After that a lot of people came to my house—asking questions—like social workers, and I went to see a therapist. There was a court case but nobody really told me or explained to me, what was going on. My parents probably thought we mustn't trouble him with all this information, where in fact I really wanted to know.

I was glad I told, because even though it caused a lot of upset in the house, and fights between my Mum and Dad, the abuse stopped. I felt responsible because I was the one who told. I had blurted out this dark secret . . .but I still think it was the right thing to do.

After that I became—kind of—introverted around my parents. That's why I didn't tell them about the bullying at school. It started off as name calling, not really physical bullying, but as time went on it got more intense. It seemed like everyone was ganging up on me. When it's everyday—it wears you down and then you begin to think, "oh, it is me". I felt alone, always alone, being the last to be picked for the team, for everything . . .I spent a lot of time alone in my room . . .I had too much time to dwell on everything that had happened, and had too much time to think negatively about myself. I tried to commit suicide by taking an overdose. It was like everything had mounted up into one big feeling of hatred for myself. I was at a really big low.

After I attempted suicide I was hospitalized and it was suggested that I see a psychiatrist. I wasn't ready to talk, I found opening up to a stranger was hard. They didn't make me feel like they wanted to listen. I was sitting in a big room and felt quite small—I felt like they were looking down on me. I didn't really open up.

I did feel some relief though because I felt that finally someone knew there was something wrong.

Box 12.3 Brian's story *(continued)*

As I got a bit older things got better. It was one summer that things just changed, before secondary school. I seemed to make more friends and when I got to secondary school, I was meeting people I had more in common with. I suppose the bullies grew up too and matured; they grew out of the mentality that because someone is different, they are an automatic target. Slowly the bullying faded away. Things started to go well for me in secondary school. I got into art and music. I was doing better academically. I found my niche a bit more.

Through school I was offered help again at a time when I was more ready to talk. For the first time it was said to me that I had depression. This really helped me to identify what was wrong. With the psychiatrist, I learned that there were things I could do to help myself more. . . . I also realized that there were a lot of people there to support me. I started getting on much better with my sister after that—she is probably one of my best friends now.

Despite all the bad things that can happen in your life, things move on and things get better, your attitudes change, relationships change and maybe you can't always see it, but there are people to help you. You should pursue that rather than staying alone. I like myself now; before I hated how I thought I was coming across to other people. I hated how I looked. I'm relaxed now and have found an image that suits me better. I have friends with similar interests who I am able to talk to about my experiences.

People like me now, I like myself.

Before, I would have been dreading the future—it all came out as self-hatred and then attempts at suicide, which was the ultimate low, but now I have a great hope for my future where I've gotten through all these bad events. I have a better life now and have a much more positive attitude. I'm able to look on the bright side of things. Though I'm not feeling very depressed now it doesn't mean I don't have problems, but I've learnt to deal with them better and that's what's important'

Discussion of Brian's story could be used to illustrate CBT concepts:

Show the link between thoughts, feelings, and behaviour

'*I felt alone, always alone, being the last to be picked for the team, for everything . . . I spent a lot of time alone in my room . . . I had too much time to dwell on everything that had happened, and had too much time to think negatively about myself*'.

Discuss the importance of telling someone if you are going through a bad time:

'*When I was younger I went through a lot. I was at school, maybe in 1st or 2nd class, when things started to get bad. I hadn't really planned it or anything, but one day my Mum asked me, "how are you?" and everything just came out*'.

Explore finding enjoyable activities:

'*Things started to go well for me in secondary school. I got into art and music*'.

Introduce the concept of taking control:

> '. . .I learned that there were things I could do to help myself more.. . .'

Show how Brian got his life back on track after being 'at rock bottom':

> 'I like myself now; before I hated how I thought I was coming across to other peo-
> ple. I hated how I looked. I'm relaxed now and have found an image that suits me
> better'.

> 'Despite all the bad things that can happen in your life things move on and things
> get better, your attitudes change, relationships change and maybe you can't always
> see it, but there are people to help you. You should pursue that rather than staying
> alone'.

In addition many of the other stories have other specific examples of cognitive–
behavioural techniques in action. For example
Susan's story has some useful advice about rumination:

> 'The worst thing you could do if you ever get upset is to stay in your room on your own,
> because it's horrible. When I'd sit in my room on my own it made me worse . . .'.

Louise's story is about gaining control of obsessive compulsive disorder, and makes
clear the concept of goal setting:

> 'I was started on a weekly programme where we set goals and targets every week,
> and then I'd try to achieve them. Little by little I was trying to spend less time on
> my routines . . .'

Each of the stories can be used in this way to bring cognitive–behavioural therapy
concepts to life.

In group work with adolescents

The 'Working Things Out' Clinical Treatment Programme is a 10 session CBT intervention with a strong focus on skills, which can be delivered in group or individual
format. The intervention is currently being evaluated as part of a 36-month research
project at the Child and Adolescent Mental Health Service (CAMHS) at the Mater
Misericordiae University Hospital, Dublin. The aim of the evaluation is to measure
the treatment effectiveness of this multimedia-enhanced CBT intervention in comparison with routine clinical care in adolescents with depressive and other comorbid
disorders attending CAMHS. In developing the programme, we have adapted some
ideas from existing treatment manuals, including the Treatment of Adolescent
Depression Study Manual (Curry, 2005) and the Adolescents Coping with Depression
Course (Clarke et al., 1990). Also relevant is the works of Wood and Harrington
(1998) in relation to CBT group treatments for adolescents. The aim in developing
this intervention was to create a flexible, modular programme that could be tailored
and used with adolescents with a broad range of disorders and comorbidities, as is
the norm in those attending adolescent mental health services (Verhulst & van der
Ende, 1997).

Participants

The intervention is suitable for young people aged 12–16 years, with a diagnosis of major depressive disorder, with or without a history of self-harm or suicidal behaviour. The majority of young people participating in the current evaluation have comorbid disorders, such as ADHD, Oppositional and Conduct Disorders, Anxiety Disorders, and Developmental and Language Disorders. These do not preclude the participation of such young people, with the exception of those with severe conduct disorders, hypomanic or manic disorders, psychotic disorders, or those in acute psychiatric crisis. This intervention would not be suitable for such young people.

The intervention

The intervention uses a blended model of narrative and CBT, which is enhanced by the use of multimedia as a way of engaging young people. It incorporates the use of the Working Things Out DVD and a related multimedia story building software, Transforming Stories (www.transformingstories.com). In the sessions, the stories are used to illustrate the thoughts, feelings, and actions of the story characters and to show how they may be able to bring about change by learning to take charge of how they think. The young people are given an opportunity to view and discuss how the story characters have coped with problems. The Transforming Stories software allows the young people to create their own stories and this is used as a way of reinforcing the skills learning aspect of the programme. This is used as a way of engaging the young people in learning new thought processes and thinking through alternative outcomes. Similar to Lewinsohn's programme, there is a focus on increasing the young person's time spent doing pleasant activities (Lewinsohn et al., 1996).

The intervention comprises a total of ten sessions, which involves one pre-group individual session with the young person and their parent/carer, eight group sessions, and one post-group individual session with the young person and their parent/carer.

The pre-group assessment session enables the young person and parent to meet the group leaders, to find out what will be involved in the group programme, and to define goals that they would like to achieve by attending the group. It allows the group leaders to evaluate the suitability of the young person for the group, and to clarify confidentiality issues.

Each of the eight group sessions lasts 90 minutes and follows a similar format:

- ◆ Welcome
- ◆ Agenda setting
- ◆ Review of what was covered in previous session and 'homework' tasks
- ◆ Feedback from participants on 'homework'
- ◆ Introduction of key topic for this session, illustrated by 'Working Things Out' story
- ◆ Exercise in small groups and skills practice
- ◆ Issues raised by the participants for the agenda

- Recap of main learning points
- Homework planning

Session outline

In the first 5 sessions of the programme, the young people are introduced to a variety of skills including step-by-step problem-solving and techniques in 'taking charge' of their thoughts. They are encouraged to develop a personalized plan in relation to which skills can be most usefully applied to their set of difficulties. The treatment approach is collaborative and there is also an emphasis on what is going well in the young person's life. In a mixed diagnosis treatment group, this collaborative approach is crucial in that the higher the level of collaboration and engagement, the better the treatment outcomes are likely to be.

Session 1 focuses on setting rules, developing a shared group philosophy, and participants are helped to define some of the difficulties that are affecting their lives. They look at what they have control over in their lives, differentiating between external and internal factors. They are encouraged to come up with specific and realistic goals and then plan the steps towards achieving these. This involves an exercise in converting problems to challenges. In Session 2, they learn problem-solving strategies and examples are used from the 'Working Things Out' stories to illustrate different ways of coping with difficulties. Sessions 3 and 4 deal with recognizing and labelling thoughts and feelings. The emphasis is on taking charge of these. We introduce mood monitoring and again, using the 'Working Things Out' stories we introduce the concept of how thoughts affect how we feel and behave. The homework tasks for these sessions involve thought and mood records. In the sessions, the participants practice replacing unhelpful thoughts with more helpful positive thoughts and monitoring the outcome in terms of feelings and behaviour. Session 5 introduces externalising as a strategy for dealing with depression, anger, anxiety, and other difficulties. We also do a series of breathing and a relaxation exercises. In Sessions 6 and 7, the young people are encouraged to apply the strategies learnt in the previous sessions. The final session reviews the course content and focuses on the theme of 'Moving On'. We look at what can be done to prevent relapse and we identify appropriate help seeking strategies.

Evaluation

The programme is being evaluated using a mixed methods approach. The desired outcomes of the intervention include reducing suicidal and self-harming thoughts and behaviours, reducing depressive symptoms, improving the young person's problem-solving and coping skills and improving ability to communicate about emotions.

An initial assessment interview is done using the KSADS-PL (Kaufman et al., 1997), which is a semi-structured standardized diagnostic interview carried out with the young person and with a parent. The K-SADS diagnostic profile gives a comprehensive overview of the young person's problem areas. The standardized questionnaires scores described below will give further information of the young person's and the parents' strengths and challenges, along with a standardized measure of the young person's level of functioning prior to the intervention.

Study participants complete the following questionnaires pre- and post-intervention, and at 6-month follow-up:

1. *The Strengths and Difficulties Questionnaire* (SDQ) (Goodman, 1997), which is a behavioural screening questionnaire that provides information on young people's behaviours, emotions, and relationships.

2. *The Children's Coping Strategies Checklist* (CCSC) (Ayers & Sandler, 1996), which is a self-rated questionnaire that provides a measure of children's coping strategies in four domains: support seeking, avoidance, active coping, and distraction.

3. *The Adolescent Well-being Scale* (Birelson et al., 1987), which is designed to pick up possible depression in older children and adolescents. The scale has eighteen questions, each relating to different aspects of an adolescent's life, and how they feel about them.

A Demographic Questionnaire is also completed to address the demographic variables of the participants, including age, gender, family composition and living circumstances.

Throughout the group sessions the Youth Session Rating Scale (Duncan et al., 2003) is used to get feedback from participant on their satisfaction with group content and process.

In addition to the quantitative data described above, qualitative data is being gathered using semi-structured interviews, focus groups, and feedback questionnaires designed to pick up the young peoples' views and feelings about process and content of the sessions.

A matched control group of adolescents attending routine clinical treatment is being used for comparative data in this study. The profile of the control group is carefully matched with the treatment group in relation to gender, age, general diagnosis, severity of difficulties, socio economic factors, previous interventions, and family factors.

To help parents understand mental health difficulties from the young person's perspective

Depressive disorders in adolescence are often characterized by an irritable mood, rather than by withdrawn behaviour or sadness (American Psychiatric Association, 1994). Such young people are not easy to live with, and cycles of negative interaction can easily develop in families in which an adolescent has a depressive disorder. Parents, siblings, and teachers often fail to recognize that the young person is suffering from depression, seeing him rather as someone with an 'attitude' or 'behaviour' problem. In such families, parental anger and criticism may be marked, and may lead to worsening of depressive symptoms in the young person. Several studies have shown an association between 'expressed emotion' and depressive disorders in young people, with some suggesting a protective effect of low 'expressed emotion' (McCleary & Sanford, 2002; Asarnow et al., 1994; Nelson et al., 2003; Miklowitz et al., 2006).

Inviting parents to view 'Working Things Out' stories can help them to better understand what their son/daughter is experiencing. This was first suggested by an adolescent with a depressive disorder with whom one of the 'Working Things Out' stories was being used in therapy. The experience was very helpful in that situation, and is now often used in our clinical practice in situations where the young person and the parent consider it might be helpful. Whether this has a role to play in reducing 'expressed emotion' has not been evaluated.

Child and adolescent mental health professionals are often asked to address Support Groups for parents of young people with a variety of mental health difficulties. 'Working Things Out' stories can bring these talks to life by giving a voice to the experiences of 'real' young people.

As a mental health resource in classroom settings

> It is clear that schools remain a crucial social institution for the education of children in preparation for life. But they need to be more involved in a broader educational role fostering healthy social and emotional development of pupils.
>
> (World Health Organization Fact Sheet No. 220)

The World Health Organization makes explicit reference to the importance of schools as important sites for socialisation and primary health promotion activities. The development of the European Network of Health Promoting Schools (ENHPS) movement has also highlighted the role of schools in promoting good health (WHO, 1996). Recent years have witnessed an expanding role for schools and teachers in promoting good health practices, with increasing recognition of the complexities of this process (Rowling & Jeffreys, 2006). For professionals wishing to promote positive mental health in young people, schools provide a unique opportunity to carry out such work, through provision of a 'captive audience' (Rutter et al., 1979).

There is a growing evidence-base on what schools need to do to promote mental health effectively (Weare & Markham, 2005). The most effective mental health promotion programmes in schools are multi-dimensional and use a 'whole school' approach, which creates a supportive climate of warmth, empathy, positive expectations, and clear boundaries. Such programmes involve teachers, pupils, and parents in their development and implementation, and provide effective training and support for those who deliver the programmes. Programmes that respect adolescents' own coping styles, rather than imposing adults' views of 'healthy coping' are more effective, as are those that include an element of peer modelling (Oliver et al., 2006).

In Ireland, the Social Personal and Health Education Programme, under the auspices of the Department of Education and Science, is part of the curriculum for all Primary schools, and for the first three years in Post-primary schools, with plans to extend it throughout the Post-primary cycle (Social Personal and Health Education, 2000). It involves a whole school approach to the promotion of positive personal development, including general health and mental health. While time is set aside each week within the curriculum for discussion of aspects of the SPHE programme, teachers are encouraged to use opportunities presented throughout the school day to explore and foster personal development. Strands of the programme ('Myself', 'Myself and Others', 'Myself and the Wider World') are taught throughout the student's school life, using an approach that is consistent with the developmental level of the students. 'Working Things Out' stories are being used to bring aspects of the SPHE programme to life, by showing young people talking about the effects of bullying and how they coped (Sam's story and Kevin's story), the importance of communication (Jack's story), and when and how to seek help for emotional difficulties (Linda's story, Ciara's story and Jack's story).

Evaluation

To examine the effectiveness of enhancing SPHE by using 'Working Things Out' stories, a pilot study was conducted over two years in seven post-primary schools in the Dublin area. The schools (2 all-female, 2 all-male, and 3 co-educational) were randomly assigned to control and enhanced conditions. Those in the control group received standard SPHE instruction, while those in the enhanced group received the WTO resource materials as well as teacher training and ongoing support. The Children's Coping Strategy Checklist (CCSC; Ayers, 1996) and the Strengths and Difficulties Questionnaire (SDQ; Goodman, 1997) were administered to 306 students at pre-, post-, and 6–8 month follow-up. Pupils were also asked to listen to two audio vignettes and answer a number of questions around problem identification, emotions, and help-seeking. Students experiencing the highest level of difficulty (borderline-clinical range on SDQ) were found to gain most benefit from the programme. Schools, teachers, and pupils all reported positive gains from this work, particularly in the areas of mental health awareness and information, teacher comfort in discussing 'sensitive' topics and in schools' commitment to a whole-school health approach. This pilot study confirmed previous promising findings about the usefulness of schools' mental health promotion work. While the results of this pilot are very promising, the refinement of both teaching approaches and the evaluation methodologies used remains an ongoing challenge for workers in the schools' mental health area.

Conclusion

'Working Things Out' is an interactive CD-ROM/DVD that tells the stories of eleven young people who have overcome depression and other mental health difficulties. It is a resource for professionals working with young people with depressive disorders and other mental health difficulties. This chapter describes how it may be used in a variety of mental health clinical and community settings. Further information is available at www.parentsplus.ie

Acknowledgements

We wish to acknowledge the young people whose stories form the basis of 'Working Things Out'. They most generously gave their time and enthusiasm to the project, and we want to thank them and their parents.

Special thanks go to the multimedia design team who worked hard on making this project a success. They are Bernadette McCarthy, Ciara Devine, Pilar Valencia, Hugh

O' Neill, Peter McCormack, and John Stapleton. We are particularly indebted to our funders (The Northern Area Health Board, The National Suicide Review Group, The Mater Foundation, Parents Plus Charity, The Ireland Funds the Health Research Board) for making this project possible. Thanks also to our colleagues at the Mater Misericordiae University Hospital, Dublin, and the many others who supported the project.

References

American Psychiatric Association (1994). *Diagnostic and Statistical Manual of Mental Disorders* (4th ed.) Washington, DC: American Psychiatric Association.

Asarnow, J.R., Tompson, M., Hamilton, E.B., Goldstein, M.J., & Guthrie, D. (1994). Family-expressed emotion, childhood-onset depression, and childhood-onset schizophrenia spectrum disorders: is expressed emotion a nonspecific correlate of child psychopathology or a specific risk factor for depression? *Journal of Abnormal Child Psychology, 22(2),* 129–46.

Ayers, T. & Sandler, S. (1996). *Manual for the children's coping strategies checklist.* Arizona: Arizona State University Program for Prevention Research.

Birelson, P., Hudson, I., Buchanan, D.G., & Wolff, S. (1987). Clinical evaluation of self-rating scale for depressive disorder in childhood. *Journal of Child Psychology and Psychiatry, 28,* 43–60.

Brent, D., Holden, D., Kolko, D., Birmaher, B., Baugher, M., Roth, C., et al. (1997). A clinical psychotherapy trial for adolescent depression comparing cognitive, family and supportive treatments. *Archives of General Psychiatry, 54,* 877–885.

Brosnan, E., Sharry, J., Fitzpatrick, C., & Boyle, R. (2005). Transforming Stories. *Annual Review of Cybertherapy and Telemedicine, 3,* 224–225.

Clarke, G.N., Hops, H., Lewinsohn, P.M., Andrew, J., & Williams, J. (1992). Cognitive behavioural group treatment of adolescent depression. *Behavioural Therapy, 23,* 341–354.

Clarke, G., Hornbook, M., Lynch, F., Polen, M., Gale, J., O'Connor, E., et al. (2002). Group cognitive–behavioural treatment for depressed adolescent offspring of depressed parents in a health maintenance organization. *Journal of the American Academy of Child and Adolescent Psychiatry, 41,* 305–313.

Clarke, G.N., Lewinsohn, P.M., & Hops, H. (1990). *Instructor's manual for the adolescent coping with depression course* (4th ed.). Eugene, OR: Castalia Press.

Clarke, G. N., Rohde, P., Lewinsohn, P. M., Hops, H., & Seeley J. R. (1999). Cognitive behavioural treatment of adolescent depression: efficacy of acute group treatment and booster sessions. *Journal of the American Academy of Child and Adolescent Psychiatry, 38,* 272–279.

Compton, S.N., March, J.S., Brent, D., Albano, A.M., 5th, Weersing, R., & Curry, J. (2004). Cognitive–behavioral psychotherapy for anxiety and depressive disorders in children and adolescents: An evidence-based review. *Journal of the American Academy of Child and Adolescent Psychiatry, 43,* 930–959.

Conduit, T., Byrne, S., Court, J., & Stefanovic, S. (2004). Non-attendance at a university-based psychology clinic: Telephone appointment reminders versus no reminders. *Australian Psychologist, 39,* 68–75.

Curry, J. (2005). Treatment for Adolescents with Depression Study (TADS). *Cognitive behaviour therapy manual.* Durham, NC: Duke University Medical Center.

Curry, J. (2006). Predictors and moderators of acute outcome in the Treatment for Adolescents with Depression Study (TADS). *Journal of Child Psychology and Psychiatry, 45,* 587–595.

Diamond, G.S., Liddle, H.A., Wintersteen, M.B., Dennis, M.L., Godley, S.H., & Tims, F. (2006). Early therapeutic alliance as a predictor of treatment outcome for adolescent cannabis users in outpatient treatment. *The American Journal on Addictions, 15*, 26–33.

Duncan, B.L., Miller, S., Sparks, J.A., & Johnson L.D. (2003). Youth Session Rating Scale.

Fitzpatrick, C. & Sharry, J. (2004). *Coping with depression in young people—a guide for parents.* England: John Wiley and Sons.

Garrison, C.Z., Jackson, K.L., Addy, C.L., McKeown, R.E., & Waller, J.L. (1991). Suicidal behaviors in young adolescents. *American Journal of Epidemiology, 133*, 1005–1014.

Goodman, R. (1997). The strengths and difficulties questionnaire: A research note. *Journal of Child Psychology and Psychiatry, 38*, 581–586.

Grunbaum, J.A., Kann, L., Kinchen, S.A., Williams, B., Ross, J.G., Lowry, R., et al. (2002). Youth risk behavior surveillance—United States, 2001. *MMWR CDC Surveillance Summary, 51(SS4)*, 1–64.

Gunther, N., Slavenburg, B., Feron, F., & van Os, J. (2003). Childhood social and early developmental factors associated with mental health service use. *Social Psychiatry and Psychiatric Epidemiology, 38*, 101–108.

Heppell, S. (1994). Multimedia and learning: Normal children, normal lives and real change. In J. Underwood (Ed.), *Computer based learning, potential into practice* (pp. 56–62). London: David Fulton.

Hoare, P., Norton, B., Chisolm, D., & Parry-Jones, W. (1996). An audit of 7000 successive child and adolescent psychiatry referrals in Scotland. *Clinical Child Psychology and Psychiatry, 1*, 229–249.

Kaufman, J., Birmaher, B., Brent, D., Rao, U., Flynn, C., Moreci, P., et al. (1997). Schedule for affective disorders and schizophrenia for school-aged children—Present and lifetime (K-SADS-PL): Initial reliability and validity data. *Journal of the American Academy of Child and Adolescent Psychiatry, 36*, 980–988.

Kazdin, A.E. (1996). Dropping out of child psychotherapy: Issues for research and implications for practice. *Clinical Child Psychology and Psychiatry, 1*, 133–156.

Kennard, B., Silva, S., Vitiello, B., Curry, J., Kratochvil, C., Simons, A., et al. (2006). Remission and residual symptoms after short-term treatment in the Treatment of Adolescents with Depression Study (TADS). *Journal of the American Academy of Child and Adolescent Psychiatry, 45*, 1404–1411.

Krupnick, J.L., Sotsky, S.M., Elkin, I., Simmens, S., Moyer, J., Watkins, J., et al. (1996). The role of the therapeutic alliance in psychotherapy and pharmacotherapy outcome: Findings in the National Institute of Mental Health Treatment of Depression Collaborative Research Program. *Journal of Consulting and Clinical Psychology, 64*, 532–539.

Lewinsohn, P.M., Clarke, G.N., Rohde, P., Hops, H., & Seeley, J.R. (1996). A course in coping: A cognitive–behavioural approach in the treatment of adolescent depression. In E.D. Hibbs & P.S. Jensen (Eds.). *Psychosocial treatments for child and adolescent disorders: Empirically based strategies for clinical practice.* Washington DC: American Psychiatric Association.

Liu, X., Gentzler, A.L., Tepper, P., Kiss, E., Kothencne, V.O., Tamas, Z., et al. (2006). Clinical features of depressed children and adolescents with various forms of suicidality. *Journal of Clinical Psychiatry, 67*, 1442–1450.

Lynch F., Mills, C., Daly, I., & Fitzpatrick, C. (2004). Challenging Times: a study to detect Irish adolescents at risk of psychiatric disorders and suicidal ideation. *Journal of Adolescence, 27*, 441–451.

Lynch, F., Mills, C., Daly, I., & Fitzpatrick, C. (2006). Challenging times: Prevalence of psychiatric disorders and suicidal behaviours in Irish adolescents. *Journal of Adolescence, 29*, 555–573.

Mann, J.J., Apter, A., Bertolote, J., Beautrais, A., Currier, D., Haas, A., et al. (2005). Suicide prevention strategies: A systematic review. *Journal of the American Medical Association, 294*, 2064–2074.

March, J., Silva, S., Vitiello, B., & TADS Team (2006). The treatment of adolescents with depression study (TADS): Methods and message at 12 weeks. *Journal of the American Academy of Child and Adolescent Psychiatry, 45*, 1393–403.

McCleary, L. & Sanford, M. (2002). Parental expressed emotion in depressed adolescents: prediction of clinical course and relationship to comorbid disorders and social functioning. *Journal of Child Psychology and Psychiatry, 43*, 587–595.

McKay, M.M., Stoewe, J., McCadam, K., & Gonzales, J. (1998). Increasing access to child mental health services for inner city children and their caretakers. *Health and Social Work, 23*, 9–15.

Miklowitz, D.J., Biuckians, A., & Richards, J.A. (2006). Early-onset bipolar disorder: A family treatment perspective. *Developmental Psychopathology, 18*, 1247–65.

Monk, G. & Winsdale, J. (1997). *Narrative therapy in practice: The archaeology of hope.* San Francisco: Wiley & Sons.

Murray, J. & Cartwright-Hatton, S. (2006). NICE guidelines on treatment of depression in childhood and adolescence: Implications from a CBT perspective. *Behavioural and Cognitive Psychotherapy, 34*, 129–137.

National Institute for Health and Clinical Excellence (2005). *Depression in children and young people: Identification and management in primary, community and secondary care.* London: National Institute for Health and Clinical Excellence.

Nelson, D.R., Hammen, C., Brennan, P.A., & Ullman, J.B.(2003). The impact of maternal depression on adolescent adjustment: The role of expressed emotion. *Journal of Consulting and Clinical Psychology, 71*, 935–944.

Oliver, K.G., Collin, P., Burns, J., & Nicholas, J. (2006). Building resilience in young people through meaningful participation. *Australian e-Journal for the Advancement of Mental Health (AeJAMH), 5*, 1–7.

Papert, S. (1996). *The connected family. Bridging the digital generation gap.* Atlanta: Longstreet Press.

Rowling, L. & Jeffreys, V. (2006). Capturing complexity: integrating health and education research to inform health-promoting schools policy and practice. *Health Education Research, 21*, 705–18.

Rutter, M., Maughan, B., Mortimore, P., Ouston, J., & Smith, A. (1979). *Fifteen thousand hours: Secondary schools and their effects on children.* London: Open Books.

Schunk, D.H. (1987). Peer models and children's behavioral change. *Review of Education Research, 57*, 149–174.

Social, Personal and Health Education; Junior Cycle (2000). Dublin: Government Publications Office.

Tuisku, V., Pelkonen, M., Karlsson, L., Kiviruusu, O., Holi, M., Ruuttu, T., et al. (2006). Suicidal ideation, deliberate self-harm behaviour and suicide attempts among adolescent outpatients with depressive mood disorders and comorbid axis 1 disorders. *European Child and Adolescent Psychiatry, 15*, 199–206.

Verhulst, F.C. & van der Ende, J. (1997). Factors associated with child mental health service use in the community. *Journal of the American Academy of Child and Adolescent Psychiatry, 36,* 901–909.

Weare, K. & Markham, W. (2005). What do we know about promoting mental health through schools? *Promotion and Education, 12,* 118–122.

Weisz, J.R., Southam-Gerow, M.A., Gordis, E.B., & Connors-Smith, J. (1997). The Primary and Secondary Control Enhancement Training (PASCET). In A.E. Kazdin & J.R. Weisz (Eds.) (2003), *Evidence-based psychotherapies for children and adolescents.* New York: Guilford Press.

WHO (1996). *Regional guidelines: Development of health promoting schools—A Framework for action.* WHO Regional Office for the Western Pacific: Manila, The Philippines.

Wood, A., Harrington, R., & Moore, A. (1996). Controlled trial of a brief cognitive–behavioural intervention in adolescent patients with depressive disorders. *Journal of Child Psychology and Psychiatry and Allied Disciplines, 37,* 737–746.

Part 5

Epilogue

Chapter 13

Progress and unresolved issues in the treatment of adolescent depression

Cecilia A. Essau

Depression is increasingly recognized as a common and debilitating condition in adolescents. Up to 20% of the adolescents in the general population meet the diagnosis of depressive disorders (MDD) some times in their life (Lewinsohn et al., 1993). MDD in adolescence is often chronic or recurrent, persisting into adulthood (Harrington et al., 1990; Rao et al., 1995), and that it has serious negative psychosocial consequences (Kovacs et al., 1997; Lewinsohn et al., 2003; Rao et al., 1995). Given the significant acute and chronic burden associated with this disorder, much effort has been invested in developing effective treatments. As presented in chapters 4–12 in this volume, numerous prevention and intervention programs have been developed in recent years. Consequently, the number of studies that examined the effectiveness of these programs has been increasing at a fast pace. As a result of this increased research attention, a number of progresses have been achieved in the treatment of adolescent depression. However, there are also a number of unresolved issues and challenges that deserve investigations. The goal of this chapter is to discuss some of the progress and unresolved issues in the treatment of adolescent depression.

Prevention and intervention programs for adolescent depression

Psychopharmacotherapy

Psychotropic drugs, including antidepressant, are prescribed to adolescents with increasing frequency (Zito & Riddle, 1995). The widespread use of psychotropic drugs raises the possibility that some adolescents may be inappropriately given medication when other types of intervention may be more desirable. Three broad types of antidepressants commonly used in depressed youths include tricyclic antidepressants, serotonin specific reuptake inhibitors, and monoamine oxidase inhibitors (see also chapter 10 in this volume). Unlike studies of adults, studies of adolescents have not been able to show clinical efficacy of antidepressants (e.g., imipramine, nortriptyline, desipramine, amitriptyline) and the typical monoamine oxidase inhibitors (e.g., phenelzine, tranylcypromine). Furthermore, most studies that examined the efficacy of these medications are problematic due to methodological limitations, including lack of double-blind, placebo-controlled studies. Most studies are open trials with a small sample size and, therefore, lack the statistical power to complete moderate medication effects. Standardized diagnostic procedure, well-defined outcome measures, and the use of a systematic side effect assessment have rarely been used. In addition to these methodological constraints, tricyclic antidepressant have potential negative side effects (e.g., dry mouth, sweating, constipation), which limit their use in children and adolescents. Additionally, little is known about the impact of chronic use of antidepresant. Although long-term use may produce long-term benefits and therefore improve prognosis, longer exposure to treatment may have negative influences on the child/adolescent cognitive, behaviour, and physical development (Vitiello & Jensen, 1995).

Psychological intervention

Recent years have seen the development of several psychological intervention programs for adolescents with depression (see chapters 4–12 in this volume). Most of these programs used cognitive–behavioural therapy or family-based approaches. As reviewed in chapters 4–12, these intervention programs have proved to be effective in reducing depressive symptoms and associated impairments. However, little information is known why they work for some adolescents, but not for others. Furthermore, most treatment outcome studies have major limitations, including small samples, use of a waiting-list control instead of comparing the test intervention with alternative or placebo treatment, wide range of the children, and adolescent's age. Both the generalization of treatment across settings and their maintenance over time upon ending the treatment have rarely been demonstrated. Additionally, most studies did not consider the presence of comorbid disorders or the co-occurring family problems.

In addition to these methodological problems, almost all the outcome treatment studies have been conducted within the so-called 'research therapy', which were conducted among volunteers with some predetermined inclusion and exclusion criteria in university clinics. Given differences between the real world of the clinic and the laboratory (Weisz et al., 1995), one must be cautious in interpreting the findings of the 'research therapy'. Another characteristics of the research therapy is its preference in using group as a format of delivery, probably due to their ease of administration, and also due to the fact that many studies are done in school settings. Research therapy generally uses manuals, which makes the treatment process rather inflexible. Some opponents of using manual argue that manuals are often too rigid, and a tendency to ignore individual differences. Differences in the approach used, the presence of comorbid disorders, and the severity and chronicity of depression seen in 'research therapy' and 'clinical therapy' make it difficult to compare findings obtained in these two types of studies. Therefore, treatments that are found effective for motivated adolescents and parents may not prove to show the same effect when offered to families in community clinical settings.

A crucial part of treatment research is to decide as to where to carry out the treatment, the type of treatment modality, and the duration of delivering the treatment. Given the high attrition rates in children and adolescents, it may be useful to have a treatment of short duration. On the other hand, brief intervention for depression produce a rather weak outcome, and that maximum impact can be achieved when the treatment is of longer duration. As argued by Kazdin (1997), progress in developing an effective treatment is hindered by the way in which studies are conducted, including the brief and time-limited nature of treatment of nonclinical adolescents, which are usually done in university settings.

With the introduction of managed cares that mandates time-limited therapies with proven effectiveness, we are expected to develop empirically supported treatments. Unfortunately, the criteria to determine whether the treatment is well-enough established to be considered as efficacious do not seem to match the reality of the world of the clinics.

Another challenge involves the implementation and evaluation of prevention programs. The first issue is to determine in which developmental stage of the children/adolescents the program should be started. There does not seem to be any known optimal periods for starting prevention, although a common recommendation has been to start as early as possible. The second issue is related to the strategies needed to prevent MDD, given numerous risk factors of MDD. This makes it difficult to pin-point the specific risk factors that need to be the focus of prevention. In selected prevention programs, there is a need to be clear about how the 'at-risk' children are defined. Another issue is related to putting the prevention program into practice. While most programs have been conducted in schools, schools are often over-burdened with academic curriculum demands. By adding a separate, multi-session curriculum to prevent depression, in addition to the program to prevent, for example, anxiety or conduct problems would swamp the schools. Finally, little is known about the cost of running a prevention program. Therefore, an area of future research would be to provide cost-benefit analyses, specifically, in terms of the cost of providing prevention compared to the reduction in cost of treatment for MDD. It may also be worth investigating in future studies the role of health promotion strategies such as physical health promotion, the presence of after-school-care, positive parenting, and positive coping in the reduction of MDD.

Another challenge is how to reach those who need the help the most. A large proportion of the adolescents with MDD in the community do not receive the professional help they need (Essau, 2005). Even if the adolescents with MDD start taking part in treatment, between 40–60% of families terminate the treatment prematurely (Kazdin, 1997). Another important fact is that it is usually not the child/adolescent him/herself who decides that behaviour needs attention and consequently makes the decision about referral, but an adult. Parent's likelihood to seek help for their children may be influenced by the extent to which the adolescent's behaviour is noticeable and bothersome, as well as by parent's mental health status and treatment history, family stress, and perceived benefits of treatment (Mash & Krahn, 1995). Other determinants of mental health services utilization include the severity and chronicity of depression, presence of comorbid disorders, psychosocial impairment, sociodemographic characteristics, the availability of services, as well as the cost and mechanism of financing. Weisz and Eastman (1995), in their 'adult-distress threshold model', proposed that cultural factors influence adults' expectancies and beliefs about the adolescents, which in turn influence how distressing the adolescent behaviour will be, and the type of actions that will take in response. In testing this model, perception of the seriousness of over- and under-controlled problems by using different vignettes was compared among adults in Thailand and in the USA. The Thai compared to American adults rated the adolescent's behavioural and emotional problem as less serious, unusual, and less likely to worry (Weisz et al., 1988). Adults in these 2 cultures also differ in the way in which they referred their children to clinics. The main reasons for clinic referral among Americans were that of externalizing problems, whereas among Thais this was related to internalizing problems (Weisz et al., 1988). Parents who are likely to seek help for their children may be influenced by the extent to which the child's behaviour is noticeable and bothersome, as well as by parent's mental health status and treatment history, and perceived benefits of treatment (Mash & Krahn, 1995). Thus, when summarizing this and other findings, factors that effect the adolescent's referral can be divided to include the adolescent, parents, and other's characteristics.

Several models (e.g., Goldberg & Huexley, 1980) have also been developed in an attempt to better understand the pathway to mental health services utilization. According to the Goldberg and Huxley's model (1980), there are several levels and filters that individuals with psychiatric disorders (including depression) have to go through until they come for specialist care:

- Level 1 refers to the presence of depressive and other psychiatric disorders in the general population. The presence of depressive symptoms and associated features would lead to help-seeking behaviour; however, most of those with the disorder will consult a general practitioner.

- Level 2 consists of the presentation of depressive psychiatric disorders to general practitioners, most of which may not be detected by the general practitioner.

- Level 3 ('conspicuous psychiatric morbidity') consists of those who are identified and recognized by the general practitioner as having depression and other disorders. The general practitioner may decide to help the adolescent themselves, or refer the adolescent to the specialist psychiatric services. The decision to choose from any two of these alternatives may be determined by the availability of services, kind of insurance system, and characteristics of the primary care workers (Verhulst, 1995).

- Levels 4 and 5 represent adolescents who are treated for their depression in psychiatric facilities.

The complexity of outcome measurement

To make progress towards developing an effective treatment, including that of depression, the followings have been proposed (Kazdin, 1997):

- Learning about factors related to the onset, maintenance, offset, and recurrence of depression;

- Trying to understand how the techniques used in treatment influence the process involved in depression, or counteract these influences through the development of new behaviour;

- Operationalizing treatment in manual form, which contains the content of each session, progress of treatment, and as to when and how to continue certain tasks and themes;
- Examining the impact of treatment on depressive symptoms and associated impairment;
- Identifying the components of treatment that produce or facilitate changes; and
- Examining factors that influence the effectiveness of treatment.

In addition to Kazdin's proposal (1997), there is an urgent need to develop outcome measurement. Outcome measurement of adolescent depression is complex and concerns a wide range of domains that may be considered pertinent to the evaluation of specific programs.

The symptomatic or diagnostic level: Adolescents are referred to treatment because of their depressive symptoms and associated impairment in specific life domains. In most studies, depressive symptom reduction is the main criterion for a good outcome (Kazdin, 2000), and many authors used categorical (Angold & Costello, 1995) and dimensional checklist-based (Achenbach, 1991) assessments that are completed by the adolescents themselves, their parents, or teachers. An unresolved issue is that the data from different informants often do not agree, causing difficulties in the interpretation of results. Authors differ in their view as to which information should be used. Angold et al. (1987), for example, recommended that the children's report be used to judge the accuracy of adult's report, whereas others have recommended the use of parents' report as the primary criterion (Rapee et al, 1994).

The assessment of treatment involves repeated assessments. In studies that use repeated ratings, levels of psychopathology on the second occasion tend to be lower than those in the first assessment (e.g., Boyle et al., 1987). This underscores the importance of using well-matched control groups and for supplementing symptom ratings with other assessments. Major problem with this approach is that although symptoms may indicate the presence of pathological processes they tell us little about the nature of the problem (Cicchetti & Cohen, 1995), and that the long-term outcomes are generally not predicted by symptom severity alone (Rutter, 1994).

The level of adaptation: The effectiveness of a particular intervention need to be judged in terms of the ability of the adolescents to adapt to the psychosocial environment, and on the extent to which treatment reduces or removes the impairment that depression imposes on the adolescent's everyday functioning. In adolescence, the critical dimensions include meeting the role demands of home and school, having adequate prosocial interactions with peers and adults.

The transactional level: Another area of concern is related to the contextual/transactional aspects of development that influences the adolescent's adaptation, and mutual accommodation between the individual and the changing environments. Because of the transactional interactions between the mental state and behavioural predispositions of the adolescents and their reactions to the environment across time (Cicchetti & Cohen, 1995), it is important to assess the quality of these transactions. Contextual/transactional measures of outcome would include the adolescent's immediate context (parent and family functioning) and life circumstances (e.g., social stressors, socioeconomic status, quality of the family's life)—all of which have been shown to moderate the effect of psychosocial interventions for children and adolescents.

The level of service utilization: The use of interventions assumes a reduction in post-treatment health services utilization. For this reason, service utilization data should be comprehensive, longitudinal, and show frequency, intensity, and duration of receipt across a wide range of services (Burns et al., 1995); a major challenge is to determine the way in which reliable data could be obtained. Such data should provide information concerning cost per service unit, total annual direct treatment costs, models of service organization, and their respective costs.

Summary

Although a number of progresses have been achieved in the treatment of adolescent depression, there are several issues that need to be resolved in the future. Some of the unresolved issues discussed in this chapter include the following: (i) which depressed adolescents benefit from what type and modality of treatment programs, (ii) whether the significant effects of therapy in 'research therapy' translate into clinically significant changes in adolescent's functioning and distress, (iii) mechanisms through which treatments achieve their effects, (iv) identification of factors that moderate and mediate treatment effect, (v) development of outcome measurement, and (vi) strategies to reach depressed adolescents who need help the most. As discussed earlier, the ultimate goal of research should ideally be the ability to cure or at least reduce the severity of MDD and the associated impairment. However, only a small proportion of those with depression actually received help. Throughout this chapter, we have attempted to discuss or present unresolved issues, with the hope of stimulating future research in the treatment of adolescent depression.

References

Achenbach, T.M. (1991). *Manual for the youth self-report and 1991 profile.* Burlington: University of Vermont Department of Psychiatry.

Angold, A. & Costello, E.J. (1995). A test-retest reliability study of child-reported psychiatric symptoms and diagnoses using the Child and Adolescent Psychiatric Assessment (CAPA-C). *Psychological Medicine, 25,* 755–762.

Angold, A., Weissman, M.M., John, K., Merikangas, K.R., Prusoff, P., Wickramaratne, G., et al. (1987). Parent and child reports of depressive symptoms in children at low and high risk of depression. *Journal of Child Psychology and Psychiatry, 28,* 901–915.

Boyle, M.H., Offord, D.R., Hofman, H.G., Catlin, G.P., Byles, J.A., Cadman, D.T., et al. (1987). Ontario Child Health Study: I. Methodology. *Archives of General Psychiatry, 44,* 826–831.

Burns, B.J., Costello, E.J., Angold, A., Tweed, D., Stangl, D., Farmer, E.M.Z., et al. (1995). Children's mental health service use across service sectors. *Health Affairs, 14,* 147–159.

Cicchetti, D. & Cohen, D.J. (1995). Perspectives on developmental psychopathology. In D. Cicchetti & D.J. Cohen (Eds.), *Developmental psychopathology. Volume 1: Theory and methods* (pp. 3–20). New York: Wiley.

Essau, C.A. (2005). Use of mental health services among adolescents with anxiety and depressive disorders. *Depression and Anxiety, 22,* 130–137.

Goldberg, D.P. & Huxley, P. (1980). *Mental illness in the community: The pathway to psychiatric care*. London: Tavistock.

Harrington, R., Fudge, H., Rutter, M., Pickles, A., & Hill, J. (1990). Adult outcomes of childhood and adolescent depression: I. Psychiatric status. *Archives of General Psychiatry, 47*, 465–473.

Kazdin, A.E. (1997). A model for developing effective treatments: Progression and interplay of theory, research, and practice. *Journal of Clinical Child Psychology, 26*, 114–129.

Kazdin, A.E. (2000). Developing a research agenda for child and adolescent psychotherapy. *Archives of General Psychiatry, 57*, 829–836.

Kovacs, M., Obrosky, D.S., Gatsonis, C., & Richards, C. (1997). First-episode major depressive and dysthymic disorder in childhood: Clinical and sociodemographic factors in recovery. *Journal of the American Academy of Child and Adolescent Psychiatry, 36*, 777–784.

Lewinsohn, P.M., Hops, H., Roberts, R.E., Seeley, J.R., & Andrews, J.A. (1993). Adolescent psychopathology: I. Prevalence and incidence of depression and other DSM-III-R disorders in high school students. *Journal of Abnormal Psychology, 102*, 133–144.

Lewinsohn, P.M., Pettit, J.W., & Joiner, T.E. Jr. (2003). The phenomenology of major depression in adolescents and young adults. *Journal of Abnormal Psychology 112*, 244–252.

Mash, E.J. & Krahn, G.L. (1995). Research strategies in child psychopathology. In M. Hersen & R.T. Hammerman (Eds.), *Advanced abnormal child psychology* (105–133). Hillsdale, NJ: Lawrence Erlbaum.

Rao, U., Ryan, N.D., Birmaher, B., Dahl, R.E., Williamson, D.E., Kaufman, J., et al. (1995). Unipolar depression in adolescents: Clinical outcome in adulthood. *Journal of the American Academy of Child and Adolescent Psychiatry, 34*, 566–578.

Rapee, R.M., Barrett, P.M., Dadds, M.R., & Evans, L. (1994). Reliability of the DSM-III-R childhood anxiety disorders using structured interview: Interrater and parent–child agreement. *Journal of the American Academy of Child and Adolescent Psychiatry, 33*, 984–992.

Rutter, M. (1994). Beyond longitudinal data: Causes, consequences, changes and continuity. *Journal of Consulting and Clinical Psychology, 62*, 928–940.

Verhulst, F.C. (1995). The epidemiology of child and adolescent psychopathology: Strengths and limitations. In F.C. Verhulst & H.M. Koot (Eds.), *The epidemiology of child and adolescent psychopathology* (pp. 1–21). Oxford: Oxford University Press.

Vitiello, B. & Jensen, P.S. (1995). Developmental perspectives in pediatric psychopharmacology. *Psychopharmacology bulletin, 31*, 75 81

Weisz, J.R. & Eastman, K.L. (1995). Cross-cultural research on child and adolescent psychopathology. In F.C. Verhulst & H.M. Koot (Eds.), *The epidemiology of child and adolescent psychopathology* (pp. 42–65). Oxford: Oxford University Press.

Weisz, J.R., Suwanlert, S., Chaiyasit, W., Weiss, B., Walter, B.R., & Anderson, W.W. (1988). Thai and American perspectives on over- and undercontrolled child behavior problems: Exploring the threshold model among parents, teachers, and psychologists. *Journal of Consulting and Clinical Psychology, 56*, 601–609.

Weisz, J.R., Donenberg, G.R., Han, S.S., & Weiss, B. (1995). Bridging the gap between laboratory and clinic in child and adolescent psychotherapy. *Journal of Consulting and Clinical Psychology, 63*, 688–701.

Zito, J.M. & Riddle, M.A. (1995). Psychiatric Pharmacoepidemiology for Children. *Child and Adolescent Psychiatric Clinics of North America, 4*, 77–95.

Index

abuse 182–3
action plan 88
action team 88
Activities that Boost Mood 107
Activities that Solve Problems 107
adapation, level of 317
adjustment disorder with depressed
    mood 279
Adolescent Well-being Scale 304
Adult-distress threshold model 315
affective training 263
age 8, 42–3
    improving care within primary care
        services 162, 163
    of onset 9–10
    and parental gender 180
    risk and vulnerability 33
agoraphobia 10
alcohol use disorder 10, 11
    see also substance use
Alliance Building Task 221, 223, 230
amitriptyline 313
anger 288, 293, 297–8
anhedonia 98
antianxiety medication 14
antidepressant medication 14, 159, 242, 313
    improving care within primary care
        services 164–5, 166, 171
    tricyclic 241, 313
    see also pharmacotherapy; and under
        specific drugs
antisocial behaviour 11
anxiety disorders 9, 10, 43, 67, 203, 302
    comorbidity 11
    duration of episodes 15
    empirically supported treatments 61, 72
    Family-based approaches 181, 184
    generalized 10
    interpersonal psychotherapy 279
    lifetime 177
    long-term course and outcome 14
anxious attachment style 219
association studies 36–7
assortative mating 181
attachment-based family therapy 189, 215–35
    adolescent development research 217–18
    anxious attachment style 219
    attachment theory 218–19
    case study 223–34
        alliance building with parent
            (task 3) 228–30

alliance building (task 2) 227–8
autonomy and competency promotion
    (task 5) 233–4
reattachment (task 4) 230–3
relational reframe (task 1) 224–7
clinical foundation 220–1
clinical structure 221–3
dismissing attachment style 218
empirically informed treatment 216
empirical support 234–5
family-based approach 215–16
repairing attachment 219–20
self of the therapist 217
theory foundation 217
treatment manual 216–17
attachment task 233
attention deficit hyperactivity disorder
    (ADHD) 61, 203, 252, 279, 285, 302
Australia 147–8, 150, 151, 152
autonomy 221, 233

Beck Depression Inventory 145
Beck Hopelessness Scale 133, 144, 148, 194
Beck's cognitive model and hopelessness
    theory 28–32
behavioural inhibition 39
behavioural parent training 195
behavioural problems 31
'behavioural responder' 68
behavioural skills 87
behavioural theory 66
behavioural therapy 61
    see also cognitive–behavioural therapy
belonging 128
bereavement 181, 196, 197–9, 200, 290
'best fit' skills 107
beyondblue schools research
    initiative 85–91, 92
    cognitive and behavioural skills taught within
        curriculum 87
    community involvement in the school,
        enhancement of 90
    individual protective skills building:
        classroom program 86
    outcomes 90–1
    supportive school environment
        building 86–8, 89
biological factors 85
bipolar disorder 254
bullying 289–91, 291–2
buproprion 252–3, 254

Calming 107–8, 129
Caregiver–child Relationship Enhancement
    Training 114–15
Care Managers 165–6, 167
Centre for Epidemiological Studies—
    Depression Scale 162, 163, 164
child abuse and neglect 182–3
Child and Adolescent Mental Health
    Service 285, 301
Children's Coping Strategies Checklist
    (CCSC) 304, 306
Children's Depression Inventory 109, 133, 144,
    148, 194
Children's Depression Rating Scale-
    Revised 109, 245–6, 250–1
Child Steps Clinic Treatment Project (CTP) 113
China 150
Choosing Healthy Actions and Thoughts (CHAT)
    program 113–14
chronic depression 242, 243
chronicity 17
citalopram 241, 243, 244, 245, 246, 253, 254
clinical factors 17
clinical mental health setting 294–5
'clinical therapy' 71–2, 314
Clinician-based program 194
clinician ratings of depression 195
closeness circle 267–8
cognitive–behavioural therapy 66
    attachment-based family therapy 235
    deployment-focused model 103
    empirically supported treatments 61
    family-based approaches 188, 189–90, 195
    improving care within primary care
        services 159, 164–5, 166, 167, 170, 171
    interpersonal psychotherapy 279
    pharmacotherapy 243, 253
    progress and unresolved issues 314
    resourceful adolescent program 123, 126–7
    School-based, universal approaches to
        prevention 91–2
    'Working Things Out' 296–301, 302
cognitive models 43
cognitive restructuring 129
cognitive skills 87
Cognitive Style Questionnaire 32
cognitive therapy 69
    see also cognitive–behavioural therapy
common elements 65
communiction analysis 270–1, 272
community involvement in the school,
    enhancement of 90
community mental health setting 294–5
comorbid disorders 12, 253, 285, 302
comorbidity 10–11, 17, 181
competency 234
Competency Promoting Task 223
Composite International Diagnostic
    Interview 162, 164
conduct disorders 10, 11, 12, 61, 285, 302

confidentiality 267
conflict reduction 89
connectedness 87
consent 92, 133
contextual factors 178
coping skills 103
core beliefs identification 106–7
'correlated consequences' model 7
cortisol 41
cultural issues and depression 8–9, 190

decision analysis 271, 272
dehydroepiandrosterone (DHEA) 41
Demographic Questionnaire 304
Deployment-focused model 97–116
    components, moderators, mediators, cost-
        benefit, system factors and fit issues 102
    effectiveness and dissemination tests 111–13
    effectiveness, implementation and
        transportability tests 101–2
    future directions 115
    goodness-of-fit, benefit and sustainability in
        practice contexts tests 102, 113–15
    initial effectiveness tests 101, 110–11
    initial efficacy trial under controlled
        conditions to establish potential for
        benefit 100, 109–10
    Single-case applications in practice settings
        with progressive adaptations to the
        protocol 100–1, 110
    theoretically and clinically guided
        construction of treatment
        protocol 99–100, 102–9
    coping skills 103
    core beliefs identification 106–7
    individualization of treatment to youth's
        'best fit' skills 107
    individual youth formulation 105–6
    initial youth session: rapport building and
        goals setting 105
    mood-boosters and teaching moments 109
    program overview 104–5
    skills emphasised in PASCET
        program 107–9
    youth practice and use of 'ACT & THINK'
        workbook 109
    youth depression as major public
        concern 97–9
depressive subtype 17
depressive symptoms 162
depressogenic attributional styles 32
desipramine 313
detection 161–4
developmental disorders 302
dexamethasone suppression test 41
diagnostic level 317
diathesis–stress models 43
differential effectiveness of
    psychosocial treatments 61–4
dismissing attachment style 218

disruptive behavioural disorder 17
'dissemination' research 73
divorce and separation of parents 184, 196, 197–9, 200
'Dodo Bird' effect 60–1
dopamine 36, 39, 40
'double depression' (major depression and dysthymia) 15, 17
drop-out rates 92
drug abuse 10, 11
   see also substance use
duloxetine 248–9, 250, 253, 254
duration of episodes 15–16
Dysfunctional Attitudes Scale 32
dysthymic disorder 4
   age of onset 9
   comorbidity 11
   deployment-focused model 98
   duration of episodes 15
   improving care within primary care services 162
   interpersonal psychotherapy 279
   prevalence 5–6
   psychosocial impairment 13
   relapse 17

early intervention program *see* resourceful adolescent program (RAP)
eating disorders 294
efficacy and effectiveness: transportability of treatments 70–3
emotionality, positive 38
emotional literacy and regulation 87
Emotionally Focused Therapy 220
emotional regulation 87
emotional support 33
empirically supported treatments 57–75
   criteria 60
   definition 59–60
   efficacy and effectiveness: transportability of treatments 70–3
   issues of concern 60–4
   manualization of psychosocial treatments 64–70
endogenous variables 42
endophenotypes 37–9, 43
environmental factors 39, 42, 254
environmental stress 37
epidemiology, comorbidity and course of depression 3–19
   age of onset 9–10
   comorbidity 10–11
   epidemiology 4–9
   health services utilization 13–14
   long-term course and outcome 14–18
   psychosocial impairment 12–13
episode indices 14
escitalopram 241, 243, 244, 245, 246, 247, 253, 254
ethics 63

ethnicity 162, 190
Europe 248
European Network of Health Promoting Schools 305
'evidence-based' decision making model 63–4
exogenous variables 42
experimental treatments 59
'explanation model' 8–9
externalizing problems 177, 178, 184, 185, 316

Family-based approaches 177–203, 314
   family climate 186–8
   parents, inclusion of in universal prevention programs 191–4
   prevention 190–1
   prevention programs, indicated 195–200
   prevention programs, selective 194–5
   targeting family functioning in treatment of other disorders 203
   transmission of maternal depression 185–6
   untested but promising strategies for prevention 200–2
   see also attachment-based family therapy; family risk factors
family climate 186–8
family conflict 127
family disruption 183–5
family factors 254
family psychoeducation 195
family risk factors 179–85
   child abuse and neglect 182–3
   family disruption 183–5
   psychopathology in family members 179–82
Family–School Partnership 191
family session 194
family therapy, short-term 189
family variables 178
father–child conflict 180
fears 288
Federal Drug Administration 251
flexibility 67–8
fluoxetine 241, 243–4, 245, 247, 253, 254
Follow-up 165
Food and Drug Administration 241
Fort Bragg Project 62, 73

gender 4, 7, 11, 33, 35, 162
genetic factors 42–3
   and depression endophenotypes 36–9
   family-based approaches 189
   family disruption 183
   risk and vulnerability 39
goals setting 105
gonadal hormones 40–1
grandiosity 128
grandparents 181–2
Gray's behavioural approach system 38, 39
grief 262, 263, 274–5
group work 301–6
   evaluation 303–4, 306

group work (*cont.*)
    helping parents understand young person's
        perspective 304–5
    intervention 302–3
    mental health resource in classroom
        settings 305–6
    participants 302
    session outline 303
growth hormone 40

Hamilton Depression Rating Scale 195, 246,
    265
health services utilization 13–14
Help from a Friend 108
help seeking 87, 89
hierarchical linear modelling 147
hope 43
hopelessness theory 28–32
5-HTTLPR polymorphism 39
hypothalamic–pituitary–adrenal axis 41

idealization 128
'idiom of distress' 9
imipramine 313
Incredible Years training program 202
indicated prevention programs 177
individualization of treatment to youth's
    'best fit' skills 107
individual protective skills building: classroom
    program 86
individual variables 178
individual youth formulation 105–6
inflammatory bowel disease 114
informed consent 92
initial youth session: rapport building and goals
    setting 105
inpatient setting 13
internalizing problems 178, 184, 185–6, 187,
    196, 316
interpersonal component 129
interpersonal deficits 262, 264, 276–7
interpersonal disputes 262, 263–4
interpersonal inventory 267–9
interpersonal loss 181
Interpersonal Psychotherapy 61, 261–81
    for adolescent children of parents with
        bipolar disorder (IPT-PA) 280
    adolescent skills training (IPT-AST) 280
    for depressed adolescents (IPT-A) 262–3,
        264, 266, 279
    Family-based approaches 188, 189
    group model (IPT-AG) 279–80
    recent empirical findings 279–80
    resourceful adolescent program 126
    see also therapeutic goals and methods
interpersonal role dispute 275
interpersonal skills training 127, 263
Interpersonal and Social Rhythm
    Therapy 280
interpersonal theory 66

intervention programs 313–18
introversion 34
Ireland 283, 305–6

language disorders 302
learned helplessness model 104
life problem solving skills 87
long-term course 14–18

major depression and dysthymia ('double
    depression') 15, 17
major depressive disorder 3–4, 19
    age of onset 8, 9–10
    comorbidity 10, 11
    deployment-focused model 97–8
    duration of episodes 15
    epidemiology 4
    family-based approaches 177, 182
    health services utilization 14
    improving care within primary care
        services 162
    interpersonal psychotherapy 279
    maternal 180
    pharmacotherapy 243, 252
    prevalence 5–6
    psychosocial impairment 12, 13
    puberty 8
    relapse 17, 18
maltreatment 33
    see also abuse; sexual abuse
manualization of psychosocial
    treatments 64–70
maternal depression 178–9, 181
    transmission of 185–6
measures of depression 42–3
medical dysfunction 31
mental health issues, awareness of 87
mental health literacy 89
mental health services utilization 14
metaphors 128–30
mood-boosters 109
mirroring 128
mirtazapine 241, 251–2, 253, 254
moderate depression 242
modular approach 69
Modular Approach to Treatment for
    Children—Anxiety, Depression and
    Conduct (MATCH-ADC) 113
monitoring 189
monoamine oxidase inhibitors 313
Montgomery-Asberg Depression Rating Scale
    (MADRS) 246
mood rating 267
Multidimensional Family Therapy 220

National Institute of Clinical Excellence 188–9
nefazadone 241–2, 250–1, 254
negative attributional style 188
negative emotionality 38–9
negative self-view 188

negative thinking 29, 30–2
neglect 182–3
Netherlands 248
neuroticism 34
neurotransmitter and neuroendocrine
    systems 39–41
New Zealand randomized blind Placebo-
    controlled trial 145
Non-directive supportive therapy 189
norepinephrine 39
No Replaying Bad Thoughts 108
norfluoxetine 243–4
nortriptyline 313
number needed to harm 242, 248
number needed to treat 242, 245, 246, 249, 250

obsessive compulsive disorder 288
oppositional defiant disorder 203, 279, 285
oppositional disorders 61, 302
Oregon Adolescent Depression Project 4
outcome 14–18
outcome measurement, complexity of 316–17
outpatient setting 13

panic disorder 10, 65
parent–adolescent session 273–4
parental conflict 184
parental depression 31, 178–81, 185–6, 193
parental gender and child age 180
parent–child relations 34–5
parents 179–81
Parents and Children series 191
parents, inclusion of in universal prevention
    programs 191–4
parent–therapist alliance 191
paroxetine 241, 243, 244–5, 246, 253
participation in pleasant events 87
participation in school 89
Partners in Care Study 161
paternal depression 180–1
Pathways component 88
patient factors 254
peer relationships 35–6
Pen Optimism Program 196
personality 34, 261
personal resource bricks 130
personal strengths 129
pharmacotherapy 14, 241–54
    buproprion 252–3
    comorbid disorders 253
    indications for 242–3
    mirtazapine 251–2
    nefazadone 250–1
    selective serotonin reuptake
        inhibitors 243–8
    serotonin norepinephrine reuptake
        inhibitors 248–50
    treatment-resistant depression 253–4
phenelzine 313
philosophy, positive 128, 130

'physiological responder' 68–9
population health argument 124
positive thinking 43–4
practice element profile 65
'prescriptive matching' 68–9
prevention programs 190–1, 313–18
    indicated 195–200
    selective 194–5
    see also resourceful adolescent program (RAP)
primary care services 159–71
    detection 161–4
    patient components 166–8
    patient outcomes 169
    quality improvement intervention 164–6
    Youth Partners in Care (YPIC) model 161
primary control skills 103, 109
primary and secondary control enhancement
    training (PASCET):
    ACT & THINK Practice Book 103, 104, 106,
        107, 108–9
    for medically ill depressed youth 114
    Physical Illness (PI) 114
    Video-guided (VG) 112, 114
    see also deployment-focused model
probable current depressive disorder 162
probable depressive disorder 162
probably efficacious treatments 59, 60, 64
problem area specific session structure 274
problem-solving 127, 129
Protecting Families Program 196
psychiatric disorders 11, 242
psychodynamic theory 66
psychoeducation 263
psychological intervention 314–17
psychological unavailability of caregiver 33
psychopathology in family members 179–82
    grandparents 181–2
    parents 179–81
    siblings 182
psychopharmacotherapy 313–14
psychosis 242
psychosocial factors 42
psychosocial impairment 12–13, 242
psychosocial treatments, manualization
    of 64–70
psychotherapy 242, 243
    see also interpersonal psychotherapy
psychotropic drugs 313
puberty 8
Puerto Rico 279

quality improvement 161, 164–6, 167, 168, 169,
    170, 171

randomized clinical trials 84, 97
    empirically supported treatments 58, 59,
        62, 71
    pharmacotherapy 241, 242, 243, 245,
        246, 247
rapport building 105

R-citalopram 244
Reattachment Task 221, 223
recognition 89
recovery 16–17
  indices 14
recruitment and reach 124–5
recurrence indices 14
recurrent depression 42, 242, 243
referral 166
Reframe Task 230
relapse 17–18
  indices 14
Relational Reframe Task 221
relationships building, positive 89
relaxation training 69, 127
remission indices 14
'research' therapy 71–2, 314
resourceful adolescent program
  (RAP) 123–53, 194
  Australia 147–8, 150, 151, 152
  'Behaviour' bubble 139
  computerization to increase teacher-
    implemented effectiveness 151–2
  dissemination and adapations 150–1
  DVD 133
  effectiveness in Mauritian school
    environment 148–9
  ethical issues 133
  family component (RAF-F) 147, 191, 194
  group composition 132
  group leaders and group processes 131–2
  Group Leader's Manual 132, 133
  indicated trial in Netherlands 149
  Indigenous Supplement (RAP-A) 150
  initial effectiveness trial 146–7
  initial efficacy trial 144–5
  'Keep Calm Bricks' 138
  'Keep the Peace' Bricks 143
  large multi-site effectiveness trial 147–8
  'Make the Peace' Bricks 143
  New Zealand 145, 150
  parallel parent (RAP-P) Program 144, 147
  Participant Workbook 132–3, 139,
    140, 142
  positive philosophy and
    metaphors 128, 130
  'Problem Solving Bricks' 140
  program structure, group size and age of
    participants 131
  'RAP house' 130
  rationale for universal approach to
    prevention 123–6
  recruitment 133
  Resource Bricks 143
  resources 132–3
  school camp structure 151
  school connectedness promotion 152
  screening 133
  Selfenometer 130–1, 134, 136, 141
  session one: getting to know you 134, 135

  session two: self-esteem building 134,
    135, 136
  session three: introduction to the RAP
    model 135, 136–7
  session four: keeping calm 135, 137–8
  session five: self-talk 135, 138–9
  session six: thinking resourcefully 135, 139
  session seven: finding solutions to
    problems 135, 139–40
  session eight: support networks 135, 140–1
  session nine: considering the other person's
    perspective 135, 141–2
  session ten: keeping the peace and making the
    peace 135, 142–3
  session eleven: putting it all together 135, 143
  skills taught 129
  summary of findings 149–50
  'Support Network Brick' 140
  for Teachers (RAP-T) 152
  'Thought Court' activity 138–9
  'Time Out' 142
rewards 89
Reynold's Adolescent Depression Scale 124,
  133, 144, 145, 148, 194
risk reduction model 178
risk and vulnerability 27–44
  Beck's cognitive model and hopelessness
    theory 28–32
  future directions 42–4
  genetics of depression and depression
    endophenotypes 36–9
  neurotransmitter and neuroendocrine
    systems 39–41
  social relationships and social support 34–6
  stressful life events 33–4
  stress generation 34
role-playing 271–2
role transitions 262, 264, 275–6

Schedule for Affective Disorders and
  Schizophrenia (K-SADS) 246, 283, 303–4
school action team 86
school-based, universal approaches 83–94, 192
  correct approach but inadequate
    implementation possibility 91–2
  inadequate research designs possibility 92
  invalidity of approach possibility 92–4
  see also beyondblue schools
    research initiative
S-citalopram 244
screening 125, 162, 163, 164
secondary control skills 103, 109
selective prevention programs 177
selective serotonin reuptake inhibitors 241,
  243–8, 253, 254, 313
  adverse effects 247–8
  efficacy 245–7
  nonresponder to treatment of 254
  pharmacokinetics 243–5
self-concept 186

self-esteem 35, 127–8, 130
self-harm 294, 295
self-object needs 128
self-worth 35
serotonin 39, 40
  norepinephrine reuptake inhibitors 248–9
  transporter gene 36, 37
  see also selective serotonin
    reuptake inhibitors
sertraline 241, 243, 244, 245, 246, 253, 254
services, linkage with 166
service utilization, level of 318
severe depression 243
sexual abuse 299–301
siblings 182
'Silver Lining', identification of 108
social functioning 261
Social, Personal and Health Education
  Programme 305–6
social phobia 10
social relationships 34–6
social services 13
social skills 87
social supports 34–6, 87
sociodemographic factors 17
specific phobias 10, 61
STEPS procedure 107
stigmatization 125
Strengths and Difficulties Questionnaire
  (SDQ) 304, 306
stress 9, 293, 297–8
  and environmental factors 186
  generation 34
  and life events 33–4
  management 127
  reduction 87
'Stress and Your Mood' brochure 165
Structural Family Therapy 220
student safety 89
subdiagnostic depressive symptoms 187
substance use disorders 10, 254
  comorbidity 11
  dependence 181
  health services utilization 14
  lifetime 177
  long-term course and outcome 14
  see also alcohol; drugs
subsyndromal depression 164
suicidal ideation/suicidality 13
  attachment-based family therapy 234–5
  family-based approaches 183, 186
  improving care within primary care
    services 159
  pharmacotherapy 242, 247–8
  'Working Things Out' 293, 296
suicide 14, 98, 177
Supporting Your Child's Education 202
supportive school environment
  building 86–8, 89
support networks 129

symptomatic level 317
symptom formation 261
syndromal depression 164
'system evaluation' research 73
systemic behavioural family therapy 189

targeted programs 84
teaching moments 109
technology and therapeutic engagement and
  motivation 285–7
temperament 34
  factors 85
  traits 38
  vulnerability 39
Temple-Wisconsin Cognitive Vulnerability
  Project (CVP) 32
termination phase 277–8
Thailand 316
therapeutic goals and methods of interpersonal
  psychotherapy 262–78
  initial phase of treatment 265–70
    session 1 265–7
    session 2 267–8
    session 3 268
    session 4 268–70
  middle phase of treatment 270–8
    grief 274–5
    interpersonal deficits 276–7
    interpersonal role dispute 275
    parent–adolescent session 273–4
    problem area specific session
      structure 274
    role transition 275–6
    sessions 5–9 270–3
    session 10 277
    session 11 277–8
    session 12 277–8
    termination phase 277–8
thinking styles, rational and constructive 87
Think Positive 108
'third person' approach 296
transactional level 317
transportability of treatments 70–3, 74
tranylcypromine 313
Treatment of Adolescent Depression
  Study 74, 171
Treatment-resistant depression 253–4
Treatment of SSRI-Resistant Depression in
  Adolescents (TORDIA) 253
'treatment as usual' 62–3, 73, 110–11
tricyclic antidepressants 241, 313
tripartite model 11
Triple-P Positive Parenting Program 201–2
tryptophan 39–40
Turn on my Positive Self 108
twinship 128
twin studies 36
two-process model of control 102–3
two-session lecture and discussion
  program 194

unipolar depressive disorder 187
United States 170, 177, 244, 248, 279, 316
universal prevention programs 124, 177
    see also school-based, universal approaches
usual care 161, 164, 169, 171

venlafaxine 241, 248–9, 250, 253, 254
verbal treatment contract 269–70
vulnerability see risk and vulnerability

wait list condition 279
well-being, benefits of
    promotion of 125
Well-established treatments 59, 60, 64
Whole-school change strategies to build
    supportive environments 89
work at home assignment 272–3
'Working Things Out' 283–306
    background to development 283–5
    character customisation palette 287
    individual stories 288–94

'joining stage' 286
limitations 294
overview of content 287
Session 1 303
Session 2 303
Session 3 303
Session 4 303
Session 5 303
story interface 286
technology and therapeutic engagement and
    motivation 285–7
'Transforming Stories' 286, 287, 302
uses 294–301
see also group work
World Health Organization 305, 306

Youth Partners in Care (YPIC) model 161, 164,
    165, 169–70, 171
youth ratings of depression (CES-D) 195
Youth Session Rating Scale 304
Youth–therapist alliance 191